Register Now for O
to Your B

SPRINGER PUBLISHING
CONNECT™

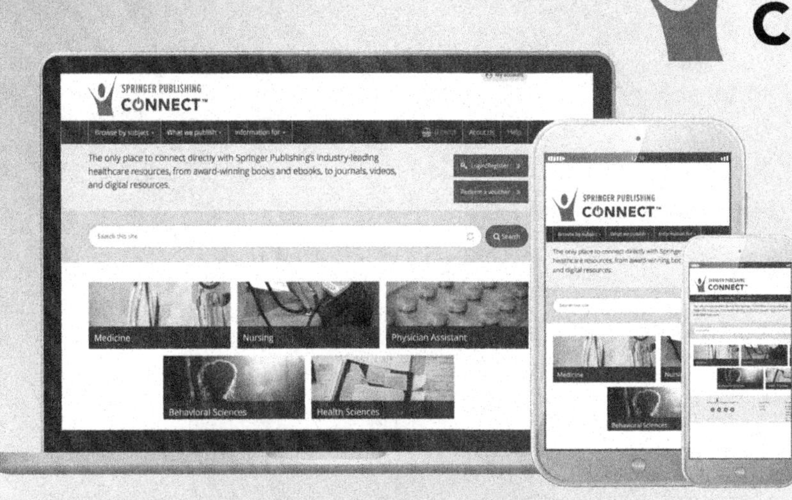

Your print purchase of *Child and Adolescent Counseling* **includes online access to the contents of your book**—increasing accessibility, portability, and searchability!

Access today at:
http://connect.springerpub.com/content/book/978-0-8261-4764-6
or scan the QR code at the right with your smartphone. Log in or register, then click "Redeem a voucher" and use the code below.

SEV8DLVC

Scan here for quick access.

Having trouble redeeming a voucher code?
Go to https://connect.springerpub.com/redeeming-voucher-code

If you are experiencing problems accessing the digital component of this product, please contact our customer service department at cs@springerpub.com

The online access with your print purchase is available at the publisher's discretion and may be removed at any time without notice.

Publisher's Note: New and used products purchased from third-party sellers are not guaranteed for quality, authenticity, or access to any included digital components.

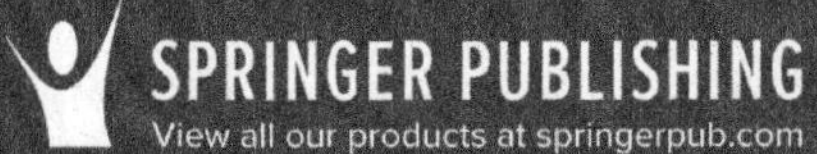

CHILD AND ADOLESCENT COUNSELING

Brenda Jones, PhD, LPC, NCC, CSC, has educational experience in the public-school system that spans over 30 years, with 9 years of high school teaching experience, over 13 years of high school professional school counseling experience, and 8 years of clinical and head counseling experience. She is a nationally certified counselor, certified school counselor, and licensed professional counselor. She earned a PhD in counseling education and supervision. This year completes her 12th year as a clinical assistant professor at the University of Texas at San Antonio. She teaches child and adolescent counseling in a system context, counseling in a multicultural setting, school counseling internship, clinical mental health internship, and practicum in counseling. She serves on the editorial board of the *Journal of Creativity in Mental Health* and the *Journal of School Counseling* and is the past president of the Texas Association of Counselor Education and Supervision, representing school counseling and clinical mental health issues. She has published and presented on related issues at the local, state, and national levels and has actively served in the American Counseling Association, Association for Multicultural Counseling and Development, and American School Counseling Association, and their related divisions. She is the recipient of the Texas Counseling Association 2017 Professional Writing Award for the book *Child and Adolescent Counseling Case Studies: Developmental, Relational, Multicultural, and Systemic Perspectives*. In 2018, along with three other authors, Avent, Robertson, and Prado, Dr. Jones became the recipient of a national award (Outstanding Article Award) from the Association for Counselor Education and Supervision.

Beth Durodoye, EdD, NCC, is professor and chair of the Department of Leadership, Technology and Human Development at Georgia Southern University. Dr. Durodoye earned her EdD in counselor education from the University of Virginia and her MA in counseling from Marshall University. She is a board-certified counselor through the National Board of Certified Counselors. During her tenure as a faculty member at the University of Texas at San Antonio, she held an appointment as a provost faculty fellow, where her responsibilities emphasized campus internationalization efforts and the recruitment, retention, and progression of underrepresented graduate students. Her research and scholarly interests include multicultural competency, race and education, and ethnic identity development. She has authored numerous international, national, and state publications, with her most recent work being her coedited book *From Disagreement to Discourse: A Chronicle of Controversies in Schooling and Education*. She is a past president of the Texas Association for Multicultural Counseling and Development and a former associate editor of the journal *Counseling and Values*. Dr. Durodoye is the cochair of the Faculty Interests and Needs Committee of the National Conference on Race and Ethnicity in American Higher Education and currently serves as a consulting elder for the *Journal of Multicultural Counseling and Development*.

CHILD AND ADOLESCENT COUNSELING

AN INTEGRATED APPROACH

Brenda Jones, PhD, LPC, NCC, CSC
Beth Durodoye, EdD, NCC

EDITORS

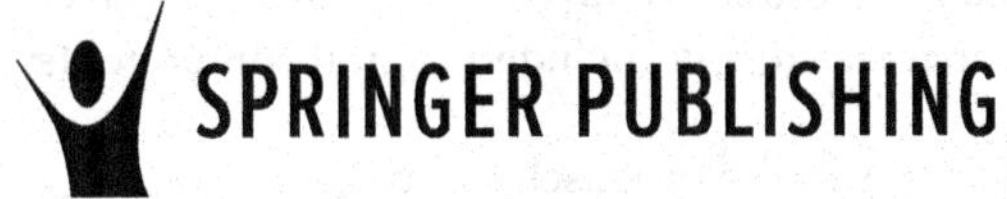

Springer Publishing Company, LLC
11 West 42nd Street, New York, NY 10036
www.springerpub.com
connect.springerpub.com/

Acquisitions Editor: Rhonda Dearborn
Compositor: Exeter Premedia Services Private Ltd.

ISBN: 978-0-8261-4763-9
ebook ISBN: 978-0-8261-4764-6
DOI: 10.1891/9780826147646

SUPPLEMENTS
Instructor Materials:
Qualified instructors may request supplements by emailing textbook@springerpub.com

Instructor's Manual ISBN: 978-0-8261-4774-5
Instructor's Test Bank ISBN: 978-0-8261-4776-9
Instructor's PowerPoints ISBN: 978-0-8261-4775-2
Instructor's Sample Syllabus ISBN: 978-0-8261-4777-6

24 25 26 / 5 4 3 2

The author and the publisher of this Work have made every effort to use sources believed to be reliable to provide information that is accurate and compatible with the standards generally accepted at the time of publication. The author and publisher shall not be liable for any special, consequential, or exemplary damages resulting, in whole or in part, from the readers' use of, or reliance on, the information contained in this book. The publisher has no responsibility for the persistence or accuracy of URLs for external or third-party Internet websites referred to in this publication and does not guarantee that any content on such websites is, or will remain, accurate or appropriate.

Library of Congress Control Number: 2021932262

Brenda Jones: https://orcid.org/0000-0001-7572-7157
Beth Durodoye: https://orcid.org/0000-0002-9127-751X

Contact sales@springerpub.com to receive discount rates on bulk purchases.

Publisher's Note: **New and used products purchased from third-party sellers are not guaranteed for quality, authenticity, or access to any included digital components.**

Printed in the United States of America by Gasch Printing.

This book honors the vast efforts of counselors-in-training, professional school counselors, and clinical mental health counselors and supervisors. Their alliances instill optimism and effect growth and possibilities for children and adolescents in their care.

Contents

Contributors

Ruby R. Bible, MsED, Professional School Counselor, Counseling Department, Ed White Middle School, San Antonio, Texas

Jennifer N. Boswell, PhD, LPC-S, NCC, RPT-S, Associate Professor, Clinical Mental Health Counseling, University of St. Thomas-Houston, Houston, Texas

Rhonda M. Bryant, PhD, LPC, NCC, NCSC, CCMHC, Associate Vice President of Student Well-Being and Dean of Students, University of the Pacific; Associate Professor of Practice, Benerd School of Education, Stockton, California

Beth Durodoye, EdD, NCC, Professor and Chair, Department of Leadership, Technology and Human Development, Georgia Southern University, Statesboro, Georgia

Irene Gomez, MA, School-Based Therapist, Family Services, Inc., Sheppard Pratt Health System, Gaithersburg, Maryland

Stacy Speedlin Gonzalez, PhD, LPC, LCDC, NCC, Professor of Practice, Department of Counseling, University of Texas at San Antonio, San Antonio, Texas

Laura A. Granato, PhD, LPC, LMFT, Executive Director, Lifestance Health, Clinical Director, Granato Group, McLean, Virginia

J. Claire Gregory, MA, LPC, LCDC, NCC, Doctoral Candidate, Department of Counseling, University of Texas at San Antonio, San Antonio, Texas

Maria Haiyasoso, PhD, LPC, RPT, NCC, Assistant Professor, Department of Counseling, Leadership, Adult Education, and School Psychology, Texas State University, San Marcos, Texas

Naderia T. Hartley, MEd, Doctoral Student, Professional School Counselor, Counseling Department, Schertz Cibolo Universal City Independent School District, Cibolo, Texas

Deborah Healy, PsyD, LP, CSC, LPC, Associate Professor, Chair, Department of Psychology, PsyD Training Director, Our Lady of the Lake University, San Antonio, Texas

Dianne P. Hengst, PsyD, Executive Director of Student Disability Services, University of Texas at San Antonio, San Antonio, Texas

Barbara Herlihy, PhD, LPC-S, NCC, Professor in Practice and Doctoral Program Director, Department of Counseling, University of Texas at San Antonio, San Antonio, Texas

Claudia G. Interiano-Shiverdecker, PhD, Assistant Professor, Department of Counseling, University of Texas at San Antonio, San Antonio, Texas

Brenda Jones, PhD, LPC, NCC, CSC, Clinical Assistant Professor, Department of Counseling, University of Texas at San Antonio, San Antonio, Texas

Tracy M. Knighton, EdD, Licensed Professional Counselor, NOVA Counseling and Consulting Services, LLC, Albany, Georgia

Jennifer Laurenza, MS, LMHC, LMFT, President/Clinical Director, Center for Creative Life Solutions, Lakeville, Massachusetts

Courtland C. Lee, PhD, Professor, Counselor Education Program, The Chicago School of Professional Psychology at Washington DC, Washington, DC

Vivian V. Lee, EdD, Associate Professor, Counseling, Johns Hopkins University, Baltimore, Maryland

Christopher Leeth, PhD, LPC-S, Assistant Professor in Practice, Department of Counseling, University of Texas at San Antonio, San Antonio, Texas

M. Elsa Soto Leggett, PhD, LPC-S, RPT-S, CSC, Professor of Counseling, CMHC & School Counseling Program Coordinator, Department of Counseling, Houston Baptist University, Houston, Texas

Mahsa Maghsoudi, PhD, LPC, NCC, Assistant Professor and Clinical Director, Department of Counseling, Educational Leadership, Educational & School Psychology, Wichita State University, Wichita, Kansas

Gretchen Eckhardt McLain, MA, CSC, Doctoral Candidate, Counseling Department, University of Texas at San Antonio, San Antonio, Texas

Crystal Morris, MEd, LPC, NCC, Doctoral Student, Graduate Research Assistant Department of Counseling, University of Texas at San Antonio, San Antonio, Texas

Kristin O'Donnell, PhD, LSSP, Associate Professor of Psychology, Psychology Department, School Psychology Program, Our Lady of the Lake University, San Antonio, Texas

Anita M. Pool, PhD, PLPC, NCC, NCSC, Assistant Professor, Department of Counseling, School of Social and Behavioral Sciences, University of the Cumberlands, Williamsburg, Kentucky

Priscilla Rose Prasath, PhD, MBA, LPC, Assistant Professor, Department of Counseling, University of Texas at San Antonio, San Antonio, Texas

Brigitte Rauschuber, MEd, CSC, Professional School Counselor, Counseling Department, Northside Independent School District, San Antonio, Texas

Devon E. Romero, PhD, NCC, Assistant Professor, Department of Counseling, University of Texas at San Antonio, San Antonio, Texas

Carol M. Smith, MACE, PhD, LPC, NCC, Professor, Counseling Program, Coordinator, Violence, Loss, and Trauma Certificate of Advanced Studies, Marshall University, South Charleston, West Virginia

Le'Ann Solmonson, PhD, LPC-S, CSC, Retired Professor, Department of Human Services, Stephen F. Austin State University, Nacogdoches, Texas

Kimberly Stewart, MEd, Instructional Support Teacher for Gifted/Talented and Advanced Academics, Northside Independent School District, San Antonio, Texas

Jane M. Webber, PhD, LPC, DRCC, Assistant Professor and Doctoral Program Coordinator, Counselor Education Department, Kean University, Bernardsville, New Jersey

Foreword

The 20th-century Irish poet William Butler Yeats is purported to have said that writing poetry was harder than breaking stones. Were Yeats to be alive today and commenting on the creation of books, his comment might be similar. Putting together a book is a long and arduous process. It involves generating ideas and breaking down concepts into clear and readable prose. It is a journey filled with late nights and early mornings, as writing, rewriting, and editing take place in the rigorous silence of composition.

Child and Adolescent Counseling: An Integrated Approach is a book that reflects the arduous procedure of breaking down thoughts into pieces that are easily comprehended and applied. It is a text that contains a wealth of information that has been refined over time to reflect the latest thinking of scholars in the field of child and adolescent mental health. This well-wrought manuscript of comprehensive chapters articulates the latest and best research in working with children and adolescents in a readable and engaging way.

Thus, this book is clinical, theoretical, and practical. It is applicable to the myriad concerns that counselors face in dealing with developmental problems and challenges. If the domain of child and adolescent counseling were a quarry, the authors of this text would not only have mined the best pieces of the literature but—with the deft help of two outstanding editors—would have built an admirable edifice out of them. This book covers developmental theorists, theoretical viewpoints, multicultural matters, counseling stages, special populations, clinical applications, and ethical and legal considerations. In other words, all of the critical factors needed to understand and become involved with members of the two major populations addressed in this work are covered.

I am impressed with the layout, the writing, and the integrative nature of this volume. It should have a long shelf life, for it is extremely comprehensive and will be relevant for years to come.

Samuel T. Gladding, PhD, LPMHC, CCMHC, NCC
Professor of Counseling
Wake Forest University
Fellow in the American Counseling Association
Past President of the American Counseling Association

Preface

OVERALL GOAL OF THE BOOK

Child and Adolescent Counseling: An Integrated Approach emphasizes the powerful interconnections that support counseling central to children and adolescents. Potential users may find that the book's appeal lies in subject matter that can be used flexibly, in both school and clinical mental health counseling settings. This textbook offers practical applications for skill and theory development supplied by an impressive roster of counselor educators with a wealth of professional and clinical expertise. Moreover, this book assists in fostering graduate students in course engagement. In addition, this book may serve as a companion textbook for *Child and Adolescent Counseling Case Studies: Developmental, Relational, Multicultural, and Systemic Perspectives*, coedited by Brenda Jones, Thelma Duffey, and Shane Haberstroh.

INTENDED AUDIENCE

This textbook is for counselor educators and counseling supervisors as they assist counselors-in-training and practicing counselors in acquiring a variety of child- and adolescent-centered theories, modalities, and methods. The book can be adopted as the main textbook for a variety of class settings and will also appeal to educators, students-in-training, and supervisors in closely related fields, including social workers and psychologists.

DISTINGUISHING FEATURES/LEARNING TOOLS

The authors of this textbook have aligned student learning objectives with accountability efforts and effectiveness in higher education and presented pedagogical elements featuring the 2009 and 2016 CACREP Standards for both school and clinical mental health counseling. This is an attractive feature to educators and program directors accredited or seeking accreditation by CACREP. The authors have included charts, graphs, tables, and figures along with infused learning pedagogy, such as case studies and activities for increased conceptualization. The authors have also included chapter summaries, points to remember, other helpful items of information for consideration, and questions for further discussion to assist students in their reflections about chapter content.

INSTRUCTOR'S RESOURCES

The book offers ancillary resources for ease of course preparation and includes sample 10- and 16-week syllabi, an Instructor's Manual, PowerPoint slides by chapter, and test bank questions, which serve as time-efficient teaching tools, which users should find practical and appealing.

ORGANIZATION OF CONTENTS

This book includes content that promotes the essence of counselor growth and theoretical grounding. A focus on skill development assists counselors-in-training to help children and adolescents in their navigation of ever-changing issues laden with personal, emotional, and social developmentally nuances. Part I of this book, Developmental, Systemic, Multicultural, and Relational Perspectives for Working With Youth Populations (Chapters 1–4), provides a holistic and integrated framework for counseling that scaffolds and threads four dimensional considerations throughout the book. This framework provides a directional path, assists the counselor in avoiding counseling mishaps, functions as a great equalizer when servicing youth, and supports optimal outcomes for young clients.

This book underscores the importance of using developmental perspectives that assist youth in successfully mastering tasks associated with various developmental milestones. Chapter 1, Developmental Theorists and Other Considerations Used When Counseling Children and Adolescents, highlights the incorporation of the self, emotional, cognitive, physical, social, and academic developmental domains. This assists counselors in assessing youth's levels of readiness and helps counselors in their quest for developmentally appropriate strategies and interventions. Chapter 2, Systemic Influences That Impact Development When Counseling Children and Adolescents, discusses the ways in which individual development interfaces with environmental milieus and provides a context reflective of how child and adolescent clients exist as part of larger systems. Unhealthy systems can inadvertently thrust youth into conundrums that may lead to harmful courses of action. Collaboration and connections with these systems remain crucial aspects for counselors when conceptualizing best recovery options. Children and adolescents develop and grow in relationships where they feel a bond with others and where they can genuinely express themselves. Counselors play an increasing role in creating relational contexts to help young people cope with the challenges of growing up. Chapter 3, Relational Considerations in Child and Adolescent Counseling, provides an understanding of youth's interpersonal and intrapersonal relations, the counselor–client therapeutic relationship, and relational cultural and attachment theories applicable to children and adolescents. Children's conceptualizations of the world emerge from culture and socialization. Given this, counselors should be trained to counsel within a multicultural framework that supports these cultural contexts. In Chapter 4, Counseling Children and Adolescents: A Cross-Cultural Perspective, the authors address cross-cultural counseling competency, diversity, and the concepts of kinship and acculturation. These perspectives honor the uniqueness of child and adolescent coping and healing traditions and serve as a model for diversity, equity, and inclusion.

Part I scaffolds Part II, Theoretical Frameworks for Working With Youths: Putting Counseling Into Practice, by providing a sound theoretical basis and structure for counseling. Part II includes Chapters 5, 6, and 7. Chapter 5, Theoretical Frameworks and Applications in Child and Adolescent Counseling, reviews a collection of counseling theories and perspectives that may be used efficiently with children and adolescents. Chapter 6, Theoretical Approaches and Modalities Used With Children and Adolescents, extends Chapter 5 to demonstrate the intersection of developmental, systemic, relational, and multicultural foci to various approaches and modalities spanning a variety of methods. Chapter 6 also includes an extensive list of research-based, best-practice creative interventions for students and instructors and a list of professional organizations and conferences for counselors related to child and adolescent counseling. Chapter 7, Counseling Sessions Involving Children and Adolescents, connects contextually to the preceding chapters and addresses in particular counselors-in-training, the various stages of counseling sessions, and the need for practical formalities for conducting a counseling session in an array of counseling settings.

Part III, Bridging Gaps: Special Populations (Children, Adolescents, and Parents), includes Chapters 8, 9, and 10 and examines current influences that spur children and adolescents to seek counseling. Chapter 8, Contemporary Issues and Counseling Tropisms: Leaning Toward Promise With Children and Adolescents, features issues regarding children at risk (or, to use an evolving term, *children at promise*) and addresses topics such as anxiety, body image, bullying, social deficits and relationships, sexual identity, sexual orientation, and engagement in the age of advanced technology and social media. Chapter 9, Addressing the Needs of Children and Adolescents With Disabilities and Those Classified as Gifted, includes a delineation of federal mandates and the identification, assessment, placement, services, and postsecondary transitions pertaining to this youth population. The authors present myriad ways that counselors may promote the personal, social, emotional, academic, career, and developmental growth of children and adolescents with disabilities and those designated as gifted. Chapter 10, Addressing the Needs of Children and Adolescents of Special Populations, speaks to the needs of children and adolescents in poverty, from ethnically diverse backgrounds, of military and changing families (including those with incarcerated parents), of same-sex parents,and with grandparents as caregivers. The authors bring to the fore children and adolescents from marginalized statuses (e.g., those with limited English proficiency; immigrants; transnationals; LGBTQ; and those from transient families, including refugees, migrants, and homeless).

Part IV, Clinical Applications for Working With Minors, encompasses Chapters 11, 12, and 13 and concentrates on therapeutic applications for children and adolescents facing issues such as child maltreatment, trauma and attachment issues, and crisis. Chapter 11, Child and Adolescent Maltreatment, focuses on the identification, signs and symptoms, and strategies to address the needs of abused and neglected children and adolescents. Other topics include adverse childhood experiences, types of abuse, reporting abuse and neglect, and child maltreatment. Chapter 12, Addressing Trauma With Child and Adolescent Clients, points to the complexity of trauma experiences and attachment issues. The authors examine the neurobiological, social, psychological, and academic impact of trauma-causing events, including cyberbullying, community violence, and human trafficking. Moreover, the authors present additional information on trauma-informed counseling, including creative interventions inspired by trauma-informed care along with trauma assessment and skills training. Chapter 13, Techniques in Crisis Management Involving School-Age Children, contrasts crisis, crisis management, and critical incidents and highlights techniques in crisis management, including prevention, planning, interventive strategies and techniques, debriefing, and multicultural considerations before, during, and following critical incidents. The chapter also presents information on the roles that professional counselors play in the creation of crisis teams and in the designing, drafting, and implementation of crisis plans. In addition, the chapter discusses the reciprocal relationship between trauma and culture and examines ways that schools and communities may promote inclusivity with a culturally sensitive focus.

Part V, Personal and Professional Concerns for Counselors, includes Chapters 14 and 15 and concentrates on additional counseling influences. Chapter 14, Ethical and Legal Considerations in Child and Adolescent Counseling, highlights significant ethical, legal, and related matters with unique applications for counseling minors, including confidentiality, consent and assent, the rights of parents and minors, custodial and noncustodial parents, the Family Educational Rights and Privacy Act (FERPA) and Health Insurance Portability and Accountability Act (HIPAA), best practices for addressing ethical issues, counselor competence and credentialing, value conflicts, dual roles and relationships, and social media. Chapter 15, Other Special Topics in Counseling Children and Adolescents: Program Identity, Essential Skills, and Counselor Wellness, addresses counselor-specific topics such as establishing and addressing barriers to effective school and clinical mental health counseling, providing access to mental health counseling through the use of an empathic framework for social justice and advocacy, detailing the evolving requirements for entrance to the school counseling profession, examining professional standards that undergird counselor preparation programs, and attending to counselor self-care and wellness.

Our vision for this book involved the creation of a text that spanned the needs of counselors-in-training, professional school counselors, clinical mental health counselors, marriage and family counselors, and supervisors in order to meet the needs of the youths they serve. We sought to create a timely text that pointedly addressed the realities that children, adolescents, and their counselors are confronted with each day. The recollection of our own optimal learning experiences motivated us to keep hands-on, concrete, and workable applications in mind. We also wanted to push readers to continue their reflections and growth beyond the bounds of the book and included resources and supplemental materials to prompt continuous personal and professional growth. Ultimately, we desired a book that assembled the contextual and interconnected information necessary for providers to address optimal recovery paths for children and adolescents.

Brenda Jones
Beth Durodoye

Acknowledgments

We respect the power of the family collectively. Its communal efforts serve to inspire and motivate our work. Brenda Jones wishes to thank her daughter, Nicole Jones; her grandson, Marcus Alexander Martin Jones; her siblings; and her late parents for their constant support and strength as she journeys to continuously provide optimal outcomes in the lives of children and adolescents. Beth Durodoye would like to express gratitude to her family, with special thanks to her mother and late father, who challenged her to make a difference to humanity through the written word.

We would like to thank each chapter contributor and our foreword author, Dr. Samuel T. Gladding, for providing the expertise that supports the best practices for counseling with children and adolescents. Their rich backgrounds and experiences provided the breadth and depth necessary for work with these populations. Their extensive work in their respective specializations is indicative of the real-world examples, practical steps, and important resources that they bring to their contributions and ultimately to the reader. We commend their efforts to provide the insight and action necessary to pointedly serve children and adolescents.

The publishing process can be likened to a jigsaw puzzle, whereby construction requires the intricate placement of parts to create a cohesive whole. We are grateful to the Springer editorial team of Rhonda Dearborn and Mehak Massand, who assisted us in putting the pieces of this process in place, remained available for questions, checked in with us at just the right times, and, most importantly, allowed us to retain our vision. We also want to thank the Springer production team (Rachel Haines and Kris Parrish) and Exeter Premedia Services Private Ltd. We are indebted to their support in the realization of our book.

PART I

Developmental, Systemic, Multicultural, and Relational Perspectives for Working With Youth Populations

CHAPTER 1

Developmental Theorists and Other Considerations Used When Counseling Children and Adolescents

Brenda Jones

LEARNING OBJECTIVES

After completing this chapter, the reader should be able to:

- Identify the relationship between social, emotional, and mental health maturation with child and adolescent development.
- Demonstrate a comprehensive understanding of how developmental theory frameworks inform crafting and integrating client-centered counseling interventions, strategies, and best-practice methods.
- Develop an awareness of counseling implications when working with children with diverse developmental histories.

CACREP STANDARDS FOR THIS CHAPTER

- CACREP 2016: 2.F.3.a., b., c., e., f., g., h., i.; F.5.f., j.; School Counseling, 5.G.2.g.; Clinical Mental Health Counseling, 5.C.2.f., g., j.
- CACREP 2009: II.G.1.c., III. a., b., c., d., f., h.; School Counseling, III.A.6, E.2.; Clinical Mental Health Counseling, III. A.9., C.8., 9., D.3., E.1., 3.

INTRODUCTION

Counselors are expected to remain mindful of the importance of incorporating a developmental perspective when counseling children and adolescents and aiding them in successfully mastering tasks set at various developmental milestones. This subsists as a long-standing, core, and essential component of counseling. Developmental considerations provide great implications for counselors. Their level of development impacts how children make sense of and act in response to critical life circumstances (Jones et al., 2017; Vernon & Schimmel, 2019). A youth's level of development impacts their readiness to adapt to a fast-changing world (Gysbers & Henderson, 2013; Jones et al., 2017; Pledge, 2004; Vernon & Schimmel, 2019). Equally significant, children's level of development affects how they respond to creative and time-efficient counseling strategies, interventions, and theoretical modalities (Jones et al., 2017; Pledge, 2004; Vernon & Schimmel, 2019). This chapter highlights the fact that empowerment begins within the child or adolescent client, making counselor efficacy crucial when dealing with developmental influences on children.

KEY ASSUMPTIONS FOR POSITIVE MENTAL HEALTH

NATURE VERSUS NURTURE

Developmental psychology includes a focus on the self, social, emotional, academic, and cognitive developmental domains. Cognitive activities comprise all the psychological processes and activities involved in thinking and knowing. This involves the mental process of knowing (awareness, perception, memory, reasoning, and judgment) and includes acquiring, processing, and organizing information. Cognitive development encompasses the study of how these processes develop in children and adolescents. Examining cognitive development provides an understanding of how youth become more efficient and effective in their mental processing, which allows them to understand their world effectively. As children develop, their thinking changes. This impacts not only their cognitive development but also their self, social, emotional, and academic development (Oakley, 2004).

Nature refers to inherited factors and includes eventful milestones that occur as children naturally mature (e.g., terrible twos, puberty, and transitioning to adulthood). *Nurture* includes those positive environmental encounters or interactions that further children's development. Long-standing debates remain as to how much nature or nurture influences development (Oakley, 2004).

Development can be defined as a maturational process that results from the optimal, two-way interaction between the child and the environment. Severe stressors, such as traumatizing events and neglect, can present developmental deficits. When vital needs become deficits, children react to these deficits contingent on their developmental level in the developmental domains listed earlier (Jones et al., 2017; Pledge, 2004; Vernon & Schimmel, 2019). Without appropriate strategies and interventions needed to minimize and overcome these deficits, children's behavioral responses may unintentionally and unknowingly impair coping choices as they tenaciously struggle to regain control over their lives. As a result of various self-defeating choices and behaviors, some children and adolescents may find themselves in overwhelming situations that may evolve into new problematic circumstances with unintended outcomes. In some instances, children and adolescents may significantly lower self-efficacy and impair their self, social, personal, emotional, and cognitive development, which could lessen academic capabilities (Jones et al., 2017; Vernon & Schimmel, 2019).

Research from various fields of knowledge provides insight into defining developmental potential and the process by which development occurs. Britto et al. (2018) stress that early childhood development (ECD) programs foster the growth and development of children's cognitive and social skills, enhance future earnings, and disrupt intergenerational cycles of poverty and lost human capital. Although developmental processes transpire fairly similarly across cultures, the development rate varies as children acquire culture-specific skills and encounter the influence of other contextual factors. Whereas science points to genetics providing the blueprint for the developing brain, many theorists posit that the child's environment molds, sculpts, and influences development. Supportive and nurturing environments foster healthy development, whereas adverse and traumatic experiences result in diminished development, which can be life changing. The inseparable components of supportive and nurturing environments (adequate health, nutrition, security and safety, responsive caregiving, and early stimulation, learning opportunities, and protection) endure as necessary elements for optimal cognitive, language, and psychosocial outcomes (Britto et al., 2018).

DEVELOPMENTAL THEORISTS

A strong theoretical framework that explains human development continues to be an important element of counseling. Developmental theories lay a strong foundation for treatment and preventive interventions (Coie et al., 1993). Additionally, by explaining how human behaviors develop, developmental theories provide a foundation for how behavior can be changed creatively and in a time-efficient manner. This informs counseling intervention, strategies, parent education, and prevention programs on which influential factors to target and when these programs can yield maximal impact (Kim et al., 2015). Many educators and counselors still subscribe to the nature-versus-nurture premise and rely on the guidance of four prominent theoretical frameworks developed by Piaget, Maslow, Vygotsky, and Bandura, who speak to the *systemic, relational,* and *multicultural* influences on development. Although not covered fully in this chapter, Bronfenbrenner's Ecological Model is examined in Chapters 2 and 8 and Erickson's Stages of Psychosocial Development are reviewed in Chapter 15. Commonalities and key elements of developments attributed to the work of these theorists detail theoretical models that continue to guide developmental research and counseling through epistemological and methodological principles. These include a developmental perspective and qualitative changes in cognition in the course of development. Again, developmental theories provide useful guides for understanding children and adolescents but will not provide a comprehensive explanation about development from diverse perspectives. Consequently, developmental generalizations may not be fully applicable to all racial, ethnic, or cultural groups.

IMPACT OF THE BRAIN ON DEVELOPMENT

Regular life stressors and traumatic event exposures may impact the development of children and adolescents. Some impacts on children's growth follow typical occurrences (e.g., milestones, such as the terrible twos, puberty, and teenage transitioning, mentioned earlier) as they affect most children at predictable ages. Other impacts appear more restricted to the individual and present life-changing events (e.g., repeated and unaddressed exposure to violence and other traumatic experiences—community violence, school shootings, death and other loss of loved ones, parental incarceration, parental divorce, parents or caregivers with mental illness, and substance abuse in the home) that may have lifelong effects on executive function (EF) and learning, adversely impacting development and academic attainments (Jones et al., 2017; King-White et al., 2019).

Professionals now pay more attention to emerging brain research. Although ill defined, the construct of EF plays an important role in understanding psychological processes involved in the conscious control of thoughts and actions (Philip & Muller, 2011). Intensive research continues to focus on a variety of other viewpoints, including the perspectives highlighted in developmental counseling and psychology, developmental psychopathology, and educational counseling and psychology. Garbarino et al. (2002) report age, social, and cognitive development as key determinants of how children respond to various stimuli. Philip and Muller further stress that developmental research on EF revealed that EF first appears early in development close to the end of the first year of life and EF develops across a broad span of ages, with significant changes transpiring between 2 and 5 years of age, with almost adult-level performance reached at approximately 12 years of age. Performance on some assessment instruments progresses to adulthood, and malfunctions of EF occur in varying situations at different ages according to the complexity of the inferences required of a particular circumstance.

Children's brains become highly susceptible to threat and trauma-related cues, which in turn can affect emotional and psychological safety, health, and development. Patterns of hyperaroused brain activity may impact children's general information processing (e.g., children experiencing trauma may misinterpret ambiguous stimuli as threatening). Traumatized children may attempt to avoid stimuli that remind them of the trauma experience, causing them to disconnect emotionally from others and show diminished interest in events that they once enjoyed. Traumatized children may also experience difficulty expressing their emotions and managing and controlling their anger (Garbarino et al., 2002). When counselors teach children and adolescents to monitor their brain's neurobiological responses, youth can better regulate their cognition and their behavior. The impact of trauma will be covered more extensively in Chapter 12.

AN OVERVIEW OF FOUR PROMINENT THEORETICAL APPROACHES

PIAGET'S COGNITIVE THEORY OF DEVELOPMENT

Piaget's theory stands as the most detailed theory of cognitive development. Piaget developed a keen interest in the nature of human knowledge and how this knowledge changed over time. This included how individuals acquired, processed, and organized information. He described human intelligence as a process of adaptation: "There is a continual construction of novelty" (Piaget, 1970, p. 11). This definitive, creative, ingenious thought continues as the formidable theoretical assumption of Piaget's theory (Ginsburg & Opper, 1979; Oakley, 2004; Piaget, 1983). Piaget emphasized the central role of individual experience as a critical mechanism of development and illuminated the importance of the developing and transformative cognition in children and adolescents. Using this theoretical approach, professionals began to examine individuals' experiences and the impact these experiences present to children's and adolescents' cognitive development (Opter &

Gelman, 2011). Piaget used two guiding principles—assimilation and accommodation—to assist professionals in understanding children's and adolescents' developing cognition.

Assimilation and Accommodation

Piaget presents the role of active experience (*assimilation and accommodation*) as agents in development. He also introduced a variety of developmental tasks (e.g., *object permanence, animism, reversibility, egocentrism, centration, conservation, and equilibrium*) as critical elements of this theoretical approach. These tasks will be discussed more fully later in the chapter. Piaget defines *schemata* as the ongoing cognitive or mental structures by which individuals intellectually adapt to and organize their environments. Schemata assist individuals in processing and identifying stimuli, which enables one to make generalizations. Through numerous transactions with the environment and reflections on these transactions, children move in an orderly fashion from an understanding of the world based on action schemata, to one based on representations, to one based on internalized, organized operations (Dodd & Crosbie, 2011; Piaget, 1983). Piaget posits that clear links exist between children's cognitive development and the natural biological maturation of the brain; and that each stage of development takes place as the brain matures. Piaget saw interaction with the environment as an important factor in cognitive development (Oakley, 2004; Piaget, 1983).

ASSIMILATION

Piaget characterizes *assimilation* as the process of using knowledge and connecting this reality into one's *current* cognitive structure. Children's current cognitive makeup can limit or determine the quality of their thoughts. Distortion in thinking inevitably occurs as children attempt to integrate, comprehend, or understand this experience. Through assimilation, children continuously filter these experiences through their current ways of understanding (Dodd & Crosbie, 2011; Piaget, 1983).

ACCOMMODATION

Conversely, *accommodation* refers to advanced modifications in cognitive organization that result from new environmental experiences. The developing restructuring of thought leads to a different and more satisfactory assimilation of the experience. Consequently, assimilation and accommodation coexist in a series of progressions through development. As a result, by fully understanding objects, events, and experiences through assimilation, children accommodate by making small cognitive adjustments, bringing them to a slightly more advanced cognitive level. However, this new cognitive level makes them aware of other inconsistencies and furthers the continuing cycle of assimilation–accommodation. For Piaget, this continues as the main process and progression of development (Dodd & Crosbie, 2011; Piaget, 1983). As children proceed through the progression of assimilation and accommodation, their brains develop through the natural process of maturation. This cultivates their understanding of the world and enhances their ability to accurately interpret and make predictions of their world (Oakley, 2004; Piaget, 1983).

Piaget's most general definition of intelligence involves the child's ability to physically and mentally adapt to the environment. This includes *systemic, relational,* and *multicultural* influences on these adaptations. Bold and controversial, Piaget's assertion is that every "normal" individual's cognitive development progresses from childhood to adolescence and occurs along a continuum through a series of four broad stages—*sensorimotor, preoperational, concrete operational,* and *formal operational* (summarized in Tables 1.1–1.4). He categorized these stages as periods of time during which a child's thinking and behavior, carried out in a variety of situations, tends to reflect a particular type of underlying mental logical structure or a general way of thinking. The stages reveal the different ways children adapt to their environment, which involve the corresponding processes of assimilation and accommodation. Each stage characterizes logical capabilities of complex growth in which development evolves gradually through a cumulative more advanced process. Each stage denotes a step, and each step typifies logical capacities for multifaceted growth in which development evolves gradually through an accumulative more advanced process (Morra et al., 2008; Piaget, 1983). Each age-related but unfixed stage entails a set of mental actions, which make available a particular type of interaction between the child and the environment, providing a fundamentally different view of the world. Piaget defines *equilibrium* as an adaptive need whereby the child continuously pursues throughout life a state of cognitive balance between assimilation and accommodation. Piaget proposed that stages follow a universal sequence, with each stage deriving from the previous stage, integrating, transforming, and readying for the next stage. Piaget also posits four broad interactive factors that impact cognitive development: (a) maturation, (b) active experience, (c) social interaction, and (d) a general progression of equilibrium (Piaget, 1961).

SENSORIMOTOR INTELLIGENCE (0 TO 2 YEARS)

Piaget's view of a child's behavior during this stage largely focuses on motor skills. Children in this stage typically demonstrate no concept of a sense of rules. Even though cognitive development occurs as schemata, the child does not interpret events by thinking abstractly. Infants come into existence with no knowledge or ability to make cognitions about their new world. At birth, they navigate their world with a set of simple sensorimotor coordinations called *reflexes* (e.g., grabbing, sucking, and observing). New coordinations emerge from those present at birth by sequences of "re-equilibrations" and the development of "compensated" schemes representing the process of development.

In explaining distinctive observations of the stages, Piaget views the child in the sensorimotor stage as manipulating objects. Through changes in schemata as a result of ongoing assimilation and accommodation, a child at age 2 possesses a more refined range of cognition and affective schemata than a newborn through changes in schemata as a result of ongoing assimilation and accommodation. The child begins to display simplistic planning by anticipating events (e.g., a child requests to be picked up in anticipation that the caregiver will be leaving [Piaget, 1983; Singer & Revenson, 1996; Wadsworth, 1979, 1989]). Piaget (1983) explains *object permanence* as the understanding that objects exist even when one cannot see, feel, or hear them. As an example, infants (with no object permanence development) who see an object placed in a box will act as though the object no longer exists because they can no longer see the object.

Between 1 and 4 months, the development of hand–mouth and eye–ear coordination occurs. Around 8 to 12 months of age, infants become cognizant of using means to acquire an end. Piaget states that the child possesses the ability to combine behaviors previously learned in order to attain goals. Infants begin communicating cooperatively through pointing gestures. Primarily, these forms of communication signify infants' social-cognitive ability to direct and understand the attention of others. Subsequently, the infant must make inferences (or provoke others to make inferences) about the needed attention

TABLE 1.1 SENSORIMOTOR INTELLIGENCE: 0 TO 2 YEARS

Stage of Development	Cognitive Development *(Relational, Systemic, and Multicultural Influences)*	Social Development *(Relational, Systemic, and Multicultural Influences)*	Emotional Development *(Relational, Systemic, and Multicultural Influences)*	Self/Physical Development *(Relational, Systemic, and Multicultural Influences)*
Sensorimotor: 0–2 years	Restricted intellectual development Enhanced imagination, but not able to discern reality Schemata dependent on overt physical actions on their world	Behavior largely between sensation and motor relationships Social experimentation (mostly through play and simple imitations) Totally egocentric, unaware of causality to simple determination of causation, and no concept of rules	Experimentation and demonstration of primary emotions and interpersonal skills Reliance on early parent–child relationships, interactions, and attachment to foster feelings of trust and security Assume parent's emotional response to vague situations	No differentiation of self from other objects Navigates world with a set of simple reflexes and gross/fine motor skills (i.e., grabbing, hand-to-mouth coordination, and eye-to-hand coordination), which becomes complex, intentional, and organized Heavy reliance on parent/caregiver High level of energy

Source: Data from Jimerson, S. R., Sharkey, J. D., Nyborg, V., & Furlong, M. J. (2004). Strength-based assessment and school psychology: A summary and synthesis. *California School Psychologist, 9*, 9–19. https://doi.org/10.1007/BF03340903; Miller, P. H. (2010). Piaget's theory: Past, present, and future. In U. Goswami (Ed.), *The Wiley-Blackwell handbook of childhood cognitive development* (2nd ed.). Wiley-Blackwell; Piaget, J. (1983). Piaget's theory. In P. H. Mussen (Series Ed.) & W. Kessen (Vol. Ed.), *Handbook of child psychology: Vol 1. History, theory, and methods* (4th ed.). Wiley; Thomson, K. C., Oberle, E., Gadermann, A. M., Guhn, M., Rowcliffe, P., & Schonert-Reichi, K. A. (2018). Measuring social-emotional development in middle childhood: The middle years development instrument. *Journal of Applied Developmental Psychology, 55*, 107–118. https://doi.org/10.1016/j.appdev.2017.03.005; Wadsworth, B. J. (1979). *Piaget's theory of cognitive and affective development.* (2nd ed.). Longman; Wadsworth, B. J. (1989). *Piaget's theory of cognitive and affective development* (4th ed.). Longman.

(Bruner, 1983; Piaget, 1952), making these types of social-cognitive abilities foundational to all forms of human communication (Opter & Gelman, 2011).

Piaget categorizes the emerging cognitive structures during infancy as schemata—an organized pattern of behavior for interacting with the environment (e.g., a sucking scheme). Dodd and Crosbie (2011); Piaget (1983); Singer and Revenson (1996); and Wadsworth (1979, 1989) expanded further on this developing scheme by indicating that as the scheme develops and becomes more distinguished, children classify objects into *suckables* and *nonsuckables*, with various subgroups such as *hard suckables*, *soft suckables*, and *tasty suckables*. These schemes become progressively organized (e.g., when the sucking and grasping schemes evolve into a higher-order structure where the child demonstrates coordinated reaching for an object and taking the object to the mouth to suck). In other words, new schemata incorporate prior schemata. They do not replace them. For example, if a young girl perceives a flower to be food, at some later time, she no longer views the flower as food but as a new object called a *flower*. She does not *replace* schemata. She creates a new schema (accommodation) for "flower," while retaining her old, but now modified, schema for food (Piaget, 1983; Singer & Revenson, 1996; Wadsworth, 1979, 1989).

One-year-old infants make their first budding attempt to produce the language they hear in order to communicate more effectively with others. In a few years, they build up a collection of linguistics items through imitative, cultural learning. This imitative, cultural aspect becomes the foundational process for more complex learning even though this factor cannot account for children's acquisition of the more abstract and grammatical dimensions of language (Tomasello, 2011).

Due to undeveloped cognitions, young children may not be able to discern between real and false acts. When observing someone pretending about something novel to them, the infant's ability to interpret the act as pretense may be especially mystifying. Young children seem to assume the parent's emotional response to a vague situation and act accordingly (Lillard & Witherington, 2004).

PREOPERATIONAL THOUGHT: 2 TO 7 YEARS

Piaget (1963) states that "the individual is not born social, but progressively becomes it" (p. 6). Piaget believes that the child's interactions with the environment foster social development and that affective development interacts interchangeably with social and cognitive development. This presents huge implications for counselors. Understanding, conceptualizing, fostering, and nurturing age-appropriate and developmentally appropriate counseling strategies and interventions remain critical when providing avenues for learning, coping, and success. Practically, this can provide important information for the timing of preventive interventions across youth development.

During the preoperational stage, the child progresses from primarily functioning in a sensorimotor mode to one who increasingly thinks about navigating the environment. The child also becomes more aware of rules. The dominance of perception over reasoning further characterizes the preoperational child. The development of language and other forms of representation or symbols (e.g., deferred imitation, symbolic play, drawing, mental images, and spoken language) starts during this stage although logical reasoning is absent. Through socialization, the child masters the use of spoken language by age 4. This becomes pivotal in allowing children to further navigate their world (Piaget, 1945/1962, 1983; Singer & Revenson, 1996; Wadsworth, 1979, 1989).

Piaget sees the preoperational characteristics of *egocentrism*, *centration*, *reversibility*, and *conservation* as necessary for cognitive development. They simultaneously serve as obstacles to the child's ability to display complete logical thoughts and restrict development. In *egocentrism*, the child cannot perceive the viewpoint or assume the role of others. Instead, the child perceives that everyone thinks and views the world as the child does. Consequently, the child never processes or evaluates their thoughts and actions and perceives others to be illogical and incorrect, allowing behavior to be dictated by this premise. At around 6 or 7 years of age, the child encounters conflict, judgment, and social pressures and begins to accommodate others during these interactions. Repeated conflict, judgment, and social pressures prompt the child to evaluate the effectiveness of their thoughts and actions in comparison to others' causing a dissolution to this cognitive egocentrism. As the child matures developmentally, egocentrism slowly diminishes and exists reconstructed when new cognitive structures develop (Piaget, 1983).

Being able to discern what appears to be real becomes an important cue for development. By age 4, children also tend to be able to distinguish between what appears real and pretense (e.g., a child playing with a baby doll might understand that placing the doll on a shelf for storage does not cause long-term harm to the doll, as it would for a real baby [Lillard & Witherington, 2004; Piaget, 1983]).

Piaget describes *animism* as the notion that inanimate objects appear alive to children with undeveloped cognitive processing. They ascribe life, for example, to cartoons and characters such as those on the television show *Sesame Street* (Elmo, Big Bird, Oscar the Grouch, Cookie Monster, Grover, Bert, Kermit the Frog, and Miss Piggy) as well as to objects and forces of nature (e.g., wind, rivers, clouds, and the sun).

Centration refers to the child's inability to examine all properties or appearances of a visual stimulus. When presented with a stimulus, the child tends to be fixated on a narrow perceptual viewpoint of the stimulus. This affects the child's ability to effectively and fully assimilate (e.g., a child given two same-length pieces of yarn to compare will state that one piece of yarn curled half way appears shorter than the other piece of yarn that remains straight). This occurs even after the child first sees both pieces of yarn spread out straight appearing at exact length. Time and experience enhance perceptual growth in this area (Piaget, 1983).

Reversibility, according to Piaget (1963), "starts in the preoperational stage and fully occurs when a child can reverse operations. Closely related to centration, it represents the most clearly defined characteristic of intelligence" (p. 41), when children acquire the capacity to reverse a series of steps using basic reasoning. When individuals reverse thoughts, they can follow the line of reasoning back to where the thought started. In the first 18 months of life, children start to acquire reversibility during the sensorimotor level; however, it is not yet represented in thought. Reversibility develops gradually up to the age of 7; but children can express objects and situations in thought and action even up to the age of 11. Full reversibility emerges in thought, imagination, or hypotheticals, enabling the child to take on the qualities of mature logical and scientific thinking (Piaget, 1983).

Perhaps the most famous task, *conservation* (i.e., of number, weight, length), used by Piaget to assess children's levels of conceptual development, relates to how well children, using a logical mathematical structure, conceptualize the amount or quantity of matter remaining the same regardless of the dimension of the container that holds the matter (e.g., a child, when given the same amount of blue liquid to be poured in a short, wider container and a narrower, more slender container, will say that the liquid in the short, wider container appears less). When a counselor shows preoperational children two rows of the same number of objects with one right above the other, the children agree that both rows appear identical. After spreading out one row while the second row remains in the same position, the child agrees that the expanded row contains more. Typically, children cannot conserve during the preoperational stage. Conservation tends to develop by the end of this stage, around the age of 7 (Piaget, 1983). Piaget would say that preoperational children fail the tasks listed previously, because they lack reversible mental operations, which characterizes the next stage: concrete operations.

TABLE 1.2 PREOPERATIONAL: 2 TO 7 YEARS

Stage of Development	**Cognitive Development** *(Relational, Systemic, and Multicultural Influences)*	**Social Development** *(Relational, Systemic, and Multicultural Influences)*	**Emotional Development** *(Relational, Systemic, and Multicultural Influences)*	**Self/Physical Development** *(Relational, Systemic, and Multicultural Influences)*
Preoperational: **2–7 years**	Thoughts characterized by emerging use of symbols and gestures, more advanced than sensorimotor, but intellectual development still restricted by perceptual activities and obstacles, including egocentrism, centration, animism, reversibility, and limited attention span Rare reflections on rigid thoughts and mostly not motivated to question own thinking but can reflect on causes Rapid language development Steady movement of cognitive development through assimilation and accommodation with limited understanding of abuse, death, and divorce	Display simple imitations Social behavior restrained by level of reasoning and knowledge (limited understanding of feelings and appreciation of social concepts such as honesty, cheating, accidents, social cues, and other's emotions) Advancing verbal and communicative behavior Progressive socialization rather than regressive with engagement in cooperative play, games, and competition with an emerging understanding of rules Emerging concerns about fitting in and belonging through personal expressions and dress	Social skills formation and successive creation of meaningful peer relationships continuously cultivated by early parent–child relationships, interactions, child-rearing practices, and attachment	Waning egocentrism that revives during the attainment of new cognitive structures High energy levels

Source: Data from Jimerson, S. R., Sharkey, J. D., Nyborg, V., & Furlong, M. J. (2004). Strength-based assessment and school psychology: A summary and synthesis. *California School Psychologist, 9*, 9–19. https://doi.org/10.1007/BF03340903; Piaget, J. (1983). Piaget's theory. In P. H. Mussen (Series Ed.) & W. Kessen (Vol. Ed.), *Handbook of child psychology: Vol 1. History, theory, and methods* (4th ed.). Wiley; Thomson, K. C., Oberle, E., Gadermann, A. M., Guhn, M., Rowcliffe, P., & Schonert-Reichi, K. A. (2018). Measuring social-emotional development in middle childhood: The middle years development instrument. *Journal of Applied Developmental Psychology, 55*, 107–118. https://doi.org/10.1016/j.appdev.2017.03.005; Wadsworth, B. J. (1979). *Piaget's theory of cognitive and affective development* (2nd ed.). Longman; Wadsworth, B. J. (1989). *Piaget's theory of cognitive and affective development* (4th ed.). Longman.

CONCRETE OPERATIONS: 7 TO 11 YEARS

In contrast to the preoperational child, the concrete operations child begins to apply cognitive and affective reasoning and logical thoughts to concrete circumstances. Logical thoughts provide the means to organize experiences (schemata) that appear more developed than previous experiences. Their thoughts appear reversible, allowing them to develop the ability to reverse operations (Piaget, 1981). Around the ages of 7 to 12, they become more adept at solving centration and conservation problems. This fosters concrete reasoning, which explains thoughts and actions. Language becomes the primary mode of communication. The child demonstrates an increased ability in understanding concepts such as causality, space, time, and speed. This evolution of cognitive development surpasses that in children functioning in the preoperational stage, although they cannot yet apply knowledge to hypothetical situations, as done in the last stage of development: formal operation (Piaget, 1972).

Conservation of feelings also occurs where children become able to organize and manage their affective thoughts from one event to another. Acts of accommodation appear more developed. They tend to view situations from others' points of view; they evaluate their own reasoning and seek validation of their own thoughts (primarily through social interactions with their peers). This makes them appear less egocentric. When encountering conflicts between perception and reasoning, they make judgments based on reasoning. They possess the ability to communicate more effectively due to enhanced language development (Piaget, 1983; Singer & Revenson, 1996; Wadsworth, 1979, 1989).

Children's morality during the preoperational stage appears to be that of obedience rather than an evaluation of their own thoughts and actions. Obedience to authority serves as the vehicle to guide and determine their sense of right and wrong. Through more developed reasoning, they begin to start making their own moral judgments around the ages of 7 or 8. Children in the concrete operational stage begin to understand the implications, consequences, and impact of rules. Cooperation during social interactions becomes more pronounced (Piaget, 1983; Singer & Revenson, 1996; Wadsworth, 1979, 1989). In the last stage—formal operation—children perform operations on generating possible outcomes while evaluating them in light of evidence (Dodd & Crosbie, 2011; Piaget, 1983).

FORMAL OPERATIONS: 11 TO 15 YEARS

Formal operations begin around the age of 11 or 12. Compared to concrete operations, children in this stage display a much greater range of application and logic in their thought processes. During this time, children's cognitive development surpasses that of the concrete operations stage to evolve into the highest level of reasoning and logic. They display a highly developed understanding of causation and can handle complex verbal problems involving propositions and hypotheticals. In essence, they can employ theories or hypotheses. At this stage, children perform cognitive processes that appear almost the same as those in adults. They come up with their own autonomous views and possess a more advanced understanding of rules. The content and function of thought vary freely and continue to improve after this stage, which explains the differences between adolescent and adult processes. They can reason effectively about the present, past, and future. However, adolescents many times cannot differentiate between the logical world and the real world. The development of schemata (new areas of knowledge) does not stop at this stage. Schematic processes continue as individuals encounter new experiences. In summary, through assimilation, accommodation, and brain maturation, adolescents

TABLE 1.3 CONCRETE OPERATIONAL: 7 TO 11 YEARS

Stage of Development	Cognitive Development *(Relational, Systemic, and Multicultural Influences)*	Social Development *(Relational, Systemic, and Multicultural Influences)*	Emotional Development *(Relational, Systemic, and Multicultural Influences)*	Self/Physical Development *(Relational, Systemic, and Multicultural Influences)*
Concrete operational: **7–11 years**	Acts of accommodation more developed Thoughts more advanced than preoperational, with improved concepts of centration, reversibility, conservation, causality, space, time, and speed, yet the highest level of use of logical operation not attained—cannot apply logic to hypothetical, purely verbal, or purely abstract Gradual reasoning processes that become more logical with real, observable objects or events; can solve conservation and centration problems and attain reversibility Limited judgment made based on undeveloped reasoning, which may result in behavioral difficulties Language becomes communicative in function	Waning egocentrism primarily through social interactions with peers (succumbing to peer pressure and acceptance) Evaluate own reasoning with evolving perspective taking, and come to seek validation of personal thoughts by showing respect for others Through social interactions, verify or deny concepts through improved sense of causality, where cooperation becomes more pronounced Heightened concerns about personal expressions and dress	Self-awareness of one's own emotions through self-reflections Able to organize and manage affective thoughts from one event to another	Nonegocentric communication evolves Awareness that others can come to conclusions different from own

Source: Data from Jimerson, S. R., Sharkey, J. D., Nyborg, V., & Furlong, M. J. (2004). Strength-based assessment and school psychology: A summary and synthesis. *California School Psychologist, 9*, 9–19. https://doi.org/10.1007/BF03340903; Piaget, J. (1983). Piaget's theory. In P. H. Mussen (Series Ed.) & W. Kessen (Vol. Ed.), *Handbook of child psychology: Vol 1. History, theory, and methods* (4th ed.). Wiley; Thomson, K. C., Oberle, E., Gadermann, A. M., Guhn, M., Rowcliffe, P., & Schonert-Reichi, K. A. (2018). Measuring social-emotional development in middle childhood: The middle years development instrument. *Journal of Applied Developmental Psychology, 55*, 107–118. https://doi.org/10.1016/j.appdev.2017.03.005; Wadsworth, B. J. (1979). *Piaget's theory of cognitive and affective development* (2nd ed.). Longman; Wadsworth, B. J. (1989). *Piaget's theory of cognitive and affective development* (4th ed.). Longman.

TABLE 1.4 FORMAL OPERATIONAL: 11+ YEARS

Stage of Development	Cognitive Development *(Relational, Systemic, and Multicultural Influences)*	Social Development *(Relational, Systemic, and Multicultural Influences)*	Emotional Development *(Relational, Systemic, and Multicultural Influences)*	Self/Physical Development *(Relational, Systemic, and Multicultural Influences)*
Formal operational: **11+ years**	A much larger range of application of logical operations as compared to concrete operation Mature cognitive structure equipped almost as well as adults with assimilation and accommodation producing schematic changes throughout life Sometimes seek instant gratification with illogical thoughts and feelings of being invincible Can process a myriad of complex hypothetical and verbal problems in present, past, and future contexts Can employ theories in problem-solving in an integrated manner with a true understanding of causation	Obtain a comprehensive understanding of social norms for behavior Evolving autonomy from parents/caregivers with increased experimentation, explorations, challenging, and testing of adult beliefs Continuing concerns about personal expressions and dress	Display variations of emotions presenting increased and varying levels of stress, anxiety, tension, rebellion, and self-consciousness Can be impulsive without an awareness of future consequences Sometimes resent the boundaries that adults present	Evaluation and reflection skills more pronounced with advanced personal, moral, and ethical responsibilities Rapid growth and physical and biological changes during puberty with clear differences between males and females

Source: Data from Jimerson, S. R., Sharkey, J. D., Nyborg, V., & Furlong, M. J. (2004). Strength-based assessment and school psychology: A summary and synthesis. *California School Psychologist, 9*, 9–19. https://doi.org/10.1007/BF03340903; Piaget, J. (1983). Piaget's theory. In P. H. Mussen (Series Ed.) & W. Kessen (Vol. Ed.), *Handbook of child psychology: Vol 1. History, theory, and methods* (4th ed.). Wiley; Thomson, K. C., Oberle, E., Gadermann, A. M., Guhn, M., Rowcliffe, P., & Schonert-Reichi, K. A. (2018). Measuring social-emotional development in middle childhood: The middle years development instrument. *Journal of Applied Developmental Psychology, 55*, 107–118. https://doi.org/10.1016/j.appdev.2017.03.005; Wadsworth, B. J. (1979). *Piaget's theory of cognitive and affective development* (2nd ed.). Longman; Wadsworth, B. J. (1989). *Piaget's theory of cognitive and affective development* (4th ed.). Longman.

organize their external world and give it structure. Schemata become the products of this organization and structure throughout the life span. The process of adaptation occurs when the individual feels a need, value, or a motivation to do so. Piaget calls this need for adaptation *disequilibrium,* an imbalance between assimilation and accommodation. During disequilibrium, the child strives to seek equilibrium to further assimilation or accommodation. *Equilibrium,* a state of cognitive balance, becomes the necessary mechanism toward which individuals constantly seek. Ultimately, assimilation and accommodation account for the growth and development of cognitive structures. The concept of equilibrium and disequilibrium presents major implications for counseling children and adolescents (Piaget, 1983; Singer & Revenson, 1996; Wadsworth, 1979, 1989).

MASLOW'S HIERARCHY OF NEEDS

Maslow's (1962) hierarchy of needs theory (as depicted in Figure 1.1) provided major contributions to numerous professions. Rather than moderating behavior to an environmental stimulus, Maslow (1970), a humanistic psychologist, adopts a holistic approach to education, learning, and development by looking at the complexities of individuals' physical, emotional, social, and intellectual qualities and the impact on learning and development. Applications of Maslow's hierarchy theory to the work of counselors appear obvious. Maslow (1943) originally stated that individuals must fulfill lower-level deficit needs before progressing on to meet higher-level growth needs. He later refined his position by stating that satisfaction of a need cannot be viewed as an "all-or-none" phenomenon and admitted that his earlier statements tended toward *"the false impression that a need must be satisfied 100 percent before the next need emerges"* (Maslow, 1987, p. 69). For example, before clients' cognitive needs (higher-level needs) can be met, they must first satisfy their basic and salient physiological needs (lower-level needs; McLeod, 2018; Piaget, 1983). For example, a hungry, tired young client living in unsafe emotional and physical environments might not always resort to giving up but might continuously and resiliently struggle to focus in the moment on educational, counseling, and therapeutic interventions.

Maslow's theoretical model posits that children's needs and the fulfillment of these needs lead to healthy development and a strong foundation for the future. Maslow (1962, 1971) and Maslow et al. (1998) focused on human potentials. Maslow believed that individuals strive to reach their highest level of competence in many areas. Maslow divides this five-stage model into *deficiency needs* and *growth needs,* with the first four levels referred to as *deficiency needs* and the top level as *growth needs.* Deficiency needs, which appear most potent, result from deprivation and motivate people when deprived needs go unmet. Personal motivation to fulfill such needs becomes stronger until the need becomes fulfilled (e.g., school-age children with low self-esteem will not improve academically at an optimal pace until their level of self-esteem has increased). Also, children become less motivated to satisfy higher level needs when they continuously experience unmet lower level needs. If children do not feel a sense of safety, they sometimes become anxious, fearful, or withdrawn and lose their innate motivation to explore and learn (Wellhousen, 2019).

Maslow (1970, 1971) describes level one—the most basic needs—as *physiologic or survival needs* (e.g., food, air, water, sleep, protection, shelter, and clothing). Maslow describes level two, *safety from physical and psychological harm,* as freedom from fear, anxiety, pain, and chaos in the present moment and a trust in a predictable future in an organized world. *Love and belonging,* Maslow's level three need in the hierarchy, includes a need to be loved and to love, a belief in seeking to overcome loneliness and alienation by gaining a sense

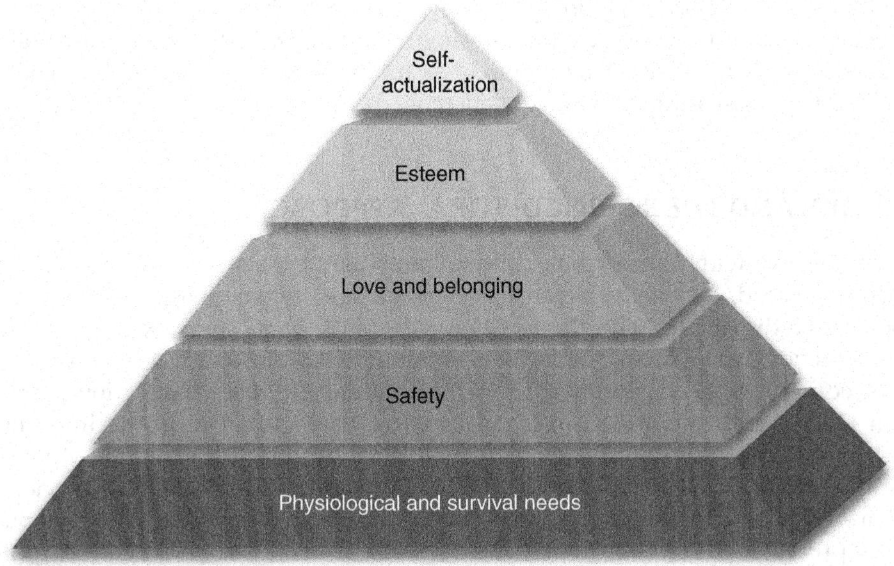

FIGURE 1.1 Maslow's hierarchy of needs.

Source: Data from Maslow, A. H. (1943). A theory of human motivation. *Psychological Review, 50*(4), 370–396. https://doi.org/10.1037/h0054346; Maslow, A. H. (1962). *Toward a psychology of being*. D. Van Nostrand Company; Maslow, A. (1970). *Motivation and personality* (2nd ed.). Harper & Row; Maslow, A. (1971). *The farther reaches of human nature*. Viking; Maslow, A. H. (1987). *Motivation and personality* (3rd ed.). Pearson Education.

of inclusion and validation. When an individual satisfies the first three levels, the need for *esteem*, level four, becomes a focus (e.g., respect, self-confidence, reputation, dignity, appreciation, prestige, achievement, and recognition). When experiencing unmet needs, people may perceive themselves as inferior or worthless.

Maslow (1970), along with McLeod (2018) and Wellhousen (2019), states that growth needs (e.g., fulfillment of goals and dreams, employment, resources, health, a realization of one's full potential) do not stem from deprivation but rather from a desire to grow as an individual. When individuals satisfy the foregoing needs, they become capable of reaching level five—the highest level need—*self-actualization*. Self-actualization needs signify the fulfillment of one's nature. "A musician must make music, an artist must paint, a poet must write, if he is to be ultimately at peace with himself. What a man can be, he must be. He must be true to his own nature" (Maslow, 1970, p. 44). Maslow believed that people do not move forward toward self-actualization when they continuously face societal hindrances (Maslow, 1970). Unfortunately, failure to meet lower level needs interrupts this progression. Lived experiences (e.g., divorce, incarceration, job loss, discrimination, the impact of a crisis such as the coronavirus disease 2019 [COVID-19] pandemic, death of a love one, and virtual grief expressions) may cause an individual to vacillate between the levels of the hierarchy. Consequently, not everyone will move through the hierarchy in a one-directional manner; some may fluctuate between the different hierarchical levels based on types of needs experienced. However, culture may present an intervening factor regarding this premise. In environments that have large numbers of people living in poverty, individuals appear capable of higher order needs, such as love and belongingness, despite deprivation, which should not occur per Maslow. Many know of individuals (e.g., Mother Teresa and Nelson Mandela) who faced innumerable deficiency needs over a large portion of their lifetime; however, they achieved self-actualization. Psychologists now conceptualize motivation as a mediating behavior, whereby needs may operate on many levels simultaneously. A person may be motivated by higher growth needs while simultaneously possessing lower level deficit needs (McLeod, 2018).

VYGOTSKY AND THE SOCIOCULTURAL APPROACH

Vygotsky agreed with Piaget that children and adolescents do not passively absorb knowledge. Instead, they actively construct knowledge. Vygotsky differed with Piaget in that he drew a distinction with the fact that children acquire complex thinking through social interactions, in particular with "expert others" (*systemic* and *relational* influences by teachers, counselors, peers, parents). Learning results from these interactions. Opter and Gelman (2011) point to cultural and social experiences as central to the importance of Vygotsky's theory of psychological development and chronicle the evolution of Vygotsky's theory into *sociocultural theory* and *activity theory*. The interconnection between sociocultural theory and the work of Vygotsky provides an interpretation of learning and development as mediated processes in that both approaches strive to theorize and investigate the processes by which social, cultural, and historical factors shape human functioning and development (Daniels, 2011). Vygotsky (1978) posits that "intermental" (social) experience shapes "intramental" (psychological) development through the aid of culturally produced artifacts (e.g., forms of talk, representations in the form of ideas and beliefs, signs and symbols). Professionals understand this to be "a mediated process produced and shaped by culture and human engagement with the world" (Vygotsky, 1934/1987, p. 78). Vygotsky further argues that cultural tools and practices produce a formative effect on development: "Every function in the child's cultural development appears twice: first, on the social level, and later, on the individual level: first between people (interpsychological), and then inside the child (intrapsychological)" (Vygotsky, 1934/1987, p. 57).

Vygotsky posits a clear relationship between language and thoughts. He further states that communication fosters individuals' social understanding (Daniels, 2011). Oakley (2004) presents the following implications regarding Vygotsky's theory for education and counseling: Vygotsky highlighted the importance of culture. Considering children and adolescents from a cultural context enhances one's understanding of their cognitive, social, emotional, and self-development. Counseling conceptualizations, assessments, and diagnoses can be flawed with a myriad of inaccurate understandings of the child without this consideration. Vygotsky believed that youth learn through their own exploration and promoted the idea that youth should be given opportunities for the use of language to enhance that exploration. Professionals should encourage youth to listen to and discuss ideas with others. This assists them in evolving their current ideas to more developed ones, thereby allowing them to come to an understanding of new ideas.

BANDURA'S SOCIAL-EMOTIONAL LEARNING THEORY

Social-cognitive theory endorses a casual structure grounded in triadic give-and-take interconnections (Bandura, 1986). In this triadic codetermination, human functioning derives from the interchange of intrapersonal influences, the individual's behavior, and the environmental forces that impact them. Again, this includes *systemic, relational,* and *multicultural* influences. Because intrapersonal influences and self-efficacy remain integral parts of the causal situations in this dynamic interchange, individuals play a large part in shaping events that take place in their lives. Founded as an agentic perspective, social-cognitive theory exerts purposeful influence over an individual's performance and the progression of experiences by one's actions. This theory provides an integrated theory of personality that speaks to the complexities of one's self-development, adaptation, and change (Bandura, 1999, 2000, 2002).

Bandura's social-cognitive theory adopts an additional perspective. Bandura (2002) offers an explanation of how the growing primacy of the symbolic environment and the expanded opportunities this theory affords enable people to exercise greater influence on how they communicate, educate themselves, carry out their work, relate to each other, and conduct their business and daily affairs. Individuals use their influence through different agencies deep-rooted in corresponding types of efficacy beliefs (Bandura, 1997, 2000). In the *personal agency* realm, individuals' influence depends on what they can control directly. However, in many areas of functioning, individuals may not possess direct control over conditions that impact their lives. They may employ what Bandura calls the *proxy agency,* instead. In this case, individuals influence others to provide resources, knowledge, and means to act on their behalf to secure the outcomes they desire. Ultimately, people do not live their lives in social isolation. Many times, in order to achieve, they must work together with others.

Self-Efficacy

Self-efficacy as a component of social-cognitive theory speaks to the foundation of self-efficacy beliefs, their structure and functional properties, their varied effects, the manner in which they work, and the progression by which one enlists such beliefs for personal and social change. Children make choices based on their self-perceptions and competence. Therefore, children perform better and appear more motivated to select increasingly challenging tasks when they believe that they hold the ability to accomplish a particular task (Bandura, 1997, 2000, 2001). Research provides abundant information on the different attributes of self-efficacy theory. Bandura states that people's beliefs regarding their capabilities vary across activities and situational circumstances, rather than manifesting uniformly across tasks and contexts. He further posits that people's beliefs in their capabilities develop in four ways and become the foundations of self-efficacy. This provides enormous implications for counseling. The first—mastery experiences—can be explained as follows: If people's attainments appear continuously easy, they come to expect quick results, which causes certain discouragement when they experience setbacks and failures. In order to develop resiliency, self-efficacy requires experience in prevailing over obstacles through perseverance. Resilience can be maintained by learning how to manage failure, in that failure becomes informative, as opposed to being intimidating and disheartening.

Second, social modeling (also known as *subconscious learning*—one of the hallmarks of social-cognitive theory, which is heavily impacted by *developmental, systemic, relational,* and *multicultural* influences) plays an influential role in developing self-efficacy through the acquisition of attitudes, values, and styles of behavior. Watching someone succeed simply through perseverance increases one's aspirations and beliefs in their own potentials. Third, Bandura lists social persuasion as a mode of influence. Being persuaded to believe in oneself increases perseverance in times when one faces struggles. This can be accomplished when the individual reduces traits such as anxiety and depression and capitalizes on physical strength and stamina, thereby acquiring a more positive self-assessment of their capabilities. Self-efficacy beliefs and coping abilities play a pivotal role in the regulation of emotional states; impact the quality of cognitive, motivational, affective, and decision-making functioning; and determine whether individuals develop a pessimistic or optimistic orientation, thereby affecting the quality of their lives (Bandura, 1986, 1997, 2001; Bandura & Huston, 1961).

Last, Bandura (1997, 2001) suggests that self-efficacy beliefs contribute to self-development. Such beliefs impact the array of options people may consider and the choices they make when deciding on setting the course of their life paths.

The Impact of Social Media on Social Learning Theory

Social learning theory posits that learning occurs through the observation, imitation, and modeling of the behavior of others (LearningTheories.com, n.d.). Deaton (2015) states that

> *social media transformed individuals' interactions and experiences. This transformation . . . changed communication, a crucial tool that fosters social learning, to a multifaceted mechanism that remains interactive, immersive, and omnipresent.* (p. 2)

Deaton further states:

> *Facebook, Twitter, Instagram, and a variety of other services are now synonymous with daily social interaction; and for the first time in human history, all the world is truly a stage . . . human interaction and learning have expanded greatly.* (p. 1)

Social media offers visual and auditory impacts that provide tactile stimuli through the physical process of interacting technological interchanges. In doing so, this multisensory approach to information sharing experienced in a social learning context provides unique avenues for symbolization and memory creation (Deaton, 2015). In essence, social media causes youth to continuously deal continuously with the complexities of our contemporary society, which presents issues far beyond their control, comprehension, and levels of developmental.

Social-Emotional Learning

Social-emotional learning (SEL) provides many implications for counselors. Some SEL interventions, grounded in Social Learning Theories, focus on how children interpret social cues and respond to social challenges. For social learning to occur, children and adolescents must exchange knowledge in an interactive environment. Within Bandura's framework for social learning, self-efficacy plays a pivotal role. In terms of social learning, children and adolescents remain steadfast in achieving a social outcome if they believe in their own capacity to achieve that outcome. Long-standing differences between self-concept and self-efficacy exist. Self-concept, as per Bong and Clark (1999), seems more strongly influenced by comparisons made in social contexts. Conversely, self-efficacy remains focused primarily on mastery. Both relate to individuals' perceptions of their abilities and appear to be influenced by individual choices (Bong & Clark, 1999). Shavelson et al. (1976) posit that self-concept plays a crucial role in explaining the alternatives children and adolescents choose when faced with decision-making tasks. As stated earlier, Bandura's (1997) self-efficacy theory stresses that ability perception appears to have a big impact on choice behavior and defines self-efficacy as the expectation to successfully perform a behavior required for a particular task.

RISK FACTORS THAT IMPACT DEVELOPMENT

Adverse social, psychological, and emotional interactions experienced by children brought on by *systemic, relational,* and *multicultural* influences incite risk factors that affect their development. The literature presents various causes of developmental communication disorders—environmental, physiological, or psychological—although most children experience difficulties for which no known etiology exists (Dodd & Crosbie, 2011). Many risk factors (e.g., inappropriate childhood discipline practices, emotional or psychological abuse, physical abuse, sexual abuse, neglect, divorce, blended family situations, military deployment, human trafficking, teenage parenting, and foster care) can provide lasting negative impacts and present asymmetrical rather than symmetrical development (Akmatov, 2011). The author of this chapter briefly examines these risk factors here; this discussion is expanded upon in other chapters.

SOCIAL, CULTURAL, AND BIOLOGICAL CONSIDERATIONS

Caregivers *systemically* and *relationally* play an important role in their children's development in diverse ways (Efevbera et al., 2017). Caregivers from poor households can devote limited resources (including time) to furthering and protecting ECD (Maggi et al., 2010). Yousafzai et al. (2018) indicate that more than 250 million children experience deficits in cognitive developmental potentials in the first 5 years of life. Research on parenting, stimulation, and early childhood education reports consistent medium to high statistical effect sizes on ECD and children's schooling outcomes.

CHILD ABUSE AND NEGLECT

From a *developmental, systemic, relational,* and *multicultural* perspective, the look in children's eyes upon encountering their caregiver many times displays anticipation as to whether this will be a positive (or a negative) interaction between the child and the caregiver. Negative interactions, collectively called *child maltreatment,* may start during early childhood, with lingering effects that may continue into adolescence. Long-standing research asserts that such maltreatment (e.g., harsh physical punishment, low nurturance, neglect, acculturation stress, historical oppression, intergenerational trauma, and ongoing marginalization) presents a number of mental health problems, including internalizing and externalizing problems as well as other maladaptive developmental problems (Maccoby & Martin, 1983; Zabin et al., 2005). Trickett et al. (2011) found that sexually abused females appear to develop earlier and have an earlier age of menarche than non-abused females, which can present many undesirable outcomes. This topic is discussed more fully in Chapter 11.

SOCIAL INFLUENCES

Although all systems (e.g., family, peer group, and media) participate in youth development, gender seems to be one social influence that impacts youths' abilities and interests (Galambos et al., 2009). Bussey and Bandura's (1999) social-cognitive theory of gender development suggests that complex social subsystems as well as cognitive processes influence gender development. They argue that boys and girls encounter different kinds of modeling and receive different feedback from their peers, families, and teachers based on their gender during their formative years. Influenced by children's immediate surroundings (e.g., parents, siblings, and caretakers), immediate settings (e.g., home and school), and external systems (e.g., workplace of parents), ECD exposure remains critical for growth (Walker et al., 2007). The home (the first and most influential environment) in which children interact and reach developmental milestones plays a significant role (Maggi et al., 2010). Therefore, a stimulating environment with nurturing, responsive, and caring parents and other caregivers (e.g., reading, singing, and playing) remains associated with language, cognitive, and social development (Black et al., 2017; Maggi et al., 2010; Yousafzai et al., 2018).

According to Perry and Pauletti (2011), females appear to outperform males on verbal tasks, and males appear to be better adept at performing spatial tasks and math word problems. In the context of attainment, females appear to choose easier tasks, avoid competition, and possess lower expectations than males and are likely to experience performance-debilitating anxiety in math. In spite of this, females currently surpass males in college enrollment, and their rate of enrollment in calculus courses appears to be similar to that of males (National Science Foundation, Division of Science Resources Statistics, 2008). In a relational context, females appear more "people oriented" and males more "things oriented" (Galambos et al., 2009). Females appear to spend a greater amount of time than males in relationship activities, whereas males appear to engage more in physical tasks, such as athletics. Females tend to prefer part-time people-oriented jobs, such as waitressing and babysitting, whereas males tend to prefer jobs that require more manual labor and working with tools. Females tend to choose more people-oriented occupations, such as teacher or social worker. Males tend to display more interest in object-oriented occupations, such as mechanic or engineer. Male competence beliefs appear higher than those of females in math, computers, and sports. Females seem stronger than males in areas such as reading, language, music, art, and social studies (Harter, 2006; Hyde, 2005). Females appear to possess poorer body image than males (Harter, 2006). Negative body image tends to foster eating disorders (anorexia, bulimia), depression, self-mutilation, low self-esteem, and appearance rumination (Ruble et al., 2006). These differences appear bigger than what probably would be expected from real differences in abilities and suggest that other factors (e.g., gender stereotypes) may contribute to this (Perry & Pauletti, 2011).

ENVIRONMENTAL FACTORS

Biological and social factors impact innate early development within the child and the wider environment of the child (Sameroff, 2006). Millions of children under age 5 in low- and middle-income areas fall short of acceptable outcomes for physical, educational, and cognitive development due to *systemic* impacts such as poverty, poor nutrition, and other social risks (Grantham-McGregor et al., 2007). A recent study estimated that many of these children show below-than-expected outcomes for socioemotional or cognitive development. Children's competencies may be inhibited with long-term consequences (Efevbera et al., 2017). Understanding the impact of factors such as poor health and nutrition remains important for early childhood developmental outcomes, because they provide the need for appropriate intervention that sets children on a positive trajectory for adulthood (Anderson et al., 2003; Engle et al., 2011).

Studies examining child and adolescent development (Jencks & Mayer, 1990; Leventhal & Brooks-Gunn, 2000) suggest that poverty provides an ecologic context that affects individuals' growth, development, and adjustment. Furthermore, poverty exacerbates family challenges in providing the experiences, resources, and services that remain essential for underprivileged youth to thrive and grow into healthy, productive adults.

Poverty- and crime-stricken neighborhoods create additional challenges for adolescents to develop positive social networks and avoid poor developmental outcomes. In addition, schools in deprived communities lack resources and social capital to provide quality education and usually evidence low student achievement, increased school failure, and dropout rates (Murry et al., 2011; Neild & Balfanz, 2006).

Conditions such as war, disaster, displacement, the chaos of forced migration, and the impact of the COVID-19 pandemic put children and adolescents at high risk for developmental difficulties. These conditions present risk of poor developmental outcomes (e.g., lower academic achievement, reduced economic earnings, and lower levels of physical and mental health) and may follow them throughout their lives.

WAYS TO ENHANCE DEVELOPMENT

Despite the enormous range of developmental challenges presented to children and adolescents, not all encounters produce maladaptive outcomes as they traverse stage-salient and other contextual tasks (as illustrated in Figure 1.2). Many children and adolescents experience dynamic *developmental, systemic, relational,* and *multicultural* interplays between

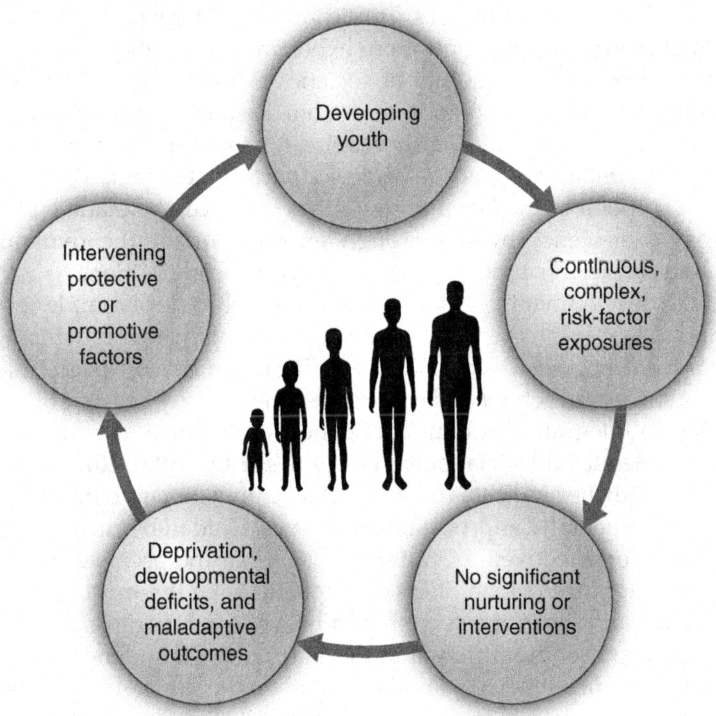

FIGURE 1.2 Cycle of healthy development.

Source: Data from Akmatov, M. K. (2011). Child abuse in 28 developing and transitional countries—results from the multiple indicator cluster surveys. *International Journal of Epidemiology, 40*, 219–227. https://doi.org/10.1093/ije/dyq168; Kim, B. K. E., Obesterle, S., Catalano, R. F., & Hawkins, J. D. (2015). Change in protective factors across adolescent development. *Journal of Applied Development Psychology, 40*, 26–37. https://doi.org/10.1016/j.appdev.2015.04.006; Search Institute. (2020). *Developmental assets.* https://www.search-institute.org/our-research/development-assets.

themselves and predictable environments, which allows them to undergo positive adjustments, in turn producing healthy social, emotional, personal, and behavioral development. Over the past 20 years, researchers and practitioners have been interested in understanding protective factors (Fraser, 2004), often referred to as *internal* or *external promotive factors* (Sameroff, 2006) or *assets* (Mannes et al., 2005), and stressed the importance of their positive function and role in youth development. These factors give children new perspectives, decrease the probability of problem behaviors, and increase the likelihood of positive outcomes. External protective factors (e.g., resources, opportunities, mentoring, social capital, and recognition) and internal protective factors (e.g., skills, resilience, motivation, desire, ability, and self-worth) occurring across multiple domains foster healthy development (Kim et al., 2015; Search Institute, 2020). Opportunities for involvement in community-based prosocial activities encourage families to increase opportunities and ensure that youth receive ample opportunities to interact with prosocial peers (Kim et al., 2015). Protective factors are discussed further in Chapter 11.

Hamre and Capella (2015) highlight the importance of schools as a central context for child and adolescent development. In the absence of a caring and nurturing environment, children may experience severe stress and psychosocial deprivation, which can lead to long-term effects on health, learning, and behavior.n the absence of a caring and nurturing environment Severe, prolonged stress and psychosocial deprivation not only affect the individual child but also may extend to subsequent generations and to the broader community through biological, behavioral, and socioeconomic processes. This leads to an intergenerational cycle of adversity, disadvantage, and trauma and the continuous exposure to inequities. These issues jeopardize the safety, social cohesion, and stability of societies (Murphy et al., 2018). Early childhood development programs and responsive care from a consistent, nurturing caregiver and community system during the child's early years may provide protection and buffer the child from negative effects and consequences while supporting healthy development. Buchmann and Steinhoff (2017) point to the fact that significant gains can be made with developmental outcomes across adolescence by a thorough examination of the dynamic interplay of opportunities and constraints linked to young people's social position.

Children with developmental issues experience a multitude of complex problems. Again, early family and systemic interventions conducive to shaping and enhancing development become imperative (Chojnacka-Synaszko, 2016). Research demonstrates that SEL remains key to children's successful school and career outcomes mostly because SEL tenets enhance children's ability to integrate thinking about their emotions and behaviors in ways that lead to positive academic and social outcomes (Jones & Doolittle, 2017; Swartz, 2017). Jones and Doolittle (2017) further indicate that SEL interventions seem to be most effective when presented as developmentally appropriate modalities. Guided by three essential principles that form the basis for effectiveness, SEL presents, first, the premise that neurologic and physical changes determine which SEL skills appear to be the most important at a given developmental state and when mastery should be achieved. For example, a shift from the ability to recognize and name different emotional states to understanding that different people can experience different emotional reactions to the same objective situation evolves and matures gradually, spanning from early childhood to adolescence. In other words, the set of skills broadens over time with some primary skills serving as the basis for later skills. Second, children's experiences (from early childhood through adolescence) outside the family and home become broader, more diverse, and influential as they grow older. Third, the method of intervention delivery must be appropriate to a child's developmental level (e.g., using play-based programs for younger children, didactic teaching and experiential activities that promote practice in middle childhood, and interventions that account for viewpoints and need for autonomy and respect for adolescents).

Additional ways to enhance development include counselors teaching youth about what happens to their brain when they encounter traumatic experiences. In the face of a crisis, older children and adolescents may use this information to "calm" their brains by taking a "mental walk" through the neurologic reactions to their bodies. In doing so, they may decrease self-sabotaging responses and outcomes. Moreover, counselors may refer youth to local university counseling services provided by the counseling clinical department or university-level counseling centers.

CASE STUDY 1.1: ADRIANA'S STORY

Adriana, an extremely emotional 16-year-old ninth-grade Hispanic female who lives in a south-central Texas city, came to the counselor's office to talk about her depressive feelings resulting from recent negative interactions with members of her peer group. Her peers confronted her about her promiscuity and unceasingly denigrated her character in a very public way. Adriana appeared confused because her mother and grandmother continuously modeled this lifestyle, which also served as a means for family income. All her life, she considered these actions to be a way of showing love and appreciation.

Over a series of counseling sessions, the counselor explored Adriana's backstory and discovered that Adriana came from a socioeconomically poor neighborhood. Adriana's mother requested that Adriana—although not fully an emancipated teen—move out, find her own apartment, and make a living for herself at the age of 15. From this, Adriana experienced encounters that most adults would struggle to navigate. From other disclosures, the counselor found out that Adriana, a new student to the campus, repeated the ninth grade due to language barriers and attendance issues while attending her previous school. Adriana enrolled as an English-Language Learner/Limited English Proficiency student. Her prior school sent recommendations to place Adriana in all remedial core courses although Adriana had earned exceedingly high grades in each of these courses.

Over the course of meeting with Adriana, the counselor integrated activities that enhanced Adriana's self-worth and her intrapersonal and interpersonal awareness regarding society's expectation of female behavior. The counselor and Adriana processed those societal behavioral expectations that appeared fair and objective as well as those that appeared to be subjective and not so fair. As Adriana's sense of self-worth, self-acceptance, and academic performance increased, the counselor met with Adriana and her core academic teachers to see if the teachers would allow Adriana to complete upper level honors and advanced placement honors courses instead of the remedial classes. All teachers agreed, and Adriana met the counselor's expectations by earning all A's. This presented clear evidence that the school, upon Adriana's entrance, inappropriately placed Adriana in courses far below her potential.

Adriana's enhanced academic performances continued through her senior year. The counselor worked collaboratively with Adriana (now 19 years old) to complete and submit admission applications and the necessary college/university-level and federal financial aid forms. The counselor also wrote letters of recommendations

(*continued*)

CASE STUDY 1.1 (*continued*)

to discreetly explain Adriana's dilemma at the beginning of her high school career and the progress and successes she later demonstrated as a graduating senior. Adriana graduated with a partial scholarship to a local university. About 15 years later, the counselor received an urgent email from Adriana, in which she invited the counselor to her university graduation ceremony. Somehow Adriana's undergraduate education was interrupted, but she persisted, switched universities, and was graduating. The counselor attended the graduation and witnessed the university president honor Adriana as the top graduate in the class! During her speech, Adriana openly recognized the counselor as a major factor that fostered her success. After graduation, Adriana started a teaching career, during which she also served as a mentor to students who encountered life experiences similar to hers.

Activity 1.1

Form small groups within the class. Participate in full discussions of the following questions. Refer to areas covered in this chapter (e.g., *nature versus nurture, developmental theories, brain development, risk factors*, and *developmental enhancers*) in your answers. Afterward, select a reporter for your group who will share answers to the full class:

- What multicultural or diversity factors would you consider for Adriana as you assess her needs?
- Assess and discuss how Adriana's personal, social, cognitive, and academic developmental levels first inhibited and later contributed to her growth, wellness, resiliency, and achievement.
- What systemic and relational approaches would you consider in your work with Adriana as a counselor?

CHAPTER SUMMARY

Developmental considerations provide great implications for counselors. Development follows a path that is continuously impacted by systemic, relational, and multicultural influences. These influences affect how children make sense out of and act in response to critical life circumstances. Incorporating a developmental perspective when counseling children and adolescents and aiding them in successfully mastering tasks at various developmental milestones continue to be an essential core component of counseling. Children's level of development affects how they respond to creative and time-efficient counseling strategies, interventions, and modalities. This makes counselor efficacy in developmental influences on children fundamental and foundational. Four prominent theoretical lenses, created by Piaget, Maslow, Vygotsky, and Bandura, serve as the framework for this chapter.

Developmental psychology includes domains such as self, social, emotional, and cognitive development and includes the process of how children and adolescents acquire, process, and organize information in order to gain a better understanding of their worlds. Long-standing debates remain as to how much nature or nurture plays a role in development. Nurture includes those positive environmental encounters that foster children's development. Although science points out that genetics provide the blueprint for the developing brain, nurture (the child's environment) molds, sculpts, and influences development. Supportive and nurturing environments foster healthy development, whereas adverse and traumatic experiences produce risk factors that can lead to asymmetrical rather than symmetrical development, which can in turn have lasting, life-changing effects.

Although developmental processes transpire similarly across cultures, the development rate varies as children acquire culture-specific skills and the influence of other contextual factors while experiencing relatable tragedies. Consequently, developmental generalizations may not be fully applicable to all racial, ethnic, or cultural groups.

POINTS TO REMEMBER

- *Development* can be defined as a maturational process that results from the optimal, two-way interaction between the child and the environment.
- Systemic, relational, and multicultural influences impact development.
- When vital needs become deficits, children react to these deficits contingent on their developmental level in the developmental self, social, emotional, academic, and cognitive domains.
- Brain research, including an understanding of EF, plays an important role in understanding psychological processes involved in the conscious control of thoughts and actions.
- When counselors teach children and adolescents to monitor their brain's neurobiological responses, youth can better regulate their cognition and their behavior.
- Despite developmental encounters presented to children and adolescents, not all challenges produce maladaptive outcomes as they traverse stage-salient and other contextual tasks.
- Early family and systemic interventions conducive to shaping and enhancing development remain imperative.

OTHER HELPFUL INFORMATION FOR CONSIDERATION

- A full summary of Piaget's theory falls beyond the scope of this chapter, and the author refers readers to other sources using the following URL: www.piaget.org
- The Search Institute's 40 Developmental Assets assists counselors, educators, and parents in their effort to foster youth development. The following link provides information and handouts in English and Spanish for various age groups: www.search-institute.org/our-research/development-assets/developmental-assets-framework
- Additional information regarding Albert Bandura's Social Learning Theory may be found at www.verywellmind.com/social-learning-theory-2795074
- Videos of Vygotsky's sociocultural theory can be found at www.bing.com/videos/search?q=vygotsky%27s+theory&qpvt=vygotsky%27s+theory&FORM=VDRE

- The Nurturing Care for Early Childhood Development framework may be found at nurturing-care.org/resources/nurturing-care-framework-toolkit
- Videos of Maslow's hierarchy of needs may be found at www.bing.com/videos/search?q=maslow%27s+hierarchy+of+needs&qpvt=maslow%27s+hierarchy+of+needs&FORM=VDRE

QUESTIONS FOR FURTHER DISCUSSION

- What ways can counselors assist parents through psychoeducational sessions in understanding stage-salient and other developmental contexts?
- How can developmental frameworks be influenced by culture-specific and other contextual factors?
- What avenues can counselors use to increase the awareness of traumatized youth to understand what happens to their brain when responding to trauma-related cues?
- In what ways can counselors assist schools and communities in providing early exposures and opportunities to enhance children's development during the formative years?
- What creative means might counselors use to foster growth in youth with asymmetrical development (e.g., children and adolescents with physical, mental, and neurologic disabilities)?

KEY REFERENCES

Only key references appear in the print edition. The full reference list appears in the digital product on Springer Publishing Connect: connect.springerpub.com/content/book/978-0-8261-4764-6/part/part01/chapter/ch01

Bandura, A. (1997). *Self-efficacy: The exercise of control.* Freeman.

Bandura, A. (2001). Social cognitive theory: An agentic perspective. *Annual Review of Psychology, 52,* 65.

Dodd, B., & Crosbie, S. (2011). Language and cognition: Evidence from disordered language. In U. Goswami (Ed.), *The Wiley-Blackwell handbook of childhood cognitive development* (2nd ed.). Wiley-Blackwell.

Jones, B., Duffey, T., & Haberstroh, S. H. (Eds.). (2017). *Case studies in child and adolescent counseling: Developmental, relational, multicultural, and systemic perspectives.* Springer Publishing Company.

Maslow, A. H. (1970). *Motivation and personality* (2nd ed.). Harper & Row.

Oakley, L. (2004). *Cognitive development.* Routledge.

Piaget, J. (1983). Piaget's theory. In P. H. Mussen (Series Ed.) & W. Kessen (Vol. Ed.), *Handbook of child psychology: Vol 1. History, theory, and methods* (4th ed., pp. 41–102). Wiley.

Vernon, A., & Schimmel, C. (2019). *Counseling children and adolescents* (5th ed.). Cognella Academic Publishing.

Vygotsky, L. S. (1987). *The collected works of L. S. Vygotsky. Vol. 1: Problems of general psychology, Including the volume "Thinking and speech"* (R. W. Rieber & A. S. Carton, Eds., N. Minick, Trans.). Plenum Press. (Originally work published 1934)

Wadsworth, B. J. (1979, 1989). *Piaget's theory of cognitive and affective development* (2nd & 4th ed.). Longman.

CHAPTER 2

Systemic Influences That Impact Development When Counseling Children and Adolescents

Laura A. Granato and Jennifer Laurenza

LEARNING OBJECTIVES

After completing this chapter, the reader should be able to:

- Identify the many systems that impact child and adolescent development.
- Describe ecological systems theory.
- Recognize the many different types of families.
- Explain how counselors in schools and mental health settings can adopt a systemic view of child and adolescents.
- Illustrate the impact of culture in the systems in which children and adolescents are embedded.
- Explain how counselors can assist in collaborating with and connecting systems for best treatment outcomes.
- Outline best practices for counselors working with children and adolescents.

CACREP STANDARDS FOR THIS CHAPTER

- CACREP 2016: 2.F.1. b, c, e, i, j, k; F.2. a, b, c, d, e, f, g, h; F.3. a, e, f, g, i; F.5. a, b, d, e, f, h, j, k, m; School Counseling: 5.G.1.d; G.2.a, b, d, g, k; G.3.h, l; Clinical Mental Health Counseling: 5.C.2. a, c, f, g, j, l; C.3. d, e.
- CACREP 2009: 2.G.1.b, c, i, j; G.2.a, b, c, d, e, f; G.3.a, c, d, f, h; G.5.a, b, c, e; School Counseling: A.2., 3, 6; B.1; C.1, 3, 5, 6; D.1, 2, 3, 5; E.1, 2, 3, 4; F.1, 2, 3, 4; G.1; H.1, 4, 5; M.1, 2, 3, 4, 5; N.1, 2, 3, 5; O.4; Clinical Mental Health Counseling: A.2, 3, 7, 9; B.1; C.1, 3, 5, 6, 8, 9; D.2, 3, 4, 5; E.1, 2, 3, 4, 5, 6; F.1, 2, 3.

INTRODUCTION

Children and adolescents depend on many systems to foster their social, emotional, personal, and developmental needs. A system consists of a network of interrelated and interdependent parts, where each part impacts the other parts positively or negatively. As mentioned in Chapter 1, some of the many systems embedded in the lives of children and adolescents include the family system, the peer system, the school system, and the community and societal systems. Changing family configurations include traditional, single parent, never married, blended, multigenerational, military, teen, LGBTQ, and foster care families. Since these larger systems encompass children and adolescents, collaboration with and connection to these systems remain crucial to the conceptualization of best approaches for treatment. When youth engage in systems that seem healthy, strong, and trusting, they develop resiliency to face rapid social changes. Counselors need to maintain a systemic perspective when working with children and adolescents in order to provide holistic care and achieve the best possible treatment outcomes.

ROLES AND INFLUENCES: SOCIAL, EMOTIONAL, PERSONAL, AND DEVELOPMENTAL

Bronfenbrenner (1917–2005), a Russian-born American psychologist and early childhood theorist, remains integral to the discussion on how systems influence children and adolescents (Ashiabi & O'Neal, 2015; Gilstrap & Zierten, 2019). As a developmental psychologist focused on human growth and development in relation to age (Eriksson et al., 2018), Bronfenbrenner developed the *human ecology theory (ecological systems theory)*, later coined the *bioecological theory*, which proposed that children develop in the context of relationships (e.g., families, friends, schools, neighborhoods, community, and society; Ashiabi & O'Neal, 2015; Gilstrap & Zierten, 2019). The *bioecological theory* stresses the role played by the individual, the impact of time, and proximal processes (the reciprocal interaction between the developing individual and other significant people in their life, such as parents or other children; Rosa & Tudge, 2013).

Bronfenbrenner proposed a reciprocal relationship between an individual and the environment: The environment influences an individual and, in turn, the individual impacts the environment (Ashiabi & O'Neal, 2015; Gilstrap & Zierten, 2019). Interdependent social systems influence and may be influenced by individuals, both directly and indirectly (Ashiabi

& O'Neal, 2015; Graves & Sheldon, 2017). Unlike other individual-focused approaches, ecological systems theory recognizes that even public policy influences development by influencing the conditions of one's life (Ashiabi & O'Neal, 2015; Gilstrap & Zierten, 2019).

Furthermore, Bronfenbrenner offered five subsystems in which human growth occurs: the microsystem, mesosystem, exosystem, macrosystem, and chronosystem (Ashiabi & O'Neal, 2015; Gilstrap & Zierten, 2019).

The *microsystem* reflects the small, immediate environment in which the child lives (Gilstrap & Zierten, 2019). Children's microsystems will include any immediate relationships or organizations they interact with, such as their immediate family or caregivers and their school or day care (Ashiabi & O'Neal, 2015; Gilstrap & Zierten, 2019). The more these groups or organizations demonstrate supportive, warm, and nurturing interactions with the child, the greater the child's opportunities for growth (Gilstrap & Zierten, 2019).

The next level, the *mesosystem*, describes how the different parts of a child's microsystem work together for the child (Gilstrap & Zierten, 2019). Two or more microsystems interacting can present a significant influence on a child's development (Gilstrap & Zierten, 2019). This might include friends interacting with parents, parents interacting with teachers, and teachers interacting with friends (Gilstrap & Zierten, 2019). For example, if a child's caregivers take an active role in a child's education (including interacting with the child's teacher), this will help promote the child's overall growth. In contrast, if the child's caregivers disagree with each other on how to parent the child or engage in high amounts of conflict, this could potentially hinder the child's growth in multiple ways (Gilstrap & Zierten, 2019).

The *exosystem* level includes the other people and places that the child may not interact with but that still present a large personal impact, such as parents' workplaces, extended family members, and the neighborhood (Gilstrap & Zierten, 2019). For example, if a child's parent becomes unemployed, the family may face financial hardship, which appears likely to present negative effects on the child; however, if the child's parent secures a new, higher-paying job, this may result in a positive effect on the child because of the family's likelihood of experiencing financial stability (Gilstrap & Zierten, 2019).

The *macrosystem* consists of the larger culture, which might include the child's personal identity, racial identity, ethnic identity, socioeconomic status, and the political and social ideologies of that culture (Gilstrap & Zierten, 2019). Lastly, the *chronosystem* encompasses major life transitions, environmental events, and historical events that occur during the child's development (Gilstrap & Zierten, 2019). Significant events (e.g., moving, a parent being deployed with the military, diagnosis of a chronic illness) in a child's life influence how the child interacts with all the other systems (Gilstrap & Zierten, 2019).

A child or adolescent's temperament influences their development and adaptability to various environments. An extroverted child, for example, may make friends easily and without much effort, while a more introverted child may struggle to make friends and may attribute this to their own deficiencies.

Francesca, for instance, an 18-year-old, navigates the transition as a first-year college student living in a residence hall 2 hours away from home. She appears to be a naturally outgoing young person living with a chronic disease, inflammatory bowel disease, seasonal depression, and anxiety that causes facial tics. However, certain protective factors, including a pleasant temperament, a tendency to seek out social interactions, an inclination toward independence and organization, and family support seem to contribute to a smoother transition than for some young adults. She summarizes her experiences in the following way:

In a nutshell, college is great. For me personally, the transition wasn't that hard. I've always been independent, so the change wasn't that dramatic for me. I've been doing my own laundry since I was 13 and am already extremely organized because I like doing everything myself. The only big change for me is almost completely living on my own and being far from my friends and family. However, I'm only 2 hours away from home so I can really go home whenever I want, and I have seen my family a lot more than I thought I would. I love the independence and freedom of being on my own. I have so much more free time and less work than I had in high school. Everyone that comes here is paying and choosing to be here, so it's taken more seriously than high school. And if someone decides to slack off and fail their classes, it's their money down the drain.

My schedule is great, and I live with all people my age. I live in the same building as most of my friends so we can literally see each other whenever we want. However, living with all your best friends and hanging out 24/7 sounds like the life to live until you all start to become sick of each other. That is the biggest downside, aside from the work, of course. It also stinks that mental illness must follow you to college, or what I like to call the happiest place on earth (Disney's got nothing on my school). Where I am, it gets cold and dark fast, so my seasonal depression came quick. And even though I am surrounded by all my friends and am loving college, I am still having those days (or even weeks) that I just need to go home and get a break from everyone. Friend groups, mental/physical health, course loads, clubs, sports, etc. are all hard to deal with, but that's life.

Mental health and mental illness play an important role in a child or adolescent's well-being, success in school, and overall outcomes. Adolescence, in particular, presents a challenging period for both children and families, characterized by many physical, social, and psychological changes. Some adolescents cope well with the stress of this developmental stage. Others experience difficulties coping and develop mental health disorders such as adjustment disorders, major depressive disorder, and generalized anxiety disorder. Some adolescents struggle with mental health challenges since childhood, which might include disorders named earlier or others such as attention deficit hyperactivity disorder (ADHD), obsessive compulsive disorder (OCD), autism spectrum disorder (ASD), and bipolar disorder. Clinicians often refer to children and adolescents with ASD as *neurodiverse* as opposed to *neurotypical* (those not diagnosed with ASD); see Armstrong (2015). These and other conditions will be expanded in subsequent chapters.

Although professionals do not universally accept the concept of neurodiversity, it appears to be increasingly supported by research (Masataka, 2018). *Neurodiversity* proposes that individuals with developmental disorders such as ASD should not be pathologized and instead should be viewed as falling into the normal variation of human behavior, while offering many strengths and gifts to society (Masataka, 2018). Although children and adolescents navigating neurodiversity and mental health challenges exhibit many strengths, they also may need support and accommodation to ensure best outcomes (Armstrong, 2015).

Mental health problems during childhood and adolescence constitute a major public health concern. Epidemiological studies show that mental health issues appear to be the first nonfatal cause of illness, ranking in the top five causes of death among adolescents and representing 16% of the global health-related burden in young people (Jiménez et al., 2019). In addition, mental health problems during adolescence remain an important predictor of socialization difficulties and absenteeism at this developmental stage, as well as one of the most significant predictors of adjustment problems and mental disorders in adulthood (Jiménez et al., 2019). Counselors need to be adequately prepared, then, with effective intervention and prevention strategies that meet the specific needs of adolescents with mental health problems (Jiménez et al., 2019).

Research supports the importance of incorporating complementary approaches targeting families in their regular services in order to adequately address the complex needs and difficulties of families of adolescents with mental health issues (Jiménez et al., 2019). Additionally, research supports a need to directly target the parental relationship and the parent–child relationship when intervening with families of adolescents with mental health problems (Jiménez et al., 2019).

FAMILY SYSTEM

Many often overlook the family to be a dynamic, complex system. Bowen (1978) introduced the *family systems theory*, which proposes that individuals can only be understood in the context of their family (Bowen Center for the Study of the Family, 2021). Families consist of systems of interconnected and interdependent individuals; family members rely on each other for support and approval and react to each other's needs, expectations, and emotional responses (Bowen Center for the Study of the Family, 2021). A change in one person's behavior usually causes corresponding changes in other members of the family (Bowen Center for the Study of the Family, 2021).

In applying family systems theory, counselors need to assess the family system, even when meeting individually with a child or adolescent client, in order to gather important contextual information. Doing so ultimately provides more effective and relevant interventions for children and adolescents. One tool for assessing the family dynamics incorporates the genogram, considered a more complex version of a family tree that typically looks at three generations of family members and identifies relationship patterns as well as mental health disorders, suicide, and substance abuse. Murray Bowen developed the concept of family diagrams as part of his family systems model. Monica McGoldrick later developed it into an important and popular therapeutic tool.

A genogram can be completed efficiently and quickly and helps open a dialogue about family relationships and dynamics (Young et al., 2018). Completing genograms with children and adolescents helps elicit important information, engage the client, build communication and rapport, and improve self-awareness, as well as guides counselors in pinpointing treatment goals (Tobias, 2017). Although genograms typically focus on historical data, more problematic interactions, and past patterns of behavior, some counselors adopt a different approach to using genograms with children and adolescents (Taylor et al., 2013). This approach involves solution-focused and narrative therapies, with a focus on current interactions, strengths, and resources tailored to the age and developmental level of the child or adolescent (Taylor et al., 2013).

Culture, Family Dynamics, and Lived Experiences

Ecological theories of child development describe how numerous systems connect to support both healthy and unhealthy development. Family networks and dynamics, including sibling relationships, remain central to early child development. Cultural factors such as socioeconomic status, race, gender roles, ethnicity, sexual orientation, gender identity, and religion as well as family history, values, and rituals significantly influence child development and the lives of families (Erdem & Safi, 2018).

Culture often refers to a group of people who share similar beliefs, spirituality, language, literature, art, science, cuisine, customs, and traditions, as well as physical objects such as clothing, artifacts, and jewelry (Mironenko & Sorokin, 2018). Family members often pass down the components of culture through the generations in a nonbiological manner (Mironenko & Sorokin, 2018). Traditions, religion, food, and even dress and clothing influence child development. Research demonstrates that racial and ethnic pride can lead to higher self-esteem; for instance, adolescents who score highly on ethnic identity also tend to demonstrate higher levels of self-esteem (Bracey et al., 2004). This highlights the importance of promoting both healthy self-esteem and positive ethnic identity development in adolescents, in clinical settings and in schools (Bracey et al., 2004).

Cultural parenting styles generally pass from generation to generation, which may influence how children learn—cognitive, social–emotional, language, self-help, and physical fine and gross motor skills. Also, children may achieve motor development milestones at different ages depending on culture (Academy of Pediatric Physical Therapy, American Physical Therapy Association, 2018). For example, cross-cultural research demonstrates that infants in Jamaica often skip crawling because of cultural beliefs that crawling is primitive (Academy of Pediatric Physical Therapy, American Physical Therapy Association, 2018). A higher percentage of 5-month-old infants living in Cameroon and Kenya are independently sitting compared to 5-month-old infants living in Argentina, Italy, South Korea, and the United States, which researchers attribute to differing emphases on upright positioning and opportunities for practicing sitting during daily activities (Academy of Pediatric Physical Therapy, American Physical Therapy Association, 2018). These differences are noteworthy because it is common for families to retain their culture-specific caregiving practices when they immigrate to a different country; thus, a child born in the United States to parents raised in another country may be raised using culture-specific practices (Academy of Pediatric Physical Therapy, American Physical Therapy Association, 2018).

People often use race and ethnicity interchangeably. However, unlike ethnicity, people base race on inherited physical traits, such as skin color and facial features. The definitions of race and ethnicity have been widely debated. As defined by society, race most often refers to physical differences that groups and cultures consider socially significant, while ethnicity refers to shared culture, such as language, ancestry, practices, and beliefs (American Sociological Association, 2020). Sociologists challenge these definitions as socially constructed and focus on how the terms "race" and "ethnicity" connect to the idea of majority and minority groups as well as the social structures of inequality and power (American Sociological Association, 2020). Race and ethnicity are connected to political and policy debates about issues such as immigration, identity formation, and racism (American Sociological Association, 2020). Likewise, researchers Eichelberger et al. (2018), in their discussion of whether race should be used as a variable in research on preterm birth, posit that in clinical research, race is often defined by fixed biological traits when in reality, race is a social construct influenced by systematic discrimination (2018).

The U.S. Census Bureau, in their data collection process, applies a narrow lens to the concepts of race and ethnicity. The U.S. Census Bureau (2020) defines race as a person's self-identification with one or more social groups. On the census, an individual can report as White, Black or African American, Asian, American Indian and Alaska Native, Native Hawaiian and Other Pacific Islander, or some other race. Survey respondents may report multiple races (U.S. Census Bureau, 2020). The Census Bureau (2020) defines ethnicity, for the purpose of the census, only in terms of whether a person identifies as Hispanic. For this reason, ethnicity divides along two lines—Hispanic or Latinx and Not Hispanic or Latinx. Hispanics may report as any race.

Considering the diversity of race and ethnicity within our communities, best practices consistently indicate that professional counselors must use culturally competent practices with their clients (Matthews et al., 2018). Multicultural counseling competence (MCC), a core requisite for professional and school counselors, requires counselors to be nonjudgmental and empathic when addressing relevant cultural issues with clients (Matthews et al., 2018). Culturally competent counselors should remain aware of their own biases and belief system and retain cultural knowledge and knowledge about power, privilege, and oppression (Matthews et al., 2018). Studies consistently demonstrate that clients experience a more positive relationship with culturally competent counselors (Matthews et al., 2018).

Religious affiliations can also present either positive or negative influences on children's development (or both). For instance, belonging to a faith community can provide a sense of belonging, shared beliefs and values, a sense of purpose and hope, a moral compass, and a sense of community. However, for some, certain religious beliefs can be restrictive (Fuist, 2016). For example, some religious groups may deny LGBTQ people and others full inclusion in their church rituals, activities, and leadership (Fuist, 2016).

Poverty and low socioeconomic status also affect the learning, behavior, emotional response, and the physical health of children (Groark et al., 2014). Poor nutrition can lead to obesity, malnutrition, and physical problems such as heart disease, high blood pressure, and diabetes (Centers for Disease Control and Prevention [CDC], 2020). The lack of affordability and accessibility to healthy foods such as fresh fruits and vegetables leads to the reliance on cheaper processed foods, which can cause physical problems and nutritional deficiencies (CDC, 2020). An unstable living environment can result in depression and poor academic performance in children (Groark et al., 2014). Shift work, multiple jobs, low-quality and/or nonaffordable childcare, and other stressors faced by low socioeconomic families all contribute to environmental stress faced by these families.

Types of Families

The profession recognizes many types of families: traditional, single parent, never married, blended, multigenerational, military, teen parenting, LGBTQ, and foster care. Family formations and configurations change over time. Fewer parents marry and divorce appears to be more common, which means that many children face transitions and possibly instability in their family lives. There appears to be an increasing number of single-parent households and blended families.

One fourth (26%) of children younger than age 18 now live with a single parent, compared to 9% in 1960 and 22% in 2000 (Pew Research Center, 2015). Five percent of children live without either parent; grandparents raise most of these children (Pew Research Center, 2015). Roughly 8 in 10 (78%) White children live with two parents, including about half (52%) with both parents in their first marriage and 19% with two parents in a remarriage; 6% live with cohabiting parents (Pew Research Center, 2015). About one in five (19%) White children live with a single parent (Pew Research Center, 2015).

Among Hispanic children, two thirds live with two parents; of these, 43% live with two parents in their first marriage, while 12% live with parents in a remarriage, and 11% live with cohabiting parents (Pew Research Center, 2015). Twenty-nine percent of Hispanic children live with a single parent (Pew Research Center, 2015).

Conversely, the majority (54%) of Black children live with a single parent. Thirty-eight percent of Black children live with two parents, including 22% living with two parents both in their first marriage (Pew Research Center, 2015). An additional 9% live with remarried parents, and 7% reside with cohabiting parents (Pew Research Center, 2015). According to the most recent data, 16% of children live in what the Census Bureau terms "blended families," a household with a stepparent, stepsibling, or half-sibling (Pew Research Center, 2015).

LGBTQ families appear to be increasingly common, more accepted, and less invisible, depending on the geographical area and community in which one lives. More children appear to be growing up with same-sex parents (Skuse et al., 2017). Medical professionals now conceive numbers of children through new reproductive technologies such as alternative insemination (AI) and in vitro fertilization (IVF) (Skuse et al., 2017). Based on 2016 household counts, an estimated 114,000 same-sex couples appear to be raising children, including 28,000 male same-sex couples and 86,000 female same-sex couples. Like male–female couples with children, the majority (68.0%) of same-sex couples with children also raise biological children. However, same-sex couples with children appear to be far more likely than male–female couples with children to adopt a child (21.4% vs. 3.0%) or a foster child (2.9% vs. 0.4%); see Goldberg and Conron (2018).

Military families face unique challenges, including frequent moves, long separations, and deployments of family members (Huebner, 2019). Military spouses often face unemployment or underemployment due to frequent moves (Huebner, 2019). Within a year of a geographic move, military youth show an increase in mental health encounters (Huebner, 2019). This presents relevance for counselors in the community since up to 50% of children of military members receive healthcare, including mental healthcare, in civilian facilities (nonmilitary treatment facilities); see Huebner (2019). Some military families become isolated from military networks and the military relocate most far away from an extended family network (Huebner, 2019). For many military families, other military families become an important social support (Huebner, 2019). Although children in military families face many stressors, some research exists showing increased resilience in military children around moving and school adjustment (Huebner, 2019). More information on military families will be presented in Chapter 10.

When working with children and adolescents, counselors must remain open and sensitive to the many different types of families. Counselors should set aside their presumption that every child or adolescent comes from a "traditional" family (i.e., nuclear family [generally thought of as two parents, stereotypically a mother and a father, and minor children living under one roof]). Counselors should use inclusive language to reflect this openness, such as asking "Tell me about your family" or "Who do you live with?" versus "What's it like living with your mom and dad?" Children and adolescents appear more likely to be open with a counselor who demonstrates acceptance of all types of families (Erford, 2008). Children and adolescents from diverse family constellations, such as LGBTQ families, foster care families, adoptive families, single-parent families, homeless families, and grandparent-headed families benefit from the counselor's help in achieving acceptance and full inclusion (Erford, 2008). Forms and handouts should be consistent with this approach. Children living in nontraditional families often feel singled out or abnormal when adults assume children or adolescents come from traditional households. An inclusive approach also remains consistent with a trauma-informed approach, to be discussed later in this chapter and in Chapters 6 and 12.

Parenting Practices and Styles

Many well-meaning parents raising healthy children may lack insight about which parenting practices appear to be most effective. In fact, many parents do not develop a plan, and they simply rely on what they believed their parents did right or wrong. In addition, no precedence for parenting practices exists in today's digital age (e.g., challenges for how parents handle their children's use of electronic devices, social media, and social networking sites).

The American Psychological Association (APA, 2017) describes three types of parenting styles: (a) *authoritative*, (b) *permissive*, and (c) *uninvolved*. The authoritative style involves nurturing, responsive, and supportive parents who set firm limits for their children (APA, 2017). They shape children's behavior by explaining rules, discussing, reasoning, and listening to their child's viewpoint (APA, 2017). Children raised with this style tend to be "friendly, energetic, cheerful, self-reliant, self-controlled, curious, cooperative, and achievement-oriented" (APA, 2017, para. 2). With the permissive parenting style, parents appear warm but can present as overly lenient; they do not set firm limits or monitor their children's activities (APA, 2017). Children raised with this parenting style tend to be "impulsive, rebellious, aimless, domineering, aggressive and low in self-reliance, self-control, and achievement" (APA, 2017, paragraph 4). An uninvolved parenting style reflects parents who seem unresponsive, unavailable, or outright rejecting (APA, 2017). Children raised with this parenting style tend to acquire low self-esteem and little self-confidence and seek other, sometimes inappropriate, role models (APA, 2017, paragraph 6).

Cultural beliefs and norms also influence the parenting style that parents utilize with their children (Bornstein, 2012). Furthermore, the outcomes of a particular parenting style vary by culture (Bornstein, 2012). For example, an *authoritative* parenting style (high warmth, high control) leads to positive outcomes in European American school children, whereas an *authoritarian* parenting style (low warmth, high control) leads to positive outcomes in African American and Hong Kong Chinese school children (Bornstein, 2012). Many studies indicate that Latinx parents are less likely to support physical discipline but that there are differences in parenting styles by acculturation levels (Ayón et al., 2015). Counselors should be aware of how culture impacts parenting practices in order to effectively help clients and families.

American parents employ many methods of discipline with their children, with *explaining inappropriate behavior to their child* being the most frequent: Three quarters of parents say they do this often, while about 4 in 10 say they often take away privileges (43%) or give a "time-out" (41% of parents with kids younger than 6); see Pew Research Center (2015). About one in five (22%) parents say they often raise their voice or yell at their kids, and 4% say they turn to spanking often as a way to discipline their children (Pew Research Center, 2015).

Some parents continue to use physical punishment, such as spanking, despite evidence that most professionals deem this practice as ineffective and harmful to children's development (Durrant & Ensom, 2012). Laws stating what constitutes physical discipline versus physical abuse vary by state, but according to the American Academy of Pediatrics, physical abuse occurs when a child is physically injured through means such as hitting, kicking, shaking, burning, or other show of force. Most physical abuse of children occurs in the context of punishment (Durrant & Ensom, 2012). Professionals associate physical punishment with slower cognitive development, lower academic achievement, and mental health problems including depression, anxiety, feelings of hopelessness, and use of drugs and alcohol (Durrant & Ensom, 2012). Most professional organizations serving children, such as the American Academy of Pediatrics, have demonstrated strong opposition to physical punishment and encourage parents to adopt alternative, nonviolent, effective, positive approaches to discipline (Durrant & Ensom, 2012). However, it is important for counselors to view parenting practices within the appropriate cultural context. For instance, one study on child discipline in African American families notes that counselors need to understand the holistic and contextual elements of child discipline in order to more clearly differentiate between discipline and abuse (Adkison-Bradley et al., 2014).

Siegel and Bryson (2016) offer an emerging parenting approach, *whole brain parenting,* that seems to be a better fit for *all* children. Siegel and Bryson (2016) explain the new science relating to the wiring of a child's brain and how the brain matures, and they provide a model that seeks to incorporate this knowledge into parenting practices. Also called peaceful parenting, positive parenting, or gentle parenting, this model suggests no yelling, threatening, or spanking. In the book *No Drama Discipline: The Whole-Brain Way to Calm the Chaos and Nurture Your Child's Developing Mind,* Siegel and Bryson describe effective discipline as "teaching skills and nurturing the connections in our children's brains that will help them make better decisions and handle themselves well in the future" (2016, p. xix). In the whole-brain approach, parents help children develop skills to manage their emotions, control their impulses, develop empathy (consider other people's feelings), think about consequences, and make thoughtful decisions (Siegel & Bryson, 2016). In their connect and redirect approach, Siegel and Bryson advocate for parents to combine deep empathic connection with clear boundaries, a consistent and predictable structure, and high, but reasonable, expectations (2016).

Similarly, Ross Greene (2014), author of *The Explosive Child, Lost at School, Lost & Found,* and *Raising Human Beings,* developed the Collaborative & Proactive Solutions (CPS) model for children experiencing trauma, children with disabilities, and neurodiverse children who do not respond to typical parenting strategies. The CPS model presents a trauma-informed parenting approach whereby parents identify the child's lagging skills and unmet expectations (unsolved problems) and then work with the child or adolescent to start solving these problems collaboratively and proactively (Greene, 2014). The premise behind this approach, which also applies to schools, highlights the fact that children want to behave well but lack the skills to meet the parent's or teacher's expectations (Greene, 2014).

Professionals commonly link parenting practices to children's development (Bornstein et al., 2017). For example, professionals associate parent limit setting with higher levels of child competence and lower levels of child disruptive behavior (Bornstein et al., 2017). Bornstein et al. (2017) associate harsh parenting and inconsistent discipline with negative behavior and delinquency. In comparison, they associate parent warmth, sensitivity, and involvement with prosocial behavior and academic achievement.

Parenting cognitions and practices appear to be more easily modifiable than factors such as family socioeconomic status, parent age, and intelligence, or even child intelligence (Bornstein et al., 2017). Early parenting programs designed to increase parents' knowledge of parenting and children's growth and development, parenting satisfaction, and positive self-talk of parenting success evidence positive effects on parenting practices and, eventually, on child behavior (Bornstein et al., 2017).

Although research-based parenting methods remain available, many factors influence a family's likelihood to seek out or gain awareness of such methods. Communities can be of help or be a deterrent depending on the resources of a particular community. Therefore, it remains essential for pediatricians, school counselors, mental health counselors, teachers, hospital programs, community centers, libraries, social media and faith centers to provide accurate parenting information and support to members of their communities.

Disciplinary Practices

In one study of disciplinary practices of parents of nonphysically abused young children presenting to pediatric EDs, researchers discovered that parental use of physical discipline seems to be significantly associated with children's aggressive behaviors and familial psychosocial risk factors (Thompson et al., 2017). The use of physical discipline relates to higher rates of reported physically aggressive behaviors in early childhood as well as with the presence of familial psychosocial risk factors (Thompson et al., 2017). Rather than reducing unwanted behaviors, physical discipline seems to model and promote child physical aggression (Thompson et al., 2017). Additionally, the use of physical discipline may indicate the presence of more serious psychosocial risk factors in the family network (Thompson et al., 2017).

Physical discipline (corporal punishment) involves the use of any physical means, such as spanking, to correct or punish behavior. The number of parents who spank their children seems to be unclear and sometimes discrepant. One study reported that more than 90% of American families report using physical discipline at some time during a child's life, although it appears to be less common in very young children (Thompson et al., 2017). In a nationally representative study, 64% of parents reported spanking children 19 to 35 months of age, and 6% of parents reported spanking infants 4 to 9 months of age (Thompson et al., 2017).

Other more effective and time-efficient parenting techniques to help children and adolescents manage behavior include the following: providing positive reinforcement and privileges; providing time-in (as opposed to time-out); helping the child understand feelings; providing natural and logical consequences (i.e., natural consequences denote the unavoidable result of the child's own actions, such as a child refusing to wear a coat and experiencing cold weather as a result, while logical consequences represent consequences imposed by a parent or caregiver that are directly related to the undesired or unsafe behavior [e.g., if a child chooses to refuse to wear a bike helmet, the child cannot ride the bike]); ignoring the behavior; holding family meetings to discuss possible logical solutions; making a plan for change with the child; developing behavioral charts; making a plan for change with the child and a professional; providing the child time-out to decompress; taking away privileges; replacing negative time with positive time; or providing alternatives for destructive acting-out behaviors; and ensuring that restitution occurs ("fix-its").

Monitoring and Supervision

Adolescents often experiment with risky behaviors, which, under insufficient parental monitoring or intervention, can escalate to problem behaviors (Bendezú et al., 2016). Youth and families living in high-risk, impoverished neighborhoods experience particular vulnerabilities given the risks associated with raising children in poverty (Bendezú et al., 2016). Parental monitoring, or parental efforts to keep track of their child's whereabouts, activities, and peer affiliations, helps prevent adolescents from engaging in problem behaviors (e.g., deviant peer affiliations, drug use, truancy) (Bendezú et al., 2016). In low-income neighborhoods, active and involved forms of parental monitoring (e.g., discussions with youth about daily activities and behavioral limit setting) that limit autonomy reduce adolescent engagement in antisocial behavior (Bendezú et al., 2016).

Families living in poor, high-risk neighborhoods can be exposed to a number of risk factors, including physical assault, inadequate housing, and failing academic institutions (Bendezú et al., 2016). In addition to these threatening conditions, parents facing poverty must also contend with poverty-related stressors that compromise psychological well-being and impair the ability to parent sensitively and attentively (Bendezú et al., 2016). When access to local resources for parenting support appears limited, effective parents resort to involved and restrictive strategies for child monitoring and supervision (Bendezú et al., 2016). These adaptive strategies appear to help protect youth from dangers looming in their communities. Thus, counselors working with youth in high-risk communities can provide psychoeducation to parents about discussing their children's daily activities as a strategy for parental monitoring (Bendezú et al., 2016).

Parental Involvement and Mental Health

In addition to ongoing monitoring and supervision of children and adolescents, parents need to be involved in their children's mental health treatment for it to be successful. However, engaging families in mental health treatment remains a serious challenge (Gopalan et al., 2010). Parental engagement generally involves the following steps: (a) recognition of children's mental health problems by parents, teachers, or other important adults; (b) connecting children and their families with a mental health resource; and (c) bringing children to mental health centers or school-based mental health providers (Gopalan et al., 2010).

Clinicians who elicit adolescents' perspectives on their own mental health symptoms to increase self-awareness may be more likely to increase adolescents' motivation for treatment (Gopalan et al., 2010). Also, resolving potential conflicts between parents and youth by finding common treatment goals may help retain clients in treatment (Gopalan et al., 2010). Making treatment available outside the traditional clinic walls through school- and home-based service delivery models can be promising for the promotion of initial engagement and service retention. Counselors can help empower parents to advocate for their children and develop the skills to do so effectively (Gopalan et al., 2010). Moreover, the use of paraprofessional family advocates and peer youth specialists appears to be gaining increasing popularity, particularly given the growing demand for consumer-led services in mental health (Gopalan et al., 2010).

Parent Consultation in Schools

Parent consultation in clinical mental health settings, as discussed previously, involves many barriers, including a waitlist at the clinic, conflicting schedules between the provider and parents (e.g., only daytime hours available), financial resources to pay for treatment, transportation, a distrust of mental health providers in general, a reluctance to acknowledge their child's mental health problems, or a reluctance to accept that parents either contribute to the problem or can be part of the solution. However, since a parent or caregiver typically signifies the one who brings a child or adolescent to counseling, counselors can often meet with the parent and child in at least the first session.

Parental absence and limited accessibility (mainly done by phone) present a greater challenge to schools, unless a school counselor requests a meeting with a parent (which can present a similar challenge as with clinical mental health counselors—it can be difficult for parents to meet during school hours). School counselors can work around these barriers by maintaining phone contact with parents or adjusting meeting times to accommodate parents, if possible.

Parent Education/Psychoeducation in Clinical Mental Health Agencies

A team approach benefits the treatment of children and adolescents with mental illness. If parents sign consent forms for all professionals working with the child to share information, each agency can work together for the benefit of the child. For example, a child's outside agency counselor can attend the child's school Individualized Education Plan (IEP) meeting and help construct a plan that best supports the child. The counselor can also report symptoms and concerns to the psychiatrist to collaborate on the best medication management. Providers can inform the school of medication regimens to increase awareness of any potential medication side effects. An in-home family therapy team usually communicates with the child's individual therapist so that care can be coordinated. Therapeutic mentors usually attend occasional family therapy meetings and consult with individual counselors to stay informed about treatment and coordinate care.

If a child enters a crisis state and requires inpatient treatment, the hospital team would consult with the outpatient team (school counselor, IEP team, individual counselor, family therapist, outpatient psychiatrist) and then provide crisis stabilization services and disseminate a discharge summary to the outpatient team. This collaboration and coordination of care can provide support and prevent a decline that could require repeat inpatient hospitalizations. Of course, access to school-based and community-based treatment depends on stigma in that community, the socioeconomic status of parents, resources available in the school and community, availability of treatment, and the availability and affordability of healthcare or health insurance.

PEER SYSTEM

Peers, especially friends, represent a well-known source of influence for children and adolescents, especially as children enter preadolescence and adolescence (Hojjat & Moyer, 2016). When children enter preadolescence and adolescence, friends become increasingly important and families often complain that friends take precedence over them. Although counselors view this as developmentally appropriate, parents struggle to understand it (Hojjat & Moyer, 2016). Friends fulfill a variety of needs that promote positive socioemotional adjustment (Hojjat & Moyer, 2016). According to Hojjat and Moyer (2016), friends provide the following critical needs in childhood and adolescence: instrumental aid (helpfulness); reliable alliance (loyalty); nurturance (comfort and support); enhancement of worth (sense of value); affection; intimacy (level of disclosure). Therefore, children and adolescents who lack friends appear to be at risk for loneliness, depression, anxiety, and low self-esteem. They might also be at higher risk for peer victimization and lower functioning at school. Students with friends also tend to be more engaged in school (Hojjat & Moyer, 2016).

The counselor can be instrumental in helping parents understand that peers and friendships denote a normal and important part of development. Counselors also continue to be uniquely equipped to help adolescents develop positive social skills, develop skills instrumental to maintaining friendships, and manage the feelings of rejection and confusion around shifting friend groups or lack of friendships. Counselors can also work with adolescents on peer-related activities, helping them make positive and responsible choices with peers, especially around sexual activity and substance use. Kiara's story provides a real-life example of how friends can impact an adolescent's school experience and how choosing age-appropriate counseling strategies can impact treatment.

> Kiara, a 15-year-old sophomore in high school in a rural town sandwiched between two industrial cities, lives in a blended family—half of the week she resides with her biological dad and during the other half she stays with her biological mom and stepmom.

> Two older biological sisters and two younger adopted siblings complete her family. She identifies some of the challenges of being 15 as "I've just given up when it comes to friends. My friend group has changed like a million times since middle school and sometimes it feels too hard to make an effort." She also says, "High school is boring and frustrating and a waste of time. I am taking pointless classes that won't help me in life and I am waiting to go to college, but it seems so far away." When questioned about her blended family, she says, "It's chill." She appears adjusted to being in a blended family, which includes parents living in a same-sex relationship. Kiara says that no one at school gives her a difficult time about it, despite living in a conservative community. "People always get so confused when I am explaining my family to them and it's really funny." Kiara struggles with mild depression, generalized anxiety, and occasional panic attacks and takes an antidepressant to help manage her anxiety. She does not want to see an outside therapist or the school counselor because she says, "I'm fine." She also experienced an uncomfortable interaction with a therapist recently. "The therapist made me color a picture of a human of where I feel my emotions." Kiara felt that the therapist treated her like a 5-year-old and did not find the counseling helpful.

Some evidence suggests that significant use of digital media (television, video games, computers, tablets, smartphones, and other device use) appears to be associated with depressive symptoms; however, additional evidence also indicates that the social benefits of digital communication can actually improve mood and offer other individual benefits (Hoge et al., 2017). The use of social media and social networking sites/apps, especially Instagram, Snapchat, Facebook, Twitter, and VSCO, now appears to be primary modes of communication among children and adolescents. Over 95% of adolescents and young adults access the internet daily; 81% report that they use social media; and 67% report using social media at least once a day (Yonker et al., 2015).

Use of social media presents advantages to adolescents, especially for those with serious mental illness (Naslund et al., 2016). For instance, individuals with serious mental illness access social media to find others with similar experiences; this provides a sense of group belonging, while maintaining anonymity (Naslund et al., 2016). Some risks of social media, however, include accessing false information and encountering hostile comments from others online (Naslund et al., 2016).

Professionals view teaching young people how to use social media responsibly and cautiously as increasingly important. They associate one negative outcome of social media with an increased risk of "desire for slimness" (DS), a well-established risk factor for eating disorders among adolescents, particularly girls (Sugimoto et al., 2019). Targeting social media use in early adolescence appears to be a promising approach to preventing DS and subsequent eating problems, particularly among girls (Sugimoto et al., 2019).

Counselors need a thorough understanding of children and adolescents' experiences with sharing electronic images; the helpful and harmful consequences of sharing images to adolescent mental health and safety, and promising interventions that allow young people to make more positive decisions and minimize their risks when sharing images through electronic devices (Cardoso et al., 2019). In one study, young people reported that they need information and advice to support their and others' online decision-making, help making situational decision-making skills for managing online interactions, and means to control information and images that can be accessed and distributed (Cardoso et al., 2019).

Researchers offer some recommendations to counselors for helping children, adolescents, and families navigate digital media use and decrease rates of depression and anxiety associated with greater use (Hoge et al., 2017). For instance, counselors can help parents monitor appropriate content (while taking into account developmental differences in their children); encourage parents to provide children opportunities for face-to-face communication (especially children with or prone to social anxiety disorder); educate parents on creating household rules for media use; and help youth with depression access social resources both in person and online (Hoge et al., 2017). The 2014 American Counseling Association (ACA) *Code of Ethics* outlines the ethical and legal responsibilities of counselors who utilize distance counseling, technology, and social media in their professional work with clients. Although technology can help better serve clients in many circumstances, counselors need to stay informed about the limitations and potential challenges of these methods, including security, confidentiality, competency, emergency procedures, and accessibility for multicultural clients and clients with disabilities (ACA, 2014).

SCHOOL SYSTEM AND SCHOOL CULTURE

As mentioned in Chapter 1, schools play a vital role in fostering the social and emotional well-being of youth (O'Dea et al., 2017). School officials define this formalized duty of care as the moral and legal obligation to ensure the well-being of their students (O'Dea et al., 2017). In addition, schools represent an ideal setting to promote mental health since adolescents spend such a considerable amount of time there (O'Dea et al., 2017). Schools naturally lend themselves to learning skills and strategies and mental health education can be integrated into the curriculum (which reduces barriers such as time, location, and cost); see O'Dea et al. (2017). Finally, schools maintain easier access to parents and families and the social context at schools allows for stigma reduction (O'Dea et al., 2017).

Although professional school counselors maintain the support of a broader range of school programs, there remains significant variability in the type, extent, quality, and evidence base of these programs (O'Dea et al., 2017). Competing responsibilities, parent disengagement, lack of support from school staff, limited resources, and significant variations in staff training serve as barriers (O'Dea et al., 2017). As a result, many schools operate under a highly reactive, disconnected, and unsystematic approach to mental health that lacks a preventive focus (O'Dea et al., 2017).

Schools focused on the "whole child" emphasize academic success as a priority; however, they also identify other public health goals in support of students, such as physical, social, and emotional health for students and families as well as safe, supportive, stable schools and communities (Diamond & Freudenberg, 2016). These types of schools result in improved student learning, stronger families, and healthier communities (Diamond & Freudenberg, 2016).

Education and health interface with one another. Healthy students demonstrate higher rates of academic success; over a lifetime, people with higher levels of education experience better health than those with less education (Diamond & Freudenberg, 2016). Specifically, professionals consistently associate more education with longer life expectancy and lower morbidity and disability, as well as decreased risky health behavior (Diamond & Freudenberg, 2016). This correlation most likely rests with the associations between education and wealth, higher levels of social support and social networks typical with more education, and the contribution of education and health to coping with stress (Diamond & Freudenberg, 2016). Substantial inequities in health and educational outcomes persist in the United States. The interactions between health and education create a cycle of disadvantage. Students in poor neighborhoods evidence worse educational outcomes leading to worse health outcomes later in life (Diamond & Freudenberg, 2016). At the same time, children in poor neighborhoods evidence worse health outcomes leading to lower educational achievement than their wealthier peers (Diamond & Freudenberg, 2016).

Parental Engagement in Schools

Many people recognize the benefits of family involvement and family engagement for students in diverse communities. *Family involvement* often includes the school (including school counselors and administration) identifying how the family can contribute to the school while family engagement tends to include listening to what parents want for their child's school experience (Ferlazzo & Hammond, 2009). Although family engagement demonstrates the best results for students, research consistently demonstrates that any kind of increased parental interest and support of students can be helpful (Ferlazzo & Hammond, 2009).

In one model of parent engagement and involvement, the Child–Parent Center Preschool to Third Grade (CPC P–3) program, each school engages a Parent Resource Teacher (PRT) (Hayakawa & Reynolds, 2016). The PRT refers to a certified teacher who serves as a liaison between families and the school system. The PRT administers a family needs assessment at the beginning of each school year, develops a parent involvement plan, and creates a parent program that solicits direct input from families (Hayakawa & Reynolds, 2016).

Families cite a variety of barriers to school involvement, such as lack of time, inconvenient times of events, lack of interest in events offered, or not believing that they can effectively contribute to the school (Hayakawa & Reynolds, 2016). The PRT strategizes to include marginalized families in school activities (Hayakawa & Reynolds, 2016). Effective strategies for addressing these barriers include personally inviting parents to events, asking about interests, creating dedicated spaces in the school for parents, and scheduling events or activities on days and times that appear to be convenient to families (Hayakawa & Reynolds, 2016). The CPC model embraces a strong school–family–community partnership that incorporates creativity, flexibility, and collaboration to develop a school-specific parent program (Hayakawa & Reynolds, 2016).

Some examples of parent activities include volunteering in the classroom, chaperoning field trips and community events, attending parent nights and open houses, attending parent–teacher conferences, "coffee hour" with school leaders, and home involvement (Hayakawa & Reynolds, 2016). Other options include participating in events on topics such as child development and parenting; language, math, and science; health, safety, and nutrition; career, education, and personal development (Hayakawa & Reynolds, 2016).

Parent–school events often involve professional school counselors. Depending on the school, they might organize psychoeducational events for parents on specific topics (e.g., suicide prevention, bullying, substance use, executive functioning skills, recognizing mental health disorders, fostering healthy peer relationships). Professional school counselors also organize parent support groups, especially for specific types of families with unique challenges (e.g., a support group for grandparents raising their grandchildren).

COMMUNITY AND SOCIETAL SYSTEMS

Psychosocial stress in children and adolescents can be accentuated by the presence of stressful, traumatic, or adverse life events (e.g., abuse, maltreatment, neglect, witnessing domestic violence, dating violence, community violence, loss events, intrafamilial problems, school and interpersonal problems) that appears to be associated with severe negative outcomes (Jiménez et al., 2019). According to the CDC (2019), adverse childhood experiences (ACEs) can impact future violence victimization and perpetration as well as lifelong health and opportunity (Figure 2.1).

Marco's Story (Age 7)

Marco, a 7-year-old Hispanic boy, spent several years in foster care before finding his adoptive family. He does not remember his birth family; but the effects of the trauma he experienced (birth parents with severe mental illness and substance abuse challenges, witnessing domestic violence, and lack of food and other necessities) remain. He displays difficulty managing frustrations, demonstrates frequent outbursts and tantrums, and does not understand safe and unsafe behaviors (running into the street, for instance, or opening the door of a moving car). However, evidence shows that he appears to be attached to his adoptive family, even though he does not understand why he could not stay with his previous foster mother. No one explained the difference between foster care and "forever families" to him while he remained in the custody of the state, which, as a result, led to confusion and acting out. However, he expresses interest in many activities, especially sports, which present a positive outlet for him to release energy and frustration and begin to develop a sense of competence and accomplishment. Marco's involvement in counseling

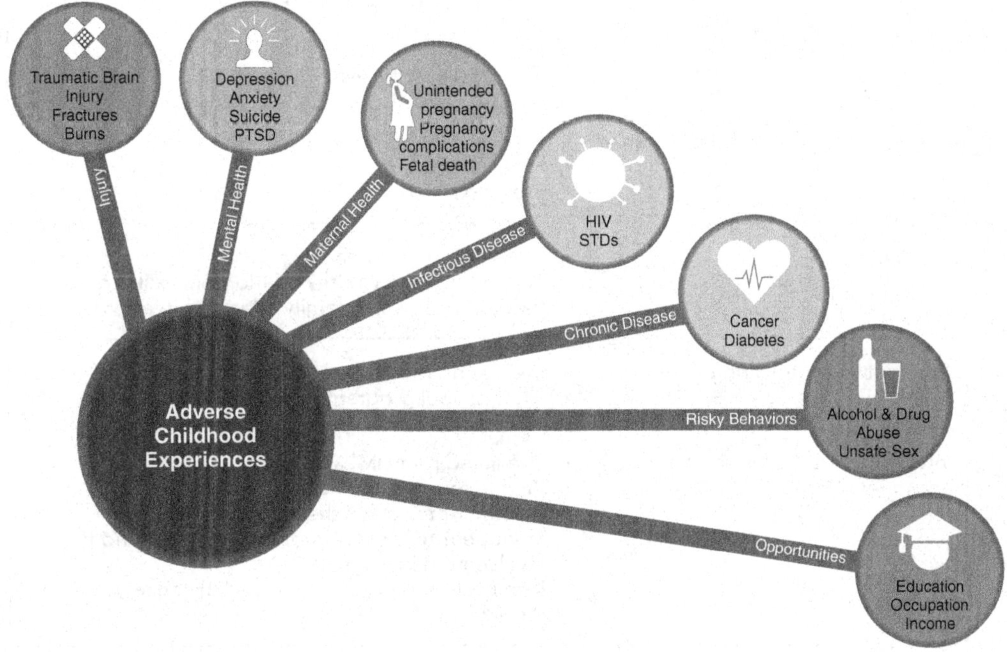

FIGURE 2.1 Early adversity has lasting impacts.

PTSD, posttraumatic stress disorder; STDs, sexually transmitted diseases.

Source: Centers for Disease Control and Prevention. (2020). Adverse Child Experiences (ACEs). https://www.cdc.gov/violenceprevention/aces/about.html

includes sessions with numerous counselors at school and in the community. The high turnover of counselors in these settings, however, led to many goodbyes and starting-over experiences, which proved difficult for him.

A child will not automatically experience poor outcomes with ACEs. However, positive experiences or protective factors can prevent children from experiencing adversity and can protect against many of the negative health and life outcomes, even after experiencing adversity. Conditions that put children and families at risk of ACEs deserve paramount attention so that providers can prevent ACEs before they happen. The CDC recommends prevention strategies outlined in Exhibit 2.1.

As part of a trauma-informed service system (as mentioned in Chapter 1), counselors can help children and adolescents develop protective factors such as self-esteem and healthy coping skills. These practices can help counteract the effects of trauma and reduce trauma

EXHIBIT 2.1

Preventing Adverse Childhood Experiences

Strategy	Approach
Strengthen economic supports to families	• Strengthening household financial security • Family-friendly work policies
Promote social norms that protect against violence and adversity	• Public education campaigns • Legislative approaches to reduce corporal punishment • Bystander approaches • Men and boys as allies in prevention
Ensure a strong start for children	• Early childhood home visitation • High-quality childcare • Preschool enrichment with family engagement
Teach skills	• Social–emotional learning • Safe dating and healthy relationship skill programs • Parenting skills and family relationship approaches
Connect youth to caring adults and activities	• Mentoring programs • After-school programs
Intervene to lessen immediate and long-term harms	• Enhanced primary care • Victim-centered services • Treatment to lessen the harms of ACEs • Treatment to prevent problem behavior and future involvement in violence • Family-centered treatment for substance use disorders

ACEs, adverse childhood experiences.

Source: From Centers for Disease Control and Prevention. (2019). *Preventing Adverse Childhood Experiences (ACEs): Leveraging the Best Available Evidence* (p. 9). https://www.cdc.gov/violenceprevention/pdf/preventingACES.pdf

responses that often manifest in internal distress or acting-out behaviors. Interventions that create protective factors include building self-esteem, employing positive coping skills, developing a healthy self-image, and learning how to manage stress and anger. The school counseling program remains a particularly effective place to advocate for and implement these trauma-informed interventions. School and clinical mental health counselors can integrate trauma-informed strategies into individual and group sessions and classroom lessons.

According to The National Child Traumatic Stress Network (NCTSN), some children who experience traumatic events handle adversity better than others (i.e., they display more resiliency [Gerrity & Folcarelli, 2008]). Protective factors that contribute to resiliency in the face of adversity include the following: the capacity for cognitive functioning; capacity for emotional regulation; presence of social supports provided by caring and competent adults; holding a positive belief about oneself; belief in the safety and fairness of one's situation; and motivation to act effectively in one's environment (Gerrity & Folcarelli, 2008, p. 17). However, responses also depend on other factors, such as the level of trauma and the number of traumatic events (Gerrity & Folcarelli, 2008). Gerrity and Folcarelli (2008, p. 17) also advocate for systemic change: "Public policies that prevent or eliminate risk factors or enhance protective factors can increase children's resilience in the face of trauma."

In the school setting, trauma-informed groups often appear to be psychoeducational, which means they help members to gain information and develop skills for challenging situations through education-based techniques. Each session should include trauma-informed group counseling strategies such as setting realistic goals and building healthy coping skills. Effective counselors demonstrate warmth, neutrality, and firmness with all children and adolescents, but these qualities seem to be especially important when facilitating a trauma-informed group as individuals with trauma often need an extra safe and structured group setting.

Trauma-informed care by school counselors include interventions that help students to feel safe, to resolve any behaviors that interfere with school success, to eat/sleep/relax healthfully, to manage overwhelming feelings, to connect with others, and to use their strengths in creating solutions for themselves. Counselors can encourage hope and normalize reactions to stress. Some helpful activities might include role plays; mindfulness lessons; specific, measurable, achievable, realistic, and time-based (SMART) goals; goal creation; art projects; coping skills application; relaxation strategies; and character education.

CASE STUDY 2.1: THE CONFIDENTIALITY DILEMMA

Michaela is a 14-year-old, Caucasian, first-year student at a medium-sized, suburban high school in the Midwest. Another student, Michaela's friend, Emma, reported to a member of the school administration that Michaela had recently disclosed to her that she had been superficially self-harming via cutting with a razor. At the administrator's request, you, the professional school counselor, meet with Michaela to discuss these reported concerns, without disclosing the name of the reporting student, and to assess Michaela's safety.

Michaela initially becomes very angry at her friend for reporting what she told her in confidence but with your gentle, nonjudgmental prodding, she eventually breaks down crying and admits that she recently started self-harming to deal with feeling depressed and anxious. She reports to you that she recently came out as

(*continued*)

CASE STUDY 2.1 (*continued*)

transgender on social media. Although many of her peers have been accepting and affirming, some of her peers have been calling her names and writing cruel things to her online. Michaela's parents do not know about her gender identity, the self-harm, or the cruel remarks from her peers. Michaela provides assurance that she is not having suicidal ideation, tells you that she is cutting herself to feel better and does not want to die, and begs you not to tell her parents either about the self-harm or about her recent coming out to her peers.

You validate her struggles and talk with her about joining the school's Gay Straight Alliance (GSA) for LGBTQ+ youth, which she did not know existed but agrees to try. You tell her that you will need to contact her parents about the self-harm, which appears to be nonsuicidal self-injurious behavior, but assure her that you will not discuss her gender identity with them. You also provide the crisis text line for both self-harm and suicide as resources and mention that an outpatient counselor in the community would be a good idea. She agrees to let you talk to her parents about setting up an appointment with a counselor in the community. You also set up a schedule to check on her regularly and tell her that you will need to consult with administration on the cyberbullying that she is experiencing outside of school. You also assure her that your office is a safe space for LGBTQ+ youth and that you will support her in any way she needs.

Activity 2.1

Form groups of three to five students and discuss the following:

1. Knowing that LGBTQ+ young people are about twice as likely to engage in self-harm, often as the result of bullying and discrimination, how can you address this important issue with (a) the student, (b) other students in the school, (c) the student's family, and (d) the school as a whole?
2. How can you learn from this situation to advocate for and promote an accepting, affirming, and safe culture for all students in your school?
3. What else could the professional school counselor do in this situation that incorporates a systems-focused and culturally competent approach to students and school culture?
4. Discuss the dilemma that counselors sometimes face regarding students' confidentiality when they are legally and ethically required to report student disclosures to guardians and school administration.

CHAPTER SUMMARY

Children and adolescents depend on many systems to foster their social, emotional, personal, and developmental needs. School leaders, school counselors, communities, families, mental health counselors, and representatives from all systems in a child's life need to collaborate and integrate care to produce the best outcomes for every child. Counselors, in particular, need to continue to advocate for better and more cohesive systems supporting youth to assist them to develop resiliency in the face of rapid social changes. In summary, counselors should maintain a systemic perspective and a high level of multicultural competence when working with children and adolescents in order to provide holistic care and achieve the best possible treatment outcomes.

POINTS TO REMEMBER

- Children and adolescents depend on many systems to foster their social, emotional, personal, and developmental needs.
- A system consists of a network of interrelated and interdependent parts, where each part impacts the other parts positively and/or negatively.
- The family system, the peer system, the school system, and the community and societal systems represent some of the many systems in which children and adolescents become embedded.
- Bronfenbrenner divided the entire ecological system in which human growth occurs into five subsystems: the microsystem, mesosystem, exosystem, macrosystem, and chronosystem.
- Involving and engaging parents in children and adolescents' treatment at schools or in clinics leads to better overall outcomes.
- ACEs consist of potentially traumatic events that occur in childhood (0–17 years) and present a significant impact on children and adolescents' development.
- Counselors must use a trauma-informed approach with *all* students and clients to ensure that students with unidentified trauma exposure receive the same support as those with identified trauma.
- Culture, race, ethnicity, religion, and socioeconomic status all impact growth and development.
- Counselors must always be mindful of the many types of families, including but not limited to LGBTQ families, military families, single-parent families, and grandparent-headed families.
- Parent education about effective parenting practices, especially with neurodiverse children and adolescents, remains an important task of counselors.
- The increase in social media use demonstrates positive and negative effects on children and adolescents. Parents may need coaching on how to support and monitor their children's social media use.

OTHER HELPFUL INFORMATION FOR CONSIDERATION

BOOKS FOR CHILD AND ADOLESCENT CLIENTS

- *A Terrible Thing Happened,* by Margaret M. Holmes
- *Enemy Pie,* by Derek Munson

- *Jenny Is Scared: When Sad Things Happen in the World,* by Carol Shuman
- *Hot Stuff to Help Kids Chill Out,* by Jerry Wilde
- *Letters to a Bullied Girl,* by Olivia Gardner
- *Stargirl,* by Jerry Spinelli (English/Edición en Español)
- *Amigas de Nunca Jamás,* by Kiki Thorpe
- *Stress Can Really Get on Your Nerves,* by Trevor Romain
- *Tear Soup/Sopa de Lagrimas,* by Pat Schwiebert
- *What on Earth Do You Do When Someone Dies?,* by Trevor Romain

WEBSITES

- ACEs Connection: https://www.acesconnection.com/blog/models-training-for-developing-trauma-informed-systems-of-care-tisc-1
- American Academy of Pediatrics: https://www.aap.org/en-us/Pages/Default.aspx
- American Counseling Association: https://www.counseling.org
- American Psychological Association: https://www.apa.org
- American School Counselor Association: https://www.schoolcounselor.org
- The National Child Traumatic Stress Network: https://www.nctsn.org
- Resources—Elementary School Counseling: http://www.elementaryschoolcounseling.org/resources.html
- School Counselor Resources: https://www.counselorresources.com

BOOK FOR COUNSELORS

McGoldrick, M., Gerson, R., & Petry, S. S. (2008). *Genograms: Assessment and intervention.* W. W. Norton & Company.

QUESTIONS FOR FURTHER DISCUSSION

- How can counselors foster collaboration among systems?
- What strategies can counselors employ with children and adolescents whose systemic support appears to be fragmented or ineffective?
- How can counselors cope with resistance among systems to collaborate?

KEY REFERENCES

Only key references appear in the print edition. The full reference list appears in the digital product on Springer Publishing Connect: connect.springerpub.com/content/book/978-0-8261-4764-6/part/part01/chapter/ch02

Ashiabi, G. S., & O'Neal, K. K. (2015). Child social development in context. *SAGE Open*, *5*(2), 215824401559084. https://doi.org/10.1177/2158244015590840

Bornstein, M. H., Putnick, D. L., & Suwalsky, J. T. D. (2017). Parenting cognitions → parenting practices → child adjustment? The standard model. *Development and Psychopathology*, *30*(2), 399–416. https://doi.org/10.1017/S0954579417000931

Diamond, C., & Freudenberg, N. (2016). Community schools: A public health opportunity to reverse urban cycles of disadvantage. *Journal of Urban Health*, *93*(6), 923–939. https://doi.org/10.1007/s11524-016-0082-5

Gilstrap, L. L., & Zierten, E. A. (2019, September 21). Urie Bronfenbrenner. https://www.britannica.com/biography/Urie-Bronfenbrenner

Jiménez, L., Hidalgo, V., Baena, S., León, A., & Lorence, B. (2019). Effectiveness of structural–strategic family therapy in the treatment of adolescents with mental health problems and their families. *International Journal of Environmental Research and Public Health*, *16*(7), 1255. https://doi.org/10.3390/ijerph16071255

Matthews, J. J., Barden, S. M., & Sherrell, R. S. (2018). Examining the relationships between multicultural counseling competence, multicultural self-efficacy, and ethnic identity development of practicing counselors. *Journal of Mental Health Counseling*, *40*(2), 129–141. https://doi.org/10.17744/mehc.40.2.03

O'Dea, B., King, C., Subotic-Kerry, M., O'Moore, K., & Christensen, H. (2017). School counselors' perspectives of a web-based stepped care mental health service for schools: Cross-sectional online survey. *Journal of Medical Internet Research Mental Health*, *4*(4), e55. https://doi.org/10.2196/mental.8369

Pew Research Center. (2015, December 17). Parenting in America. https://www.pewsocialtrends.org/2015/12/17/parenting-in-america

Siegel, D. J., & Bryson, T. P. (2016). *No-drama discipline: The whole-brain way to calm the chaos and nurture your child's developing mind*. Bantam Books.

Thompson, R., Kaczor, K., Lorenz, D. J., Bennett, B. L., Meyers, G., & Pierce, M. C. (2017). Is the use of physical discipline associated with aggressive behaviors in young children? *Academic Pediatrics*, *17*(1), 34–44. https://doi.org/10.1016/j.acap.2016.02.014

CHAPTER 3

Relational Considerations in Child and Adolescent Counseling

Maria Haiyasoso

LEARNING OBJECTIVES

After completing this chapter, the reader should be able to:

- Demonstrate an understanding of how relational contexts impact psychosocial and developmental processes for children and adolescents.
- Expand knowledge of relational-cultural and attachment-based theoretical approaches and their applicability in clinical work with youth.
- Recognize ways to apply relational considerations in clinical practice across school and clinical mental health settings.

CACREP STANDARDS FOR THIS CHAPTER

- CACREP 2016: 2.F.1.b., 2.F.2.d., 2.F.3.f., 2.F.5.f.; School Counseling, 5.G.2.a.; 5.G.3.h.; Clinical Mental Health Counseling, 5.C.2.a., j.
- CACREP 2009: II.B.1.; II.G.1.a., II.G.2.a., d., II.G.3.d., f., h., II.G.5.e.; School Counseling, III.A.3., 6.; D.1.; F.1.; Clinical Mental Health Counseling, III.A.2., 3.; B.1.; E.1., 2.; G.1.

INTRODUCTION

For years mental health professionals taught people that they could be psychologically healthy without social support, that "unless you love yourself, no one else will love you." . . . The truth is, you cannot love yourself unless you have been loved and are loved. The capacity to love cannot be built in isolation.

—Bruce D. Perry, MD, PhD & M. Szalavitz, *The Boy Who Was Raised as a Dog*

Perry and Szalavitz's (2006) quote reminds counselors of the importance of learning about child and adolescent clients' relational contexts and prioritizing the therapeutic relationship. This author recalls supervising a master's student counselor-in-training, in which the university's training clinic unexpectedly assigned the student a 7-year-old male to work with. The student left the session wide eyed, stating, "I struggled with the most basic things in that session!" After processing in the supervision session, the student asked about materials that would help her "have a successful next session" with the child client. This author replied, "Be completely present, be yourself, and remember to see the child's experience through the lens of 'we' than rather than 'me.'" The student hoped for a different response, but she eventually learned what many counselors know about working with youth: When children feel a sense of safety and connection, they tend toward success—inside and outside of counseling. This chapter comprises the understanding of child clients within relational contexts, the therapeutic relationship, and attachment-based and relational approaches suitable for counseling youth.

THE IMPACT OF CLIENTS' INTRAPERSONAL AND INTERPERSONAL PROCESSES WITHIN RELATIONAL CONTEXTS

Developmentally, children and adolescents evolve in their perception of themselves, others, and the world around them. For example, according to Piaget (1932/1997) and as mentioned in Chapter 1, children in the preoperational stage, which lasts until around 7 years of age, characteristically experience their world through egocentrism (seeing oneself as the primary, central figure and unable to take another's perspective). A counselor should select interventions and goals with their child and adolescent clients' developmental stages in mind. Yet, across all stages of development, counselors must address child and adolescent clients' intrapersonal and interpersonal processes in order to better understand clients' mental health concerns. The term *intrapersonal* refers to the process that occurs within the child, such as understanding of self and inner thoughts. Interpersonal contexts involve interactions with others. Learning about child and adolescent clients' intrapersonal skills as well as their interpersonal interactions with others provides counselors with valuable information integral to developing a holistic view of clients.

ATTENDING TO INTRAPERSONAL SKILLS

Counselors benefit from understanding intrapersonal skills or internal processes when addressing mental health concerns in children and adolescents. Children begin to demonstrate intrapersonal functions, such as experiencing primary emotions (e.g., surprise, joy, anger, sadness, fear, and disgust) from approximately 3 to 8 months of age and self-conscious emotions (e.g., empathy, jealousy, embarrassment, pride, shame, guilt) from 1.5 to 2.5 years of age (Lewis, 2002). Various factors, such as genetics, temperament, maturation processes, and observing caregivers, influence this development. Intrapersonal skills that begin early and impact how one relates to one's self and others over the life span include self-esteem, self-understanding, and self-regulation.

Counselors learn about child and adolescent clients' self-esteem, or what they think and feel about themselves, to learn more about messages they internalize, their sense of agency, and their perceived worth. Knowing about a client's self-esteem allows counselors to choose responses and interventions that target goals aligned with intrapersonal enhancement. Self-awareness encompasses the ability to recognize and to identify the self and one's internal experience as well as how one impacts others. Exploring children's self-awareness helps counselors understand how children make sense of their inner experience and external environment. Self-regulation encompasses the ability to control one's behavior and inward and outward expression. Counseling offers a prime opportunity for counselors to help children and adolescents practice noticing their internal states and managing heightened emotions or sensations. For example, a counselor might talk to a child about a time when the child felt angry using statements or questions that elicit more detail about the anger (e.g., "Point to the angry feeling in your body"; "Do you see its shape or color?"). Then, the counselor might ask the child to practice time-efficient breathing exercises to help make the angry feeling more tolerable. For a young child, a counselor can teach the child to inhale for a count of three and exhale for a count of three but on exhaling blow a pencil lying across the top of a table so that the pencil slowly rolls away from the child. For an adolescent, the counselor can teach four-square or box breathing, where the adolescent inhales for three or four counts, holds for three or four counts, exhales for three or four counts, and then repeats. If a child chronically struggles intrapersonally (e.g., feels low worth and low sense of agency, experiences regular meltdowns, or struggles to manage difficult emotions), counselors can use a variety of creative means, such as mindfulness, breathing and relaxation strategies, movement, role play, puppet play, narrative activities, and sand tray. These techniques can help the child enhance their intrapersonal skills to equip them to self-manage in contexts outside of the counseling session.

Consider the example of Lynn, a 9-year-old female raised by her maternal grandmother, Petra. Petra raised Lynn at the age of 18 months, when Lynn's mother met a man and left the home to begin a new life. Petra resented her daughter for leaving, not staying in contact, and not helping to support Lynn. No one knew Lynn's father's identity. Petra knew that only she could care for Lynn, even though she earned modest wages as a school bus driver. Petra consistently provided for Lynn but struggled to provide her with emotional support.

Petra, at the recommendation of Lynn's teacher, consented to Lynn visiting with the school counselor for weekly sessions because the teacher reported that Lynn appeared to shut down in class and did not do her work. Initially, Lynn appeared wary of the school counselor, Angie, and seemed skeptical when Angie showed interest in learning about her. Lynn did not speak to Angie, and when she did, she spoke inaudibly or in an extremely low tone. Angie explained that Lynn could choose any activity and direct the course of the session. Lynn experienced discomfort with the sole focus of an adult directed on her and felt awkward with her position of power. At the beginning of counseling, Lynn moved around Angie's office tentatively, barely grazing the toys and materials with her fingertips. Eventually, she routinely gravitated toward the puppet stand for many following sessions. Lynn consistently chose a kangaroo hand puppet with a joey in the pouch attached by an elastic string. Lynn removed the joey from the mama's pouch every time she played with the puppet. She made the mama kangaroo drive to the store, attend to chores, make meals, and talk or text on the phone. Over time, Lynn opened up to Angie and visibly enjoyed being in charge. Her animated puppet play and the themes in her play included feeling lonely, seeking protection, and wanting to be nurtured. Lynn believed that she made "things harder" for her grandmother, she "tries to stay out of the way" at home, and "feels stupid" at school. Lynn clearly saw herself as alone and as a burden.

Activities such as the puppet play in the case example of Lynn can create an opportunity for understanding intrapersonal dynamics in children and what children and adolescents perceive and believe about themselves. Consequently, play and experiential activities with youth provide counselors with data for establishing goals and crafting tailored interventions. In the case illustration, the school counselor focused on esteem-building responses to facilitate a sense of mastery and efficacy (Landreth, 2012) in Lynn. When children possess a healthy sense of self, they can navigate their social spaces with more flexibility and adaptability. In addition, the school counselor challenged Lynn to engage and interact in an unfamiliar way. The next section further discusses the importance of attending to interpersonal capacities in child and adolescent clients.

ADDRESSING INTERPERSONAL CONTEXTS

Childhood remains inherently full of rapid change, transition, and internal reorganization. However, children and adolescents, like all people, exist and develop within interpersonal contexts. For example, children begin emotional development and acquire interpersonal skills, such as social referencing (i.e., reading emotional cues in others) around 2 years of age (Thompson, 2006) and using emotional vocabulary in self and others between 2 and 4 years of age (Ridgeway et al., 1985). Adolescence produces a time of emotional ups and downs, with hormonal changes and the environment contributing to the fluctuation (Collins & Lausen, 2012). Adolescents' emotional development involves growing an ability to regulate mood, but this does not occur in a vacuum and rather impacts how adolescents engage in social contexts. Understanding the mutual influences between children and their environments throughout their development remains integral to effective treatment. When counselors explore the various contexts in which a child exists (e.g., family, peer group, school, societal/cultural), they can begin to understand the etiology and progression of mental health concerns.

Family System

Professionals view the family as the first and primary interpersonal system to which most children belong. Family members typically function in a routine or in a manner that aims to achieve a sort of systemic homeostasis (members seek to achieve balance in the family system); see Anderson and Sabatelli (2007). The notion of homeostasis depends on the idiosyncrasies and norms for a particular family. Despite having common goals (often around survival), family members maintain individual needs. Yet the manner in which children do or do not identify or express their needs depends on multiple factors. If children customarily get their needs met via nonverbal gestures, verbal requests, or crying and their caregivers respond predictably and in a healthy manner, children know what to expect from their caregivers and feel safe in those relationships. In contrast, if children do not get their needs met by caregivers or if their requests for help result in neglectful, punitive, or abusive reactions, they may seek alternative ways to meet their needs or may entirely give up going to the caregiver for help. Even worse, children may carry shame and perceive themselves as incapable, disappointing, or unworthy (Badenoch, 2018). For example, Lynn would not ask for help with reading. In Lynn's previous attempts to ask Petra for help, Petra had expressed her exhaustion after long shifts driving the school bus or indicated that Lynn needed to pay more attention in class if she experienced difficulties reading. Through these interactions, Lynn often felt embarrassed asking for help with reading and eventually ceased asking.

Related concerns emerged in Lynn's play during counseling. In the puppet play, Angie noted that Lynn did not play in a manner that the mama kangaroo acknowledged or engaged with the joey, which was removed from the pouch and dangling behind the mama kangaroo by the elastic string, as she moved from task to task. Lynn spoke rapidly and rushed when acting as the mama kangaroo. When acting as the joey, Lynn spoke quietly and despondently stated "I feel cold and want to be in the pouch" and attempted to climb in. Lynn regularly moved the mama kangaroo away from the joey and often stated, "Not now" or "In a little while." Lynn, speaking as the baby joey, displayed disappointment and frustration. She said quietly "You always say that" and did not provide a response from the mama. Lynn regularly played out this scenario in slightly variant ways, but ultimately the story line remained the same: She attempted to engage the joey and the mama in the beginning of the puppet play and quit trying by the end. In response, Angie reflected Lynn's feelings and honored her desire to be seen, heard, and closer to her grandmother. Angie conveyed warmth and acceptance, leading Lynn to feel safe in the counseling environment and counseling relationship and making the expression of those difficult emotions possible. As such, part of Angie's work then included engaging Petra in treatment.

When working with youth, counselors typically work with key individuals in a youth's interpersonal contexts—their caregivers. Counselors often find that they can involve caregivers as partners in treatment, using caregiver consultations or inviting caregivers to participate in sessions with permission from the child. Counselors should work diligently to convey respect, empathy, and credibility to the caregivers of the youth they serve. If caregivers feel heard and supported in the process of the child's treatment, their relationship with the counselor strengthens, becomes rooted in trust, and facilitates caregivers' receptivity to learning and collaboration. Receptive and invested caregivers welcome education and suggestions about how to continue treatment or practice skills at home (Landreth, 2012). For example, Angie invited Petra to meet to discuss Lynn's academic needs, and in the meeting she additionally informed Petra about Lynn practicing healthy self-expression and clear communication when discussing feelings and needs associated with homework. This created a continuous thread of care for Lynn because Angie educated Petra on the value of healthy self-expression and clear communication and tasks to work on with Lynn to help her achieve this interpersonal goal along with academic goals.

Individual family members will bear influence on one another when one member of the family system shifts or changes behavior. Again, family members seek to achieve balance in the system and when one member shifts, other members likely sense the shift and respond—even unconsciously. Therefore, counselors need to make relational considerations regarding family context and maintain ongoing check-ins with caregivers to learn about shifts in behavior and the impact, favorable and unfavorable, on the relationships in the family system.

Peer Groups

Peers become increasingly important to children's interpersonal context as they grow older. Friendships serve as cognitive and social resources for children and play a fundamental role in their emotional well-being (Sullivan, 1953). Lansford et al. (2014) found an increased likelihood in the long term for well-liked children aged 5 to 8 to possess high-quality dyadic friendships in their adulthood. Connections in youth potentially impact the ability to form bonds later in life.

Around age 12, peer groups become one of the most influential in an adolescent's life (Furman & Buhrmester, 1992). During most of adolescence, the areas of the brain responsible for self-regulation and good decision-making remain undeveloped. This may account for increased reward-seeking and risk-taking behaviors throughout this developmental period, often characterized by prevalent peer pressure (Collins & Laursen, 2012). Adolescents develop more interest in social relationships with peers and engage in more intimate relationships overall (Collins et al., 2009). Self-esteem seems to decline or become unstable for adolescents as a shift in social and romantic relationships occurs (Bee & Boyd, 2007). Yet perceived support from friendships predicts adolescents' self-worth beyond the support of parents and romantic partners (Laursen et al., 2006). Counselors working with adolescents should consider the more central role relationships play in adolescents' lives.

School System

For many children and adolescents, school remains the predominant interpersonal setting outside of the home. People may hope that school environments only provide comfortable, enriching, and growth-fostering social experiences for youth; yet realistically many youth might experience an array of distressing social interactions and events (e.g., bullying, disagreements with teachers or administrators, or academic challenges). According to the American School Counselor Association's (ASCA's) Professional Standards and Competencies (2019), professional school counselors work in tandem with families and other school personnel to foster academic, developmental, and relational wellness for pre-K–12 students. As such, professional school counselors support children and adolescents in need and ideally attend to relational and contextual factors related and unrelated to their school environment.

If students struggle in their interpersonal interactions with peers and teachers or become the subject of bullying, school counselors can create programming and provide direct and indirect services with these relational considerations in mind. This author discusses the therapeutic relationship in an upcoming section in this chapter, but it remains important to note that professional school counselors highly influence students' lives in important and lasting ways beyond their elementary and secondary education when they attend to relational considerations. They can address social justice inequities by advocating for students, attend to disruptive behaviors often associated with poor self-concept (Bidell & Deacon, 2010), and help students choose college and career paths (Shapiro et al., 2015).

For counselors practicing in community agencies and private practice, working with school-age youth requires similar considerations for their school environment and experiences. From her own private practice, this author estimates that she better served a substantial number of child and adolescent clients through collaborating with their school counselors and teachers. Students' mental health concerns can impact their academic performance, and professional school-based and community-based counselors support teachers and families to help school-age clients reach their academic and therapeutic goals.

Child and adolescent clients' families, peer groups, and schools comprise their primary interpersonal and systemic contexts. However, all people exist within a broader societal and cultural context. Counselors who invest in relational considerations acknowledge the importance of the cultural and contextual views of clients.

Cultural Context

Beyond interpersonal contexts at school and home, children and adolescents navigate their sociocultural environment and cultural identities. Culture refers to the identity of a group based on values, beliefs, norms, behaviors, and institutions (Ratts & Pederson, 2014). Culture influences perception of self, others, the world, and the relationships among people. Thus, multiculturally competent counselors show commitment to acquiring the knowledge, awareness, and skills for working with multicultural populations. They should seek to acquire information about their child and adolescent clients' concerns within the context of their cultural identities, to distinguish and account for within-group and between-group differences, and to examine their own cultural context, beliefs, and assumptions (Ratts et al., 2016).

Returning to the case example discussed previously, Lynn's grandmother, Petra, a Mexican American woman in her late 50s, comes from a low socioeconomic background. Petra married at a young age, stayed married to a mostly absent husband, and never remarried after his death. She devoted herself to raising her children. Later in life, she provided care and assistance to her mother and drove her to and from dialysis and other medical appointments. When Petra took on primary caregiving responsibilities and guardianship of Lynn, she felt an intense mix of emotions. Petra felt betrayed by her daughter, for whom she had provided all necessities and whom she had raised with values centered on the importance of family. Further, she felt angry when she paralleled her daughter's abandonment with her husband's absence and felt a sense of guilt, wondering if more could be done to model good parenting. Petra loved Lynn, but she did not anticipate starting over and raising another child.

Despite the torrent of emotions, Petra lived in a state of survival and operated in a task-oriented manner. Petra wondered, "Do I have it in me to raise another child at my age?" and "Somehow I messed up in raising her mom, but what if I don't have the energy to figure out a different way to be with Lynn?" She possessed little tolerance for her own emotional reactions to these questions but reached out to her priest and her aunt for advice. Petra did not invite emotion-filled discussions, and Lynn could not help but pick up on cues from Petra to avoid asking questions about her mom.

Unaccustomed to exploring her feelings and inner experiences, Lynn hesitated to open up in counseling, when a teacher referred her to the school counselor after Lynn appeared shut down in class and missed several assignments. In addition, Lynn felt unsafe expressing her personal reactions to academic challenges, to the lack of help at home, and to her mother's permanent absence. Lynn instinctively abided by the adage: Family business stays in the family. Angie contacted Petra to involve her in addressing Lynn's presenting concerns. Petra never considered seeking counseling for herself or Lynn and somewhat resented Angie for asking her to attend a meeting at the school.

In the case of Lynn, any counselor working with this family would do well to understand Latinxs often carry traditional values of interdependence, especially *familismo* (an emphasis on family; Calzada & Suarez-Balcazar, 2014). Some Latinx families entrust family matters to very few outside of the family (Delgado, 2000). The counselor should also consider relational dynamics between the matriarch of the family and her grandchild. Lynn follows her grandmother's lead without question and reveres her, a typical characteristic of Latinx families (Delgado, 2000). Other traditional values include *dignidad* (dignity) and *respeto* (respect), which counselors should consider when building their relationship with Petra and earning her trust. Petra appears to be prideful, but a counselor should avoid misinterpreting her reticence to explore emotion for rudeness when, in fact, she finds opening up and trusting others a lifelong challenge.

Although counselors should know general information about cultural groups based on testimonies and research, they should avoid assuming that all people within a group identically relate, behave, think, and feel in their interpersonal interactions. Instead, counselors can honor within-group differences and practice *cultural humility*, or a state of being that embodies the cultural competence that arises when counselors remain open to learning about their clients (Hook et al., 2013). For Lynn, the preceding general characteristics about Latinxs applied to her family. These applicable qualities of Latinxs could inform Angie's approach to relating to Lynn and Petra as well as frame her understanding for how they related to each other. Yet, counselors should remember that the Latinx population represents many different countries of origin, ethnicities, races (e.g., Black, White, Mestizo), socioeconomic statuses, languages, religions, and immigration and settlement trends (Calzada & Suarez-Balcazar, 2014). Moreover, culturally competent counselors must reflect on their own cultural context and assumptions. For example, if a counselor learned to value individualistic ideals associated with Western culture (e.g., autonomy and separation), then the counselor may make negative assumptions about clients from collectivistic cultures who insist on consulting with family members before making decisions. In order for counselors to relate to and learn from clients, they must evaluate their own beliefs.

In sum, counselors help clients practice healthy ways to self-manage and habituate in interpersonal and intrapersonal situations across settings and contexts. Counselors need to assess intrapersonal skills that serve as the framework for how child and adolescent clients perceive themselves and others. Counselors need to consider interpersonal contexts such as family, peer groups, and school environments, and they work toward engaging caregivers and school professionals who can help provide continuity of care and bridge counseling and the other areas of the client's life. Finally, they seek to understand the impact of culture on clients' relationships and practice cultural humility to forge strong therapeutic relationships with clients. In order to effectively treat mental health concerns and to address the needs of children and their families, counselors must take into account intrapersonal and interpersonal contexts throughout the counseling relationship.

THERAPEUTIC RELATIONSHIP

Since Freud's seminal work in the late 19th and early 20th centuries, years of theory development and empirical research continue to reveal that a positive, trusting, and collaborative therapeutic relationship positively affects treatment outcomes (Horvath, 2005). As such, clinicians and researchers continue to recognize the important role of the therapeutic relationship (Horvath & Bedi, 2002; Karver et al., 2005), which functions to produce a milieu that facilitates client change (Shirk & Saiz, 1992). Although the majority of this research previously focused on adult populations, empirical evidence similarly indicates that the therapeutic relationship between child clients and counselors is significantly and consistently associated with treatment outcomes (Kazdin et al., 2005; Shirk & Karver, 2003). In Shirk and Karver's (2003) meta-analysis of the association between relationship variables and treatment outcomes for children, the association between the therapeutic relationship and treatment outcome held regardless of type of counseling or level of child development. Child age, gender, or race did not account for a moderating effect on the relationship between therapeutic alliance and treatment outcomes.

Unlike results of studies where the measure of therapeutic alliance occurred early in treatment with adults and found more predictive of outcomes, Shirk and Karver (2003) found that alliance measures that occurred later in the treatment more reliably predicted outcomes for studies of child treatment. Relatedly, for youth with a history of maltreatment, the therapeutic alliance better predicts outcomes when it is measured later in therapeutic relationship versus early in treatment (Eltz et al., 1995). Adolescents who experienced abuse demonstrated lower positive therapeutic relationship scores in the initial phases of therapy but over time showed a pattern of improved alliance comparable to children without histories of maltreatment. Child characteristics such as emotional or functional differences, gender, or symptom severity did not account for the association. In short, it may take time to build a connected and trusting therapeutic relationship.

These findings remain particularly salient for those working with children and adolescents mandated to attend counseling or whose home environments do not promote trust and safety. Child and adolescent clients from such circumstances may not want to participate in counseling right away or may be slow to connect with the counselor. Notably, youth who consistently held low alliance scores evidenced the worst outcomes (Eltz et al., 1995), which emphasizes the greater point that investing in quality therapeutic relationships can make a difference for youth. Returning to the case of Lynn, her initial hesitancy toward counseling and unfamiliarity with the focal attention of an adult caused Angie to work diligently toward building the therapeutic relationship. In other words, Lynn eventually learned that her relationship with Angie fostered a sense of safety and trust. Lynn experienced safety in connecting with Angie, which allowed the therapeutic relationship to evolve from labored and unsteady to attuned and secure. As counselors continue to work toward strong therapeutic relationships, they should expect them to ebb and flow.

Forming the therapeutic relationship requires consistent messages of acceptance. Landreth (2012) proposed that therapists hold responsibility for conveying "four healing messages" to children: "I am here," "I hear you," "I understand," and "I care" (pp. 209–210). This helps children feel safe in the relationship. A connected and strong therapeutic relationship involves building trust over time and conveying understanding, which necessitates counselors to consider clients' relational factors. How can one develop a relationship and truly know about a child without knowing about the aforementioned intrapersonal, interpersonal, and cultural contexts? In the selected relational approaches outlined in the following section, the therapeutic relationship serves not only to create safety but also as a vehicle for new relational understanding (see Figure 3.1). New relational understanding emerges when the following occurs:

1. Counselors learn about a client's relational contexts across the intrapersonal, interpersonal, and cultural domains of experience.
2. Counselors build a therapeutic relationship rooted in understanding the aforementioned contexts and contextual factors and continue to grow their understanding.

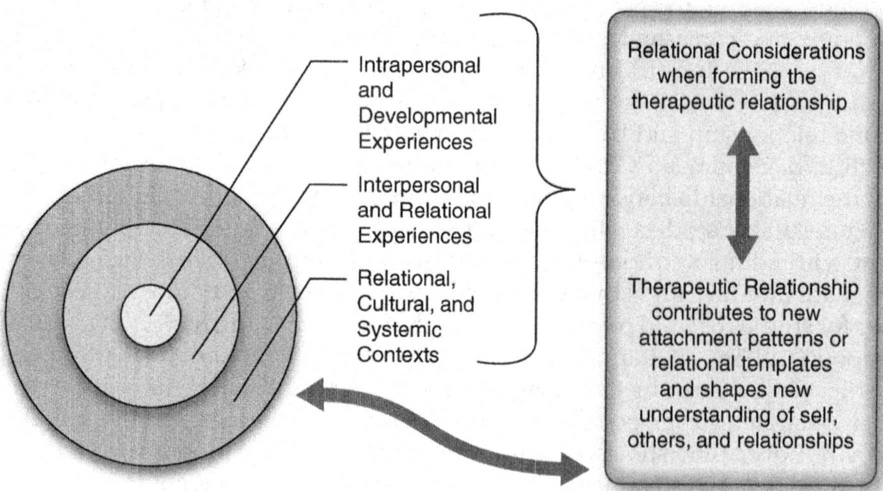

FIGURE 3.1 Forming therapeutic relationships. Relational considerations for counselors that inform a therapeutic relationship. The therapeutic relationship can contribute to new relational understanding of self and others, and the new understanding becomes integrated into their relational context.

3. Through expressed interest, acceptance, attunement, and empathy, the therapeutic relationship contributes to positive changes in the client's view of self, self-in-context, and self-in-therapeutic relationship.
4. New relational templates and self-understanding form and become integrated into the client's evolving relational contexts.

RELATIONAL APPROACHES APPLICABLE TO CHILDREN AND ADOLESCENTS

Elkins (2012) suggested that counseling involves a relationship between people rooted in a human predilection to reach out for help or to provide help to others in times of need. Humans operate hardwired for connection with other human beings (Banks, 2015), and as such counselors should stay mindful of relational considerations in approaches that work well for counseling youth. In the following, the author briefly overviews relational approaches including attachment theories and relational-cultural theory (RCT) as they pertain to working with child and adolescent clients. For more in-depth information on these theories, the author recommends consulting the resources listed in the resources section of this chapter.

ATTACHMENT THEORY

Based on studies of orphaned and homeless infants during World War II, John Bowlby (1951, 1953, 1969, 1979, 1988) concluded that infants need a consistent relationship with a primary caregiver to develop healthily. Bowlby (1973) suggested that attachment to caregivers creates a bond that plays a protective function as children explore their world. People operate using an *internal working model,* or an understanding of interpersonal relationships that constitute the basis for personality development (Bowlby, 1973). In their strange situation study, Ainsworth et al. (1978) studied the impact of brief separation on mother–infant dyad behaviors. Their observations showed three attachment styles: *secure, avoidant,* and *resistant.* Securely attached children greeted their mothers and engaged in physical contact after a separation. Children with avoidant attachment did not engage with or prefer their mothers over strangers after separation and displayed aggression toward them. Children with resistant attachment pursued physical contact but also demonstrated anger toward the mothers upon reuniting. Main and Solomon (1990) later offered a fourth attachment style—*disorganized/disoriented*—to describe children who indicated contradictory, fearful, and distressed behaviors toward their caregivers. The vast body of attachment research contributed to mental health professionals' understanding of parent–child relationships and the impact on individuals over the life span. The following section specifically includes attachment-informed therapy approaches for children.

ATTACHMENT-INFORMED APPROACHES

Attachment theory informed several clinical approaches designed for counseling children. In the 1960s, Ann Jernberg developed Theraplay, which the counseling field recognizes as one of the first approaches to integrate the principles of attachment theory for children to help with healthy attunement in parent–child interactions (Booth & Jernberg, 2010). Theraplay consists of interactive and relationship-focused activities during an intensive and short-term treatment geared to facilitate secure attachment and optimal mental health (Booth & Jernberg, 2010). Counselors use a structured play format, but they use few toys. Instead, counselors serve as the main toy and incorporate everyday items such as cotton balls, bubbles, lotion, and bouncy balls. Children receive attentive responses, and counselors intentionally engage children in eye contact and activities involving touch (Bundy-Myrow & Booth, 2009). Goals include improved attachment patterns, better coregulation, and empowered parents who continue to interact in ways that sustain positive changes in attachment and attunement (Bundy-Myrow & Booth, 2009).

Similarly, the developers of the Circle of Security (COS; Marvin et al., 2002) created an attachment-based intervention for high-risk toddlers and preschool children who experienced behavioral and emotional difficulties often related to insecure attachment with their caregivers. The COS protocol included teaching caregivers to facilitate healthy development in their children and consequently improve their attachment. To establish the attachment classification, trained clinicians coded the data from the caregivers' completed assessments, video-recorded interactions, and interviews. Marvin et al. (2002) described the following common styles and attachment patterns found in dyads: (a) *Secure (child)-Autonomous (parent)*; (b) *Insecure, Avoidant-Dismissing*; (c) *Insecure, Ambivalent-Preoccupied;* and (d) *Insecure, Disorganized or Insecure-Other.* The clinicians provided each caregiver-child dyad with feedback and interventions specific to their attachment style and internal working models. Currently, multiple forms of COS treatment exist, with the overarching goal of caregivers learning about the value of observing and appropriately responding to their child and increasing their reflecting skills to strengthen secure attachment (Marvin et al., 2002).

Another example and an evidence-based, trauma-informed model, Trust-Based Relational Intervention (TBRI), aims to address trauma through meeting attachment needs of children (Purvis et al., 2013a). Grounded in attachment theory and developmental neuroscience, the TBRI model comprises three tenets: *empowering* to address physical needs, *connecting* to build trust and set the stage for secure attachment, and *correcting* to address behavioral needs (Purvis et al., 2013a). Clinicians used the TBRI model with children across many settings, including day camps (Purvis et al., 2013b) and residential treatment facilities (Purvis et al., 2014).

When working with youth who may lack secure attachments, attachment-focused counselors should be mindful of the fact that they may be the only secure attachment in the child's life and should attend to their own internal working models and build awareness of their own attachment patterns (Wallin, 2007). Adults' attachment styles correspond to the attachment styles in children: secure (corresponds to secure in childhood), avoidant (corresponds to avoidant in childhood), preoccupied (corresponds to resistant in childhood), and fearful (corresponds to disorganized in childhood); see Alexander (1992).

Recall that Angie used experiential and play-based activities with Lynn in her sessions. Lynn's attachment style could be categorized as insecure, specifically anxious-avoidant. Her internal working model, as evidenced by her play, suggests that she finds her caregiver to be unresponsive and that she is unworthy of attention. Fortunately, counseling can provide opportunities for constructing new attachment patterns (Wallin, 2007). When counselors are consistent, congruent, and accepting, clients feel safe relying on the counselor and the therapeutic relationship. The corrective experience of a cohesive and trusting therapeutic relationship helps create new and secure attachment patterns (Wallin, 2007). In order to establish safety for paving the way to secure attachment, counselors should make sessions feel inviting, warm, predictable, and nonjudgmental and behave in congruent and culturally sensitive ways.

RELATIONAL-CULTURAL THEORY

RCT, developed by scholars at the Stone Center at Wellesley College, focuses on creating growth-fostering relationships and exploring connections and disconnections in one's life and relationships (Miller, 2008). The focus on connection in youth may seem contradictory to one of the tasks commonly associated with development in childhood: to grow more self-sufficient. However, RCT departs from the traditional notion that individuals need to separate and strive for individuation and rather promotes a focus on building and maintaining meaningful, healthy connections (Miller, 2008). Children increasingly regard interpersonal relationships as important as they mature and develop. In essence, relationships help children make sense of their world and their place in it. Thus, a focus on wellness and growth through the prism of connection allows counselors to target salient areas of child and adolescent clients' lives.

As RCT counselors address the relational considerations of intra- and interpersonal dynamics and cultural context of child and adolescent clients, they may find specific RCT tenets consistently applicable: *mutual empathy, connection, disconnection, relational images, relational resilience,* and *power.*

Mutual Empathy

The relational-cultural approach moves away from traditional views of empathy, in which empathy operates solely in one direction, from counselor to the client. RCT theorists suggest that bidirectional *mutual empathy* benefits the counseling relationship, in which both parties openly acknowledge each person's impact on the individuals and the relationship (Jordan, 2018). They also endorse self-empathy to help clients honor their experiences with compassion (Duffey & Somody, 2011). These forms of empathy allow clients to feel safe and accepted, a sense of agency and mattering, and hopefully an empathic understanding of self. Lynn, unfamiliar with mutuality, felt uncomfortable when Angie regarded her as funny and smart. Angie smiled and laughed when Lynn made clever or humorous remarks, and Angie thanked Lynn every time she taught her something new. Over time, Lynn saw her positive impact on Angie, and this augmented her view of herself and improved her relational confidence over the course of therapy.

Connection

Jean Baker Miller (2008) proposed that sense of self and worth subsists through an ability to form and maintain growth-fostering connection in relationships. Growth-fostering relationships characteristically reflect "five good things: (a) a sense of zest; (b) clarity about oneself, the other, and the relationship; (c) a sense of personal worth; (d) the capacity to be creative and productive; and (e) the desire for more connection" (Jordan, 2008, p. 2). The therapeutic relationship, from the RCT perspective, creates new relational templates for child and adolescent clients and models growth-fostering connection due to mutual empathy and empowerment. The warm and accepting presence of the counselor, the clear boundaries and expectations of the relationship, challenging negative relational images (discussed in more detail in the following section) to foster a more compassionate sense of self, and consistent and genuine interactions all culminate to form growth-fostering connection. Through the therapeutic relationship, child and adolescent clients can strive for new relational patterns characteristic of growth-fostering connection, with a sense of possibility for healthy relationships outside of the context of counseling.

Disconnection

Alongside connection, RCT theorists value disconnection as a normative and healthy part of all relationships. Disconnections occur in relationships void of empathy and mutual empowerment and may result in a person feeling disappointment, misinterpreted, violated, or a sense of danger (Jordan, 2018). Disconnection leads to stronger connection when people in the relationship experience disconnection in a manner that allows the people in the relationship to feel heard, respected, and free to be authentic (Jordan, 2008). Yet, if a person experiences invalidation or dismissive responses when disconnection occurs, one may resort to strategies of disconnection (Duffey & Somody, 2011). *Central relational paradox* represents one strategy of disconnection in which a person engages in an inauthentic way to achieve (or stay in) connection with others (Miller & Stiver, 1997). The paradox arises because people use inauthenticity as a shield to protect themselves from rejection, but inauthenticity keeps people from real connection with others (Miller, 2008).

Society may perpetuate the paradox (Miller & Stiver, 1997) through the overt or covert messages children and adolescents receive. According to several of this author's own child and adolescent clients, overt and covert messages around trauma and relational violations, substance use, familial and community values, gender roles and expectations related to behavior and appearance, academic achievement and career aspirations, interactions on social media, friendships and popularity, intimate relationships, and political climate all feed into how they create meaning of their relationships and their roles in those relationships. In Lynn's case, she protected herself by withholding her need and desire to ask questions about her parentage and to let Petra know that she yearned for her affection and attention. She hid away the part of herself that she believed created difficulty for Petra. One clearly sees Lynn's logic in self-protecting. Equally and unfortunately, one can see the impossibility of true connection with Petra as long as Lynn withholds her needs.

Relational Images

Relational images reflect the patterns of one's relational experience, which begins early in life and continues over the life span (Miller & Stiver, 1997). According to Miller and Stiver (1997), people ascribe meaning to their relational images, which informs their views of themselves, others, and the world. Lynn felt abandoned by the adults in her life, and this served as the primary basis for her relational images. She believed herself to be unworthy and bad, which allowed her to make sense of her biological parents' abandoning her and her grandmother's emotional unavailability. She felt largely ignored and learned that if she could make herself invisible, everything at home seemed less stressful for her grandmother. Before Lynn started counseling, she kept conversations with Petra light and brief, spent most of her time playing in her room, and stayed out of Petra's way as much as possible. Petra suspected and feared that Lynn experienced loneliness, but recall that Petra avoided emotional expression and discussion. Petra sidestepped Lynn's emotional needs—not out of malice but in response to her own discomfort and grief. Lynn, unaware of Petra's insight, continued to exist quietly and viewed her strategy to be successful: Staying quiet yielded positive results. The positive outcome reinforced Lynn's relational images of caregiver–child relationships. Here, one can see that the meaning the child or adolescent takes away from an experience plays a key role in determining how they function intra- and interpersonally. Thus, part of a counselor's role involves understanding the relational images and templates that guide child and adolescent clients' lived experiences and reality.

Relational Resilience

People demonstrate relational resilience when they move toward growth-fostering relationships and mutuality after experiencing disconnection (Jordan, 2013, 2018). Achieving new or renewed connection remains less relevant than actually attempting to reconnect after experiencing adversity (J. Jordan, personal communication, June 21, 2014). Many children and adolescents struggle with chronic disconnection as a result of conflict or other issues (e.g., name-calling, bullying, and severe childhood maltreatment). Some may resort to isolation to self-protect. If a child ventures out from isolation after surviving relational or physical trauma and attempts to connect with others, this connotes a sign of relational resilience.

Initially, Lynn took her time trusting her school counselor. Lynn expected her to become disinterested and to leave her behind, as others did. Over time, Lynn started to not only welcome the counseling sessions but became excited to spend time with Angie. Feeling safe in the therapeutic relationship, she allowed herself to attempt connection with Angie, sharing her perspectives of Petra (that she minimally mattered to Petra) and her wishes for a better relationship with her. During parent consultations, Angie provided feedback, psychoeducation, and homework, and she helped facilitate communication that gave Petra insight about Lynn's perceptions and feelings. Petra employed the strategies she learned in the parent consultations at home. She made concerted efforts to increase eye contact and dialogue with Lynn every day. If Lynn approached her for any reason, she committed no less than 60 seconds of her attention to Lynn's comments, question, or immediate needs. She invited Lynn to help with dinner and other manageable and developmentally appropriate tasks to increase their time together and to help with the workload. Petra reported that she needed more time to increase her comfort with discussing Lynn's mom and still struggled to increase her own emotional vocabulary and expression. Nevertheless, both Lynn and Petra reported improved mood, connection, and home life. After successful connection with Angie and improved connection with Petra, Lynn's teacher reported that Lynn made other attempts of connection with her teachers and two classmates. Lynn's attempts at connection indicated a newfound relational resilience that spanned several areas of her life.

Power

Relational-cultural theorists distinguish *power over* (i.e., control) from *power with* (i.e., empowerment) in their view of power in people's lives and society (Jordan, 2018). Power over occurs in relationships that allow people to dominate and control others, and power with involves mutual empowerment of all people in a relationship (Jordan, 2018). Counselors can offer child and adolescent clients choices and can allow them to take the lead in sessions to promote empowerment, as Lynn's counselor did in their sessions. Yet counselors also recognize that power differentials exist in child and adolescents' lives and the settings in which they live. Understanding that shared power may be unsafe or unsuitable for all situations, counselors can work with caregivers to identify appropriate opportunities for empowering their children. Caregivers can offer choices to their children whenever possible. Petra realized that the process for allowing Lynn to make choices could be simple and easy and still produce the desired outcome of shared power. She encouraged Lynn to decide the station they listened to on the way to church, to choose between two dessert options for them to enjoy after dinner, and many other daily choices. Caregivers, through communicating that children's opinions carry value, can offer moments for them to engage in decision-making that not only create immediate satisfaction but also create a sense of agency.

Many approaches target problem-solving and symptom reduction in children. Although targeting these important areas helps children, relational health influences mental health as well. Exploring the RCT concepts allows counselors using relational approaches to provide opportunities for youth to expand their self-understanding in relationships, to identify characteristics of growth-fostering relationships, and to practice establishing and maintaining healthy boundaries in relationships (Haiyasoso & Schuermann, 2018).

APPLYING RELATIONAL-CULTURAL THEORY IN COUNSELING CHILD AND ADOLESCENT CLIENTS

Counselors integrate the aforementioned RCT principles into models to target specific populations. For example, Haiyasoso and Schuermann (2018) propose RCT as an appropriate framework for counseling adolescent survivors of child sexual abuse (CSA) to address common relational concerns and to build relational health in the aftermath of abuse. Haiyasoso and Schuermann (2018) offer the Relational Health Model (RHM), which merges relational competencies and the role of power (Duffey et al., 2009) with areas in a relational model of resilience (Jordan, 2013). Tenets of the model include the following: *Shared Authenticity and Empathy, Reciprocity, Attempts to Connect, Mutual Empowerment,* and *Holistic Awareness* (see Figure 3.2). Shared Authenticity and Empathy encompasses the idea that counselors can help adolescents grow in their own awareness about areas of life where they may or may not feel safe enough to be authentic. Counselors stay mutually engaged and authentic to model a therapeutic, growth-fostering relationship in the adolescent's life. Authenticity leads to freedom to be vulnerable, and when people in interpersonal relationships can be vulnerable, true connection and shared empathy is possible. Reciprocity involves counselors modeling and highlighting that mutuality and respect can exist in relationships where all parties involved in the relationship encourage and hold space for one another. In Attempts to Connect, counselors explore the biological and social imperative of connection with adolescents and learn about their perceived relational confidence. Within the Mutual Empowerment domain, counselors focus on power as a concept that influences interactions across relational contexts. Counselors should empower adolescents to exercise their power through self-expression and effective use of their voice, and counselors should stay mindful of clients' cultural and intersectional identities that may impact their experiences with power or lack thereof. In the last tenet, Holistic Awareness, counselors can scan adolescents' previous and current social connections for the five good things. They can also explore patterns of giving and receiving support and establishing healthy boundaries. Haiyasoso and Schuermann (2018) apply the model to a case illustration to address relational, developmental, and therapeutic needs of adolescent survivors of CSA.

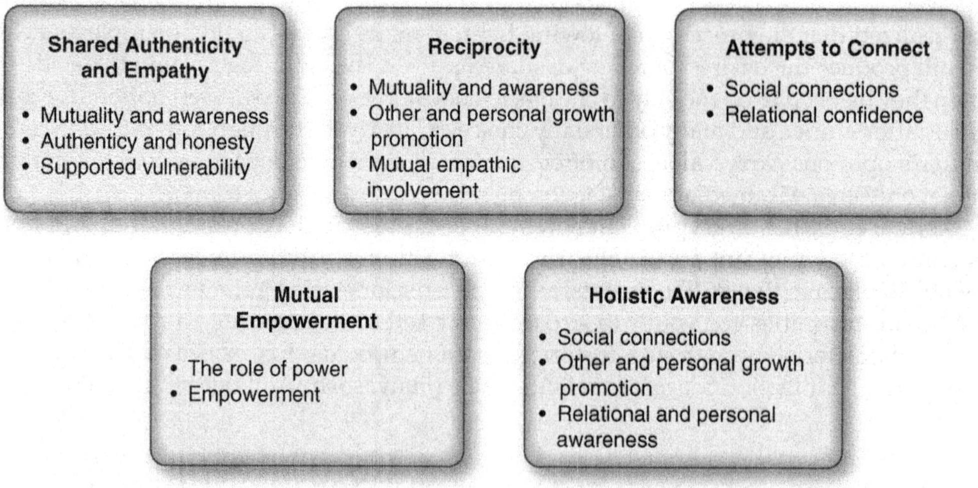

Shared Authenticity and Empathy
- Mutuality and awareness
- Authenticy and honesty
- Supported vulnerability

Reciprocity
- Mutuality and awareness
- Other and personal growth promotion
- Mutual empathic involvement

Attempts to Connect
- Social connections
- Relational confidence

Mutual Empowerment
- The role of power
- Empowerment

Holistic Awareness
- Social connections
- Other and personal growth promotion
- Relational and personal awareness

FIGURE 3.2 Relational Health Model. Relational Health Model for counselors working with survivors of child sexual abuse, merging relational competency, power (see Duffey et al., 2009), and relational resilience (see Jordan, 2013).

Source: Adapted from Haiyasoso, M., & Schuermann, H. (2018). Application of relational-cultural theory with adolescent sexual abuse survivors. *Journal of Child and Adolescent Counseling, 4,* 171. Copyright 2018 by the Association for Child and Adolescent Counseling.

PROCESSING QUESTIONS FOR EACH DOMAIN IN THE RELATIONAL HEALTH MODEL

- *Shared Authenticity and Empathy*: When and where does the client feel safe enough to be vulnerable? Can they reach out to others and avoid isolation? Am I as the counselor cultivating safety? Am I modeling authenticity? In what ways can I highlight our therapeutic relationship as an example for a healthy relational template?
- *Reciprocity*: Have I defined and demonstrated mutuality and mutual empathy well? In what relationships outside of counseling do clients experience mutuality and see their impact on others? How does this client promote self and others?
- *Attempts to Connect*: How readily does the client trust others? Do they trust themselves? How do they perceive connection with others? Knowing that mutuality bolsters relational confidence, when, where, and with whom do they experience mutuality?
- *Mutual Empowerment*: When has this client felt empowered? When has this client felt violated or disempowered? What are the cultural norms around power and expression for this client? How can I offer opportunities to empower the client in session?
- *Holistic Awareness*: Are there behaviors serving as attempts to connect with and feel connected to others? What previous relationships contain the five good things? Which relationships lack the five good things?

For youth in school settings, Tucker et al. (2011) provide a framework of the *5 Es* to foster relational skills in adolescents: encourage self-empathy, explore relational images, educate about power, explain disconnections and conflict, and expand relational capacities (p. 312). Students' social and peer relationships come fraught with challenges (e.g., relational aggression and bullying). Counselors can assist students who experience these challenges through helping them build relational skills to more effectively manage areas of concern or conflict (Tucker et al., 2011).

In another example, Vicario et al. (2013) developed relational-cultural play therapy (RCPT) through integrating the principles of trauma-focused play therapy (Gil, 2011) and the relational-cultural approach from Tucker et al. (2011). The RCPT approach addresses trauma through Gil's (2011) *3 Rs,* which include reexperiencing (i.e., recollecting traumatic events and placing blame on the offender), releasing (i.e., experiencing the trauma as an event from the past and no longer occurring), and reorganizing (i.e., experiencing the trauma as a moment in time versus a defining and focal part of the child's identity [Vicario et al., 2013]). The authors integrated the 3 Rs (reexperiencing, releasing, and reorganizing) with Tucker et al.'s (2011) 5 Es (encourage self-empathy, explore relational images, educate about power, explain disconnections and conflict, and expand relational capacities) and suggested that RCPT could be adapted to work with adolescents and adults if counselors apply the principles through other forms of counseling, such as psychodrama, art, or music therapy (Vicario et al., 2013).

Common RCT concepts exist at the core of the previously discussed relational approaches proposed for youth. Although counselors view these integrative approaches to be anecdotally effective, they lack empirical research on their effectiveness. In an effort to hone in on relational considerations and help promote growth-fostering characteristics in a developmentally appropriate manner, counselors can integrate these approaches with evidence-based practices if clients present with poor relational health and a lack of healthy connection with others.

CASE STUDY 3.1: NOEMI

Before the coronavirus disease 2019 (COVID-19) pandemic, Noemi, an 11-year-old Filipino American female, and her family lived a modest and comfortable life. Noemi's parents owned and operated a local coffee shop but temporarily closed their café when the pandemic struck. As the shutdown continued, the emotional, physical, and financial toll on her parents grew increasingly evident. Noemi overheard her parents' discussions about their financial difficulties and saw many instances of her father consoling her crying mother. Eventually, Noemi, her parents, and her three younger siblings moved into her paternal aunt's home. Despite being surrounded by people she loved, Noemi felt isolated and sad. Accustomed to her siblings, she knew how to share, wait her turn, and coexist without a lot of privacy. Yet, at her aunt's home, she had to contend not only with her siblings but also with her cousins, all younger than Noemi. She felt lost as she tried to focus on online school assignments when her school resumed remotely. She experienced difficulty with paying attention and focusing on her assignments due to the busyness around her, with all of the children and adults trying to work from home. Her typically cheery affect became blunted, and her normally open manner appeared shut down and withdrawn. She communicated with her best friend via phone calls and text messages and shared a little bit about her feelings with her best friend's mom. Noemi described feeling intense shame for feeling angry about being forced to move into her aunt's home and being required to stay home from school. Otherwise, she maintained few relationships with peers and expressed minimal emotions with others. Her mother noticed her markedly changed demeanor and contacted the school counselor. The school counselor suggested scheduling a virtual counseling session with Noemi.

Activity 3.1

The following written exercises can help bring focus to relational considerations and relational-cultural responses. Reference the preceding case example to complete the exercises.

Written Exercise 1: Intrapersonal and Interpersonal Context

Exploring the client's intrapersonal and interpersonal contexts (family, peer, school, and cultural) fosters better understanding of the client and allows the client to feel heard.

- Take 1 to 2 minutes to list the questions that first come to mind after reading the case example of Noemi and her family.
- Then, scan those questions to see which questions assess her intrapersonal functioning (e.g., self-esteem, emotional expression, and regulation) and which examine her identities, cultural groups, and family/peer interactions. Do you notice any differences in your lists?
- Refer to the processing questions for the following RHM domains (p. 69): *Attempts to Connect, Mutual Empowerment, and Holistic Awareness.* If you were the counselor, are there additional questions that you might add to learn about Noemi's intrapersonal and interpersonal contexts?

Written Exercise 2: Therapeutic Relationship

In order to cultivate mutual empathy and authenticity in the therapeutic relationship, a counselor must attempt to create a supportive environment.

- List the top three necessary qualities you want to convey to Noemi to create a sense of trust and connection.
- Briefly describe what you need to do to demonstrate mutual empathy.
- Indicate in two to three sentences how you will know that you have achieved connection and trust with Noemi.

CHAPTER SUMMARY

Relational contexts impact psychosocial and developmental processes for children and adolescents. Intrapersonally, children develop their sense of self-esteem, learn their own self-awareness, and expand their ability to self-regulate. Adolescents participate in this ongoing process and attempt to keep pace with evolving needs and hormonal changes. Interpersonally, youth reside within embedded relational contexts including family, peer groups, school settings, and the broader community. Children and adolescents increasingly value friendships and peers as they mature. Counselors should seek to understand relational contexts in their clinical work with children and adolescents because treating the whole child requires understanding of these relational and cultural influences. Knowing the integral nature of human connection and relationship, counselors working from an attachment-based or relational lens explore their child and adolescent clients' relational health and competency and encourage relational resilience. Above all, focusing on building and fostering a strong therapeutic relationship over time remains among the most important relational considerations and key to effectively connecting with child and adolescent clients.

POINTS TO REMEMBER

- Focus on the "we" instead of the "me" in clients' experiences. Children and adolescents exist and develop within relational, cultural, and systemic contexts.
- Learn about child and adolescent clients' intrapersonal and interpersonal experiences in order to conceptualize them in a holistic manner.
- Understand the mutual influences between children and their environments (familial, social, academic) throughout their development.
- Seek to form a therapeutic relationship that honors the human tendency to reach for connection in the counseling setting as well as in clients' daily lives.
- Remember that the therapeutic relationship can reshape child and adolescent clients' relational templates, which leads to an augmented understanding of self and self in context.

- In terms of relational resiliency, counselors view establishing connection or reconnection as less relevant than the actual act of attempting to reconnect. The effort, vulnerability, and courage to try matter most.

OTHER HELPFUL INFORMATION FOR CONSIDERATION

RECOMMENDED READING

Banks, A. (2016). *Wired to connect.* Tarcher/Penguin.
Coan, J. A. (2016). Toward a neuroscience of attachment. In J. Cassidy & P. R. Shaver (Eds.)., *Handbook of attachment: Theory, research, and clinical applications* (3rd ed.). Guilford Press.
Kestly, T. A. (2014). *The interpersonal neurobiology of play: Brain-building interventions for emotional well-being.* W. W. Norton & Company.
Miller, J. B. (Ed.). (1973). *Psychoanalysis and women.* Brunner/Mazel.
Munns, E. (2003). Theraplay: Attachment enhancing play therapy. In C. E. Schaefer (Ed.), *Foundations of play therapy.* Wiley.

QUESTIONS FOR FURTHER DISCUSSION

- The chapter centers on relational considerations. Appraise your own awareness of your relational contexts. How might these influence your own understanding of child and adolescent clients' presenting concerns?
- Reflect on the case of Lynn. What feelings come up for you as you reflect on Lynn and Petra? How did Petra's background and relational contexts contribute to your understanding of Petra?
- Consider the distinctions in the RCT perspective of power (*power over* vs. *power with*). In a society that values competition, how do you reconcile the relational idea of mutual empowerment (e.g., "I feel empowered when you are empowered")? Do you see yourself integrating *power with* dynamics in your therapeutic work with child and adolescent clients?
- Think of the five good things that characterized growth-fostering relationships: zest, clarity, worth, productivity and creativity, and desire for more connection. You may simply ask your child and adolescent clients to reflect developmentally on their relationships and list those that possess these qualities. However, that may not always be appropriate. What other experiential ways can you work with young clients to explore the quality of their relationships?
- The therapeutic relationship naturally experiences ups and downs. How do you envision managing this dynamic process with child and adolescent clients?

KEY REFERENCES

Only key references appear in the print edition. The full reference list appears in the digital product on Springer Publishing Connect: connect.springerpub.com/content/book/978-0-8261-4764-6/part/part01/chapter/ch03

Banks, A. (2015). *Four ways to click: Rewire your brain for stronger, more rewarding relationships.* Penguin Group.

Bowlby, J. (1988). *A secure base: Clinical applications of attachment theory.* Routledge.

Collins, W. A., & Laursen, B. P. (2012). *Relationship pathways: From adolescence to young adulthood.* SAGE Publications, Inc.

Duffey, T., & Somody, C. (2011). The role of relational-cultural theory in mental health counseling. *Journal of Mental Health Counseling, 33*(3), 223–242. https://doi.org/10.17744/mehc.33.3.c10410226u275647

Elkins, D. (2012). Toward a common focus in psychotherapy research. *Psychotherapy, 49*(4), 450–454. https://doi.org/10.1037/a0027797

Horvath, A., & Bedi, R. (2002). The alliance. In J. Norcross (Ed.), *Psychotherapy relationships that work: Therapist contributions and responsiveness to patients.* Oxford University Press.

Jordan, J. V. (2018). *Relational-cultural therapy* (2nd ed.). American Psychological Association.

Miller, J. B. (2008). VI. Connections, disconnections, and violations. *Feminism & Psychology, 18*(3), 368–380. https://doi.org/10.1177/0959353508092090

Miller, J. B., & Stiver, I. P. (1997). *The healing connection: How women form relationships in therapy and life.* Beacon Press.

Wallin, D. (2007). *Attachment in psychotherapy.* Guilford Press.

CHAPTER 4

Counseling Children and Adolescents: A Cross-Cultural Perspective

Courtland C. Lee, Vivian V. Lee, and Irene Gomez

LEARNING OBJECTIVES

After completing this chapter, the reader should be able to:

- Identify cultural factors that influence the psychosocial development of children and adolescents.
- Define the key factors of cultural competency.
- Describe what the term "counseling with culture in mind" means.
- Delineate a culturally responsive perspective on counseling with children and adolescents.

CACREP STANDARDS FOR THIS CHAPTER

- CACREP 2009: II.G.2.a., b., c., d., e., f; 3.a., c., d., f., h.; School Counseling: III.A.6; B.2; C.1., 2., 3., 5.; D.1., 2., 3.; E.1., 2., 3., 4.; F.1., 2., 3., 4.; H.1., 5.; L.1; M.1., 2., 3., 5.; N.1., 2., 3., 4., 5.; O.2.3., 4., 5.; P.1., 2, Clinical Mental Health Counseling: III.C.1., 8.; D.2; E.1., 2., 3., 5.; F.3.; H.1.
- CACREP 2016: 2.F.2.a., b., c., d., e., f., g., h; 3.a., b., c., f., g., h; 5.a., b., f., g., h; 6.g; School Counseling: 5.G.2.b; 3.d., f., h; Clinical Mental Health Counseling: 5.C.2.j.

INTRODUCTION

Counseling children and adolescents in contemporary society requires a cross-cultural perspective. Demographic trends in the racial and ethnic composition of the U.S. youth population suggest that over the past several decades, this segment of the U.S. population underwent some important shifts. From 1980 to 1999, the proportion of non-Hispanic White children in the U.S. population fell from 74% to 63%. From 2000 to 2010, the percentage of non-Hispanic White children declined from 61% to 54%. This proportion continued to decrease through 2016, reaching 51%, and is projected to fall slightly further by 2020 to 50%. The percentage of the non-Hispanic Black child population stayed relatively constant since 1980, at about 15%; this figure is expected to decline only slightly further by 2020 to 14%. Significantly, the proportion of ethnically Hispanic (Latinx) children grew steadily, from 9% in 1980 to 25% in 2016, with projections to reach 26% in 2020. The proportion of non-Hispanic Asian and Pacific Islander children grew steadily over the past few decades, from 2% of the child population in 1980 to 5.1% in 2016. The percentage of the non-Hispanic American Indian or Alaska Native U.S. child population remained relatively constant from 1980 to 2016, at around 1%. In 2016, non-Hispanic children of more than one race constituted roughly 4.2% of the total U.S. child population, an increase of two percentage points from the 2000 census. Among all children identified as being of more than one race (including Latinx children), the majority (4.4% of all children) were White combined with one other race, with 1.7% identified as White and Black, 1.1% identified as White and Asian, and 0.6% as White and American Indian or Alaska Native (Federal Interagency Forum on Child and Family Statistics, 2017).

These demographic data suggest both challenges and opportunities for the counseling profession with respect to counseling children and adolescents. These challenges and opportunities require that counselors exhibit the competency to ensure that all young people, no matter their race or ethnic background, receive counseling services that ensure they fulfill their developmental potential and are both physically and mentally healthy.

This chapter provides a cross-cultural perspective on counseling children and adolescents. The chapter begins with a conceptual overview of counseling youth across cultures. Next, the chapter presents culturally diverse perspectives on psychosocial development. The chapter concludes with case studies that provide direction for counseling children and adolescents with culture in mind.

COUNSELING YOUTH ACROSS CULTURES: A CONCEPTUAL OVERVIEW

Counseling across cultures can be perceived as a working alliance between a counselor and a child or adolescent that takes the personal dynamics of the counselor and the young person into consideration alongside the dynamics found in the cultures of both of these individuals. As a process, therefore, counseling youth cross-culturally takes into consideration their cultural background and individual experiences and how their unique developmental needs might be identified and met through counseling (Lee, 2019).

CROSS-CULTURAL COUNSELING COMPETENCY

The basis for counseling across cultures is the concept of cross-cultural competency, which outlines a set of attitudes and behaviors indicative of the ability to establish, maintain, and successfully conclude a counseling relationship with individuals from diverse cultural backgrounds (Ratts et al., 2016). Counselors who strive for cultural competency in their work with children and adolescents exhibit attitudes and behaviors that indicate heightened self-awareness, an expanded cultural knowledge base, the ability to use helping skills in a culturally responsive manner, and a commitment to actions that foster social justice for youth.

PSYCHOSOCIAL DEVELOPMENT AND CULTURAL DIVERSITY

As mentioned in Chapter 1, theorists and researchers have suggested that major aspects of human psychosocial development unfold in a series of life stages and are influenced by both heredity and environment (Erikson, 1950; Havighurst, 1972; Kohlberg, 1984; Piaget, 1972). As individuals progress through the life stages, they must master a series of developmental tasks. Mastery of tasks at one stage of life influences success with those in succeeding stages. This success contributes to the formation of all aspects of human thinking, feeling, and behaving.

When counseling with youth, the focus stays on the tasks of childhood and adolescence. Understanding the developmental dynamics of these two life stages remains basic to effective counseling with young people.

Childhood can be characterized as the stage that forms the foundation for human development across the life span. The mastery of fundamental skills such as walking and talking characterizes the early part of this period. Developing skills in reading, writing, and calculating mark the later part of the period. Childhood occurs when human beings, through family interaction, develop a sense of trust and autonomy. In addition, through mastery of basic skills, children develop a sense of initiative and industry. Childhood also comprises a time when individuals learn social skills that involve relating emotionally to the family, adults, and peers. Acquisition of such skills involves an aspect of developing attitudes toward social groups and institutions (Daehler & Bukatko, 1985; Kessen, 1979).

Adolescence, the next life stage, marks the developmental transition between childhood and adulthood. This period characterizes significant physical and psychological changes. It marks a sudden increase in body size and strength as well as a change in many physiologic functions, including reproductive capacities. Adolescence also marks major personality changes designed to attain self-identity and meaningful independence (Elkind, 1984; Erikson, 1965; Offer et al., 1981).

Although there seem to be universal aspects to the phenomenon, social and behavioral scientists indicated that the process of psychosocial development may need to be revised when considered across cultures (Mead, 1928; Munroe & Munroe, 1975; Powell et al., 1983). This process suggests considerable racial and ethnic variation in its behavioral manifestations, its symbolic meaning, and its societal responses (Rotheram & Phinney, 1987). Children and adolescents must master psychosocial developmental tasks through their socialization within a cultural context. This refers to social environments, such as family and community, and their patterns of interpersonal relationships, which impact affect, behavior, and cognition (Koss-Chioino & Vargas, 1992). Through family and community interaction, the beliefs, values, social forms, and material traits that comprise cultural realities pass from older generations to younger ones.

Cultural variation in the context of families and communities can be observed along dimensions such as the following:

1. **Notions of kinship.** There appear to be important cultural differences in the emphasis placed on bonds of interpersonal affiliation established within family and community kinship networks. In some cultural traditions, a major emphasis rests with the nuclear family and individual autonomy, while in others there remains a great importance placed on extended family kinship networks and interdependence among individuals (Höllinger & Haller, 1990; Souvatzi, 2017). This individualistic versus communalistic distinction in kinship social organization can affect the development of perceptions and attitudes regarding relationships with individuals, social groups, and institutions among young people.
2. **Roles and status.** Cultural differences exist with respect to roles and status within families and communities. This involves centrally prescribed notions or traditions concerning individual responsibilities and obligations that are based on age- and gender-defined roles and status. Children and adolescents become socialized into roles and assigned status within a family/community hierarchy based on such notions (Georgas et al., 1997; Heras & Revilla, 1994).
3. **Gender role socialization.** Cultural differences remain evident concerning perceptions of the role of males and females. Differential gender perceptions can influence the expectations considered normal for psychosocial development. Such expectations may account for fundamental differences in personality development for boys and girls in the traditions of many cultures (Block, 1973; Lee et al., 2020; Sanchez et al., 2017).
4. **Language preference.** Acquisition and use of language exist as important aspects of socialization for young people. Mastery of language often fosters success in succeeding developmental tasks. Children are socialized into a language tradition at an early age. There are, however, significant cultural differences in language traditions, as well as the value placed on specific language use (Lieven, 1994; Mohanty & Perregaux, 1997). Personality development in childhood and adolescence can be significantly impacted by distinctions in language traditions. This becomes particularly evident when conflict of cultural perceptions occurs regarding differences in language traditions and value (Geerlings et al., 2015; Lueck & Wilson, 2010).
5. **Religion/spirituality.** Religious and spiritual influences universally and importantly shape the formation of behavior and values in young people. However, significant cultural differences exist in the extent to which such influences may impact childhood and adolescent psychosocial development. The distinctions between religious and secular life vary across cultural groups. The degree of such distinctions among families and communities can significantly affect aspects of psychosocial development (King & Roeser, 2009; Saroglou & Cohen, 2013).
6. **Racial/ethnic identity.** Importantly, dynamics represented by those discussed earlier, when considered in total, contribute to the development of a racial/ethnic identity among young people. Racial/ethnic identity comprises the primary principle for understanding psychosocial development in a cultural context. According to Phinney and Rotheram (1987), "ethnic identity refers to one's sense of belonging to an ethnic group and the part of one's thinking, perceptions, feelings, and behavior that is due to ethnic group membership" (p. 13). It can be considered as the "inner vision" that one develops of oneself as an "African American," "Arab American," "Korean American," "Mexican American," "Native American," or "Italian American." Racial/ethnic identity greatly influences psychosocial development, particularly in a culturally pluralistic country like the United States. The manner in which young people come to view themselves in relation

to members of their own racial/ethnic group and members of other racial/ethnic groups can significantly impact aspects of development (Phinney & Rotheram, 1987).

7. **Poverty and discrimination.** The "culture of poverty" has long been recognized as a societal reality (Lewis, 1966). It has been theorized that sustained poverty generates a set of cultural attitudes, beliefs, values, and practices among groups of people. Poverty affects racial/ethnic groups disproportionately. In particular, for many people of color, poor housing, inadequate schooling, and low-quality healthcare impact negatively on most aspects of family and community life (Reeves et al., 2016). The forces of socioeconomic disadvantage can converge to impact negatively upon the psychosocial development of children and adolescents. Poverty can negate the cultural context and impede the emergence of a climate conducive to the successful mastery of developmental tasks.

   For children from diverse cultural backgrounds, poverty may often be compounded by discrimination—harmful actions toward others because of their race, ethnicity, religion, nationality, or language. Racism and other forms of discrimination bear considerable consequences for the psychosocial development of young people (Comer, 1989; Heard-Garris et al., 2018; Stevenson et al., 2020).

   Poverty and its intersection with discrimination tends to constrict young people's environments as well as their access to resources that help to positively nurture the mastery of the tasks considered crucial for normal physical and emotional development.

8. **Acculturation.** Acculturation, within the context of American society, refers to the degree to which an individual identifies with the attitudes, behaviors, and values of the predominant macroculture (Lee, 1991). These attitudes, behaviors, and values reflect the cultural traditions of middle-class Americans of European origin. The acculturation process differs in significant ways, again depending on the particular racial/ethnic group to which young people belong, and whether that group holds majority or minority status in society. Acculturation may present a major developmental challenge to young people of color. Social and economic success is often predicated on an individual's ability to adopt the lifestyle of the macroculture. Young people of color must master the task of balancing an ethnic identity with one that will ensure success in the macroculture. In many instances, young people can find themselves caught between two cultures. The challenges of attempting to negotiate two cultural realities often lead to acculturation stress in many children and adolescents (Ahmed et al., 2011; Gil et al., 1994).

While this list of factors that characterize cultural variations in childhood and adolescent development is by no means exhaustive, they provide key points of reflection for understanding the importance of counseling with culture in mind. Although the relevance of these dimensions may vary across young people, a working knowledge of them and how they may impact psychosocial development should frame the context of culturally competent counseling with children and adolescents.

COUNSELING CHILDREN AND ADOLESCENTS WITH CULTURE IN MIND

In order to exhibit competence in cross-cultural encounters with children and adolescents from diverse cultural backgrounds, counselors must approach the helping process with culture in mind (Vontress, 2009). This means that cultural factors must be considered in any counseling interaction. It is important to approach the helping process with the mindset that cultural differences are just that, differences. These differences do not necessarily connote deficiencies or pathologic deviations. Counseling with culture in mind entails working from a perspective that simultaneously acknowledges human similarity and celebrates human difference. Counselors must adopt a holistic philosophy that views each young person as a unique individual while, at the same time, taking into consideration their common experiences as a human being and the specific experiences that come from their cultural background. Importantly, counselors must consider each child or adolescent within a cultural group context and a broader global human perspective (Lee, 2019).

Case Studies 4.1 and 4.2 illustrate aspects of counseling with culture in mind with a child and an adolescent. The authors urge caution in generalizing the strategies addressed in these case studies to all children or adolescents from these cultural backgrounds. The ideas presented in work with these two young people exemplify guidelines for counseling with culture in mind and relate specifically to the individuals in each case.

CASE STUDY 4.1: CHILDHOOD

Cesar, a 5-year-old boy, recently arrived in the United States from Honduras. His parents immigrated to the United States when he was 2 years old, leaving him and his older brother and sister in Honduras in the care of an aunt. Cesar traveled to the United States with his brother and sister, enduring multiple hardships, in order to be reunited with his parents. Cesar was held in a detention center with his siblings for nearly a month until he was released to his parents. He is currently enrolled in kindergarten in his neighborhood elementary school. Cesar is currently in an English as a second language (ESL) class where he is surrounded by other classmates who are all experiencing a new culture and learning English for the first time. As he is in a small class, he receives the support of his teachers and peers. His parents have learned a few words in English but cannot have a conversation in the language yet. Cesar was referred to counseling by his teacher and his parents due to behavioral concerns. His teacher stated that when it is time for reading, he gets frustrated and refuses to do work. At home, his parents said that he seems to be happy and only has moments of frustration when it comes to completing his schoolwork.

COUNSELING CESAR: A CULTURALLY RESPONSIVE DEVELOPMENTAL PERSPECTIVE

Placing Cesar Into a Cultural Context

Cesar is a Latinx male who is a recent immigrant. His psychosocial development is being impacted by a number of factors. First, some issues related to his detention experience upon entering the United States clearly need to be considered. Second, he appears to be experiencing acculturation stress. As a recent immigrant, Cesar is faced with the task of balancing his Honduran identity with one that will ensure success in the United States. It appears that Cesar is in between two cultures. Third,

(continued)

CASE STUDY 4.1 (*continued*)

a crucial element of acculturation stress for Cesar seems to be his challenges with English language proficiency, which appear to be contributing to his behavioral issues.

Counseling Cesar With Culture in Mind

Given his age and language ability, counseling with Cesar may need to be focused on a nonverbal activity approach. This might include a combination of play and art therapy. Play and artistic expression cross all cultures and are good ways to allow for nonverbal expression of feelings among children (Gil & Pfeifer, 2016; Gonzalez & Bell, 2016). Providing Cesar with the opportunity to engage in play activities in addition to encouraging him to engage in artistic endeavors, such as drawing, can offer him outlets for expressing the emotions associated with the trauma of his immigration and detention experiences. Such activities can also be a way for him to express his frustration with the challenges of learning to read in a new language and in adapting to a new culture. When verbal exchanges occur, it may be important to have Cesar speak in Spanish since, at the present time, this is his language of preference.

A culturally competent counseling approach with Cesar would also involve assuming an advocate role. It may be necessary to consult with Cesar's teachers to help them more fully understand the factors behind his behavioral issues, namely immigration trauma and acculturation stress.

This advocacy may need to extend to work with Cesar's parents. Perhaps in working with a translator, it would be important to address the family's acculturation process. One aspect of this process might be helping the parents understand the dynamics of acculturation stress and its impact on Cesar's psychosocial development. Another important aspect might be exploring resources to help the parents strengthen their English language proficiency. If the parents become more proficient in English, they may serve as important role models for their son.

CASE STUDY 4.2: ADOLESCENCE

Thomas is Cesar's 16-year-old brother. Upon arriving in the United States, he was enrolled in the ninth grade in high school because lack of English precluded him from being placed in a higher grade. He is currently receiving ESL classes to help him in learning English. Since he is in high school, his classes are much larger and, therefore, he is unable to get the individual attention needed to improve his English. He is surrounded by peers who have similar experiences and are all learning English. However, due to the lack of support from his teachers, Thomas does not care to learn the language or care about his studies. Thomas is having difficulty adjusting to the new culture that is present in the United States. In Honduras, he was a good student and was persistent in his studies. His parents

(*continued*)

CASE STUDY 4.2 (*continued*)

are concerned about his sudden shift in behavior and therefore referred him to receive counseling. They worry that he is holding in his emotions and that doing so will lead him to be around the wrong crowd at school and jeopardize his success. They want Thomas to take all of the opportunities that he can being in the United States. At home, his parents state that he has isolated himself and does not really communicate with them anymore.

COUNSELING THOMAS: A CULTURALLY RESPONSIVE PERSPECTIVE

Placing Thomas Into a Cultural Context

Like his younger brother Cesar, Thomas is a Latinx male who is a recent immigrant. As with Cesar, evidence of acculturation stress is evident in Thomas's behavior. Thomas is trying to adapt to a new country and culture at a crucial developmental stage. He is at the important life stage of adolescence, and there are two key factors that appear to be impacting his psychosocial development. First, he seems to be challenged by the crucial task of developing an identity. In Honduras, his identity was reinforced by his academic success. Since arriving in the United States, however, he struggled academically, which seems to negatively impact his self-concept. His academic struggles, fueled by his challenges with English language proficiency, leave Thomas grappling with the crucial developmental question of adolescence, "Who am I?"

Second, Thomas is likely turning to his peers for support and validation. He is no doubt attracted to a peer group whose members, like him, are struggling with acculturation stress, identity issues, and English proficiency challenges. The appeal of his peers becomes reinforced by Thomas's perception of the demands placed on him by his parents. The increasing importance of peers in an adolescent's life remains an important milestone of this developmental stage.

Counseling Thomas With Culture in Mind

Helping Thomas relieve his acculturation stress will involve getting him to talk about his feelings. It would be important to help him process the detention experience and its impact on him—likewise, to help him to explore his identity and his struggles to balance between Honduran and U.S. culture. Part of this would be to help him answer the question, "Who am I?" This might entail helping him explore how he can become the type of student he was in Honduras. Encouraging him to process his feelings about his parents' expectations would be an important part of the process. It would be important to encourage him to explore respectful ways to communicate with his parents about his acculturation struggles.

In addition to individual counseling, another strategy that might be particularly helpful in getting him to articulate his feelings would involve inviting Thomas to

(*continued*)

CASE STUDY 4.2 (*continued*)

join a psychoeducational group with some of his Latinx peers who underwent similar immigration experiences. Such a group experience could provide a forum for Thomas and his peers to discuss problems, issues, and concerns they encounter at school and at home. The group could also help participants explore where they fit in their new culture and who they are as individuals. Importantly, the group members could decide on how and when to communicate in either Spanish or English (Hipolito-Delgado & Diaz, 2013).

The following conditions can help make the group a success for Thomas. This experience would provide him with a safe space to talk about his life experiences in the United States and his experience of being a Latinx high school student. It is crucial that the group facilitator develop a personal relationship with Thomas in order to earn his trust and respect. This trust should allow the facilitator to challenge Thomas and his peers to dig deeper into feelings related to their acculturation challenges.

As with his brother, advocating with Thomas's parents is important. The nature of advocacy efforts on Thomas's behalf should focus on helping his parents understand the nature of acculturation stress from an adolescent developmental perspective. Importantly, the counselor can assist the parents to process Thomas's attempts to balance between two cultural identities and answer the question, "Who am I?" As a part of this processing, it will also be important for the parents to assess the expectations they hold for Thomas as the eldest child in their new homeland. Taking advantage of opportunities in his new home country remains key for Thomas; however, his parents should monitor their expectations for him and avoid contributing to his acculturation stress by putting undue pressure on him to succeed and be a family trailblazer in the United States.

CHAPTER SUMMARY

Changing demographics suggest ever-increasing cultural diversity among children and adolescents in American society. This reality presents important challenges and opportunities for the profession of counseling. No longer can counseling practice with young people in schools or mental health settings be considered exclusively within the confines of one cultural perspective. Instead, important aspects of cultural diversity, such as race/ethnicity, must be factored into effective counseling practice. Therefore, if counselors are to have an impact on the mental health and well-being of increasingly diverse groups of children and adolescents, then counseling practice must be grounded in cultural competency. This process involves acquiring not only the awareness and knowledge, but also the skills for effective counseling intervention with young people from diverse cultural backgrounds. To begin with, counselor awareness must be grounded in an exploration of one's own cultural heritage with an emphasis on its impact on their own childhood and adolescent development. In addition, one must examine biases and preconceived notions they hold about people who are different.

Next, counselor knowledge must include an exploration of racial/ethnic variation in child and adolescent psychosocial development. One should become knowledgeable of how cultural variation in the context of families and communities with respect to factors such as notions of kinship, family roles and status, gender role socialization, language preference, religion/spirituality, racial/ethnic identity, acculturation, and poverty and discrimination exerts an important influence on the developmental tasks associated with childhood and adolescence.

Finally, a counselor who exhibits cultural competency when working with a child or adolescent must be able to "counsel with culture in mind." They should possess the skill to place a young person and their presenting issue into a cultural context while still seeing them as a unique individual. In addition, counseling with culture in mind would entail engaging in interactions with young people that incorporate their unique worldviews, values, social identities, and family dynamics. Importantly, as appropriate, one must be able to advocate for young people with parents or teachers to ensure that they remain allies in promoting mental health and well-being.

POINTS TO REMEMBER

- Changing population demographics require that professional counselors view their interventions with children and adolescents from a perspective that emphasizes cultural competency.
- Professional counselors should always view their interventions with young people from a developmental perspective. An important aspect of such a perspective is considering how cultural influences impact the mastery of developmental tasks in childhood and adolescence.
- "Counseling with culture in mind" suggests considering each child or adolescent within a cultural group context and a broader global human perspective.

OTHER HELPFUL INFORMATION FOR CONSIDERATION

- American Counseling Association: https://www.counseling.org
- American School Counselor Association: https://www.schoolcounselor.org
- Association for Multicultural Counseling and Development: https://multiculturalcounselingdevelopment.org
- Multicultural and Social Justice Counseling Competencies: https://www.counseling.org/docs/default-source/competencies/multicultural-and-social-justice-counseling-competencies.pdf?sfvrsn=20

QUESTIONS FOR FURTHER DISCUSSION

- What kinds of training do you believe to be important for professional counselors in order to assure that they are able to exhibit cultural competency in their work with children and adolescents?

- Think back to your own childhood and teenage years. What factors from your cultural background do you think influenced your development?
- How can you avoid engaging in cultural stereotypes in counseling interventions with young people from diverse backgrounds?
- While counseling a teenage boy, he says to you, "How can you help me, you're not Black!" What would you do?
- What personal qualities do you feel you would need to be an effective advocate for young people from diverse cultural backgrounds in helping them confront systemic forces that appear to stifle their development?

KEY REFERENCES

Only key references appear in the print edition. The full reference list appears in the digital product on Springer Publishing Connect: connect.springerpub.com/content/book/978-0-8261-4764-6/part/part01/chapter/ch04

Erikson, E. (1950). *Childhood and society*. W. W. Norton & Company.

Federal Interagency Forum on Child and Family Statistics. (2017). *America's children: Key national indicators of well-being, 2017*. Author. http://www.childstats.gov/americaschildren/tables.asp

Geerlings, J., Verkuyten, M., & Thijs, J. (2015). Changes in ethnic self-identification and heritage language preference in adolescence: A cross-lagged panel study. *Journal of Language and Social Psychology, 34*(5), 501–520. https://doi.org/10.1177/0261927X14564467

Gil, A. G., Vega, W. A., & Dimas, J. M. (1994). Acculturative stress and personal adjustment among Hispanic adolescent boys. *Journal of Community Psychology, 22*(1), 43–54. https://doi.org/10.1002/1520-6629(199401)22:1<43::AID-JCOP2290220106>3.0.CO;2-T

Lee, C. C. (1991). Cultural dynamics: Their importance in multicultural counseling. In C. C. Lee & B. L. Richardson (Eds.), *Multicultural issues in counseling: new approaches to diversity* (pp. 11–17). American Counseling Association.

Lee, C. C. (2019). Multicultural competency: A conceptual framework for counseling across cultures. In C. C. Lee (Ed.), *Multicultural issues in counseling: New approaches to diversity* (5th ed., pp. 3–13). American Counseling Association.

Munroe, R. L., & Munroe, R. H. (1975). *Cross-cultural human development*. Brooks/Cole.

Phinney, J. S., & Rotheram, M. J. (1987) *Children's ethnic socialization: Pluralism and development*. Sage Publications.

Reeves, R., Rodrigue, E., & Kneebone, E. (2016). Five evils: Multidimensional poverty and race in America. *Economic Studies at Brookings Report, 1*, 1–22.

Stevenson, M. C., Bottoms, B. L., & Burke, K. C. (Eds.). (2020). *The legacy of racism for children: Psychology, law, and public policy*. Oxford University Press.

PART II

Theoretical Frameworks for Working With Youths: Putting Counseling Into Practice

CHAPTER 5

Theoretical Frameworks and Applications in Child and Adolescent Counseling

M. Elsa Soto Leggett and Jennifer N. Boswell

LEARNING OBJECTIVES

After completing this chapter, the reader should be able to:

- Describe the different theoretical frameworks commonly used in child and adolescent counseling.
- Identify specific reasons why these theories effectively work with children and adolescents.
- Apply interventions appropriate to the guiding theoretical framework.

CACREP STANDARDS FOR THIS CHAPTER

- CACREP 2016: 2.F.5.a; F.5.b; F.5.j.; School Counseling: None; Clinical Mental Health Counseling: 5.C.1.b; 3.b.
- CACREP 2009: 2.G.2.d; 3.b., d., h.; 5.b., c., d., e; School Counseling: C.1; Clinical Mental Health Counseling: C.8; E.3.

INTRODUCTION

The Centers for Disease Control and Prevention (CDC) report that nearly one in five children exhibits a mental health, emotional, or behavioral problem. Of this number, only 20% receive treatment (CDC, 2015). Meeting the mental health needs of children and adolescents presents unique challenges, especially when considering a theoretical viewpoint. Research indicates that there appear to be more than 400 approaches to address the clinical needs of this population, each with a level of effectiveness when compared to no treatment (Ziomek-Daigle, 2017). The wide range of therapeutic approaches often scales down adult-based theories to fit the child or adolescent client. However, limited verbal and linguistic development notably differentiates adult approaches and those addressing children and adolescents. Important considerations are necessary when addressing the mental health needs of children and adolescents. This includes distinct developmental stages from infancy to adolescence. Children and adolescents also exhibit limited understanding of situations or their ramifications. Moreover, they display a limited ability to generate effective coping strategies (Vernon & Schimmel, 2019). An additional consideration continues in that counselors in all settings work with young clients from diverse backgrounds. Therefore, adding to the requirement of competency to developmental levels includes the requirement of awareness of various ethnic and cultural groups. Clinicians consider the acculturation process and identity development models as required knowledge and proficiency (Davis-Gage, 2019).

Counselors should begin their work with children and adolescents by exploring their personal theories of orientation and practice (Table 5.1). Counselors need an identified theoretical orientation that serves as the foundation for their interaction with clients. This exploration should lead counselors to understand the appropriateness of their theory with this specified population, as well as the client's culture. This includes the appropriate incorporation of creative, expressive, and play approaches to suit a client's verbal, linguistic, cognitive development, and cultural background. Attention to this area supports the American Counseling Association (ACA) Code of Ethics (ACA, 2014, Section A.2.c.), pointing to counselors' ethical obligation to communicate with a client in a developmentally appropriate manner, as well as the ACA Code of Ethics preamble to "honor diversity" (ACA, 2014, p. 3).

ADLERIAN THERAPY

OVERVIEW

Alfred Adler, born in 1870 in Austria, worked alongside Freud in the Vienna Psycho-Analytical Society. Over time, he found himself at odds with Freud's understanding of the mind and behaviors. Eventually, he separated himself from the society and developed the Society for Individual Psychology. Adler's strong belief in social interest led him to invite teachers, mental health workers, medical physicians, and other professionals into the Society. Adlerian therapy or individual psychology, whether with adults or children, encompasses a holistic, goal-oriented, phenomenological approach (Carlson et al., 2006), differing from Freud's belief in sexual impulses as the root of psychological development.

Adlerian counseling consists of four phases that the client and counselor move through as treatment progresses. These phases consist of (a) building a safe, therapeutic relationship; (b) exploring the client's style of life; (c) assisting the client in gaining insight into their style

TABLE 5.1 THEORIES ACROSS AGES

Theory	Birth and Infancy 0–3	Early Childhood 3–5	Middle Childhood 6–11	Early Adolescence 11–14	Middle Adolescence 15–Early Adult
Adlerian		√	√	√	√
Choice (reality) therapy			√	√	√
Cognitive behavioral therapy			√	√	√
Dialectical behavior therapy			√	√	√
Family and family systems	√	√	√	√	√
Gestalt therapy			√	√	√
Narrative therapy			√	√	√
Play therapy	√	√	√	√	√
Rational emotive behavior therapy			√	√	√
Solution-focused therapy		√	√	√	√

of life; and (d) reorienting and reeducating the client to view other alternatives to their behavior. These phases provide counselors with four overarching goals: (a) decrease the client's symptoms, (b) increase healthy functioning, (c) increase the client's sense of humor, and (d) produce a change in the client's perspective (Carlson et al., 2006). The beginning of all Adlerian counseling centers on the relationship between the counselor and client. All other components of the therapeutic relationship continue to be built around and through this alliance. Adlerian clinicians continually explore how clients view themselves, others, and the world. As clinicians aid clients in understanding these views and making changes to socially useless or unhelpful views, clients begin to recognize and make small changes to their thinking and behaving. Adlerian counselors, especially when working with children and adolescents, typically develop relationships with parents, caregivers, teachers, and other important persons centered on consultation, education, and parent feedback. This is typically done as the counselor seeks to understand the client's style of life or the client's way of making sense of the world and navigating life's challenges. During this second phase, the counselor uses a variety of assessments such as family constellations, birth order, dreams, assessment of feelings of inferiority and superiority, and early recollections to understand the client's childhood and family influences and important memories. During the third phase, the focus shifts to helping the client gain insight into their style of life. In this phase, the counselor focuses on developing client awareness of faulty logic about self, others, and the world and recognizing the choices and consequences for chosen ideas and behaviors. In the fourth and final phase of counseling, treatment centers on teaching and using new behaviors and skills that aid in breaking old patterns. Counselors use role-playing, guided imagery, encouragement, and other action-oriented interventions to help the client take specific steps toward change and growth; and design these changes to help foster an increased sense of self-worth, cooperation, and connection with others leading to a new, healthier style of life.

Specifically when working with children and adolescents, Adlerian counselors engage in the following processes: (a) establish a working, egalitarian relationship with the client, parents, and other significant persons in the client's world; (b) explore the client's thoughts, feelings, perceptions, and experiences of self, significant people in the client's life, and of the world; (c) create a client conceptualization and treatment plan identifying important needs of the client and the dynamics between the client and significant others; (d) aid the client in gaining insight and exploring personal values and interpersonal dynamics; and (e) help the client practice and use new decision-making skills that meet client needs in a more socially appropriate way (Kottman & Meany-Walen, 2015).

BASIC CONCEPTS

Adler based individual psychology on four different constructs, which see people as (a) socially embedded, (b) goal directed, (c) creative, and (d) subjective in the manner in which they hold views of the world (Carlson et al., 2006). The core values and tenets of Adlerian therapy include understanding that people should be viewed within a social context, individuals display goal-directed and purposeful behavior, and a person's perception of reality remains vital to their understanding of the world and the development of their style of life.

SOCIAL EMBEDDEDNESS AND SOCIAL INTEREST

Adler believed that all people, regardless of age, come into this world with a desire to connect and relate to others in their world. Even though all persons hold this ability, individuals must still be taught how to make these connections in positive, healthy ways (Adler, 1956). Social embeddedness means that all people strive to belong and connect to others in the world. From an early age, people find ways to fit into the world and in their relationships with others. Often, when people cannot experience success in finding connection or a place in their world, they will go about finding connection through negative, unhealthy, or socially useless ways. Adler also believed that a person's lifestyle, or style of life, solidifies by age seven or eight. By this time, a person's personality and perceptions of self along with an understanding of others and the world become solidified. A person's style of life creates a pathway to navigate life and relationships and typically remains out of awareness. Carlson et al. (2006) defined style of life as "the characteristic way we act, think, and perceive and the way we live" (p. 12). This way of perceiving oneself and others remains consistent and stable throughout the life span. When the person lives a negative or unhealthy style of life, mental health treatment often becomes necessary to create cognitive and behavioral change. Healthy social adjustment and embeddedness lead to feelings of belonging and connectedness. This connection and a sense of belonging foster social interest. Watts (2014) explained that social interest, or *gemeinschaftsgefühl,* emphasizes the key relational and social-contextual features of individual psychology. Watts and Eckstein (2009) further expand this emphasis: "True community feeling (i.e., sense of belonging, empathy, caring, compassion, acceptance of others, etc) results in social interest (i.e., thoughts and behaviors that contribute to the common good, the good of the whole at both micro- and macro-systemic levels)" (Watts & Eckstein, 2009, p. 282).

GOALS

In addition to being socially embedded, this theoretical approach posits all persons to be goal-directed. This means that Adler views all behavior to be purposeful and directed toward personal goals. Adler and Adlerian counselors believe all people to be motivated by a desire to meet life goals and specifically choose behaviors that they believe will aid in achieving these goals (Kottman & Meany-Walen, 2015). Through counseling, clients gain an understanding of their life goals and address how their behaviors help or hinder them in achieving those goals. People come to learn that their own faulty thinking or logic impairs healthy functioning and growth.

Rudolph Dreikurs, a psychiatrist and educator, continued Adler's work through the 1970s. He developed a way to understand the goals of children's misbehavior and ways clinicians, parents, and educators could work with children to not only identify the goals of the misbehavior but also aid the child in developing more healthy and useful ways of meeting those goals. He identified four common goals of misbehavior: (a) attention seeking, (b) power seeking, (c) revenge seeking, and (d) displaying inadequacy. Therefore, by aiding a client in understanding the faulty logic behind behaviors and thinking, a counselor can help a client decrease feelings of inferiority and failure and move toward greater self-efficacy, confidence, and social interest.

CREATIVITY AND SUBJECTIVITY

The two remaining components of Adler's theory include creativity and subjectivity. Adler believed all people to be creative in the way they move through life and their perception of the world around them. Therefore, each person views their lifestyle to be unique. Adlerian clinicians also believe a person's understanding of the world, and how they find belonging and meaning in the world, to be subjective. Therefore, a person's subjective interpretation of themselves and the world around them appears more important than objective reality. Understanding a client's creative means of behaving and interacting with the world (lifestyle), along with their subjective reality, helps clinicians understand the private logic and core beliefs that impact their client's behaviors and relationships with others.

THEORETICAL APPLICATION

Adlerian counselors working with children and adolescents integrate the concepts found in individual psychology with an understanding of child development and common techniques found in play therapy. Adlerian therapists often use toys, books, stories, puppets, drawings, role-playing, and other techniques as a means of communication with the client. Often, counselors use toys and materials to communicate with the client. Simultaneously, the counselor uses the Adlerian framework to conceptualize the client and presenting problem. Within Adlerian counseling, especially with children and adolescents, a focus subsists on identifying and valuing the child or adolescent's uniqueness, imagination, and creativity (Kottman & Meany-Walen, 2015).

Family Constellation

Adlerian counselors use family constellations as a means of understanding a client's perception of belonging and connection with the family system. A family constellation takes into account the client's birth order and how it impacts the client's perception of behaviors and attitudes about self and others. The family constellation also provides information related to the family atmosphere, relationship patterns, hierarchy, and overall structure of the system.

Encouragement

Counselors consider Adlerian counseling to be a holistic, growth, and wellness model. As such, Adlerian clinicians view clients through a hopeful and optimistic lens where they see clients as unique, creative, capable, and responsible. Adlerian counseling emphasizes prevention, optimism and hope, resilience and growth, competence, creativity and resourcefulness, social consciousness, and meaning making and a sense of community in relationship (Watts, 2014). Consequently, Adlerian counselors use encouragement both as a technique to foster client growth and change and as a way of being with clients to model *gemeinschaftsgefühl*, or community feeling and social interest toward others. In his work, Alfred Adler stressed encouragement as a vital aspect of therapy. He stated "Altogether, in every step of treatment, we must not deviate from the path of encouragement" (p. 342). Kottman and Meany-Walen (2015) also highlight encouragement as a central tenet of Adlerian counseling with children and teens. They stressed that encouragement, as a technique, consists of eight elements including (a) conveying unconditional acceptance of the child, (b) showing faith in the child's abilities, (c) giving recognition for efforts, (d) focusing on strengths, (e) giving credit for positive aspects of work and ignoring parts that do not meet standards, (f) demonstrating care, (g) modeling the courage to be imperfect and make mistakes, and (h) teaching a child to learn from mistakes (2015).

Acting As If

Adler created the technique *acting as if* for use in the later phases of counseling and used it to help encourage clients to act as if they exist as the person they want to be, such as being a confident or assertive person. By doing this, the person may consider new, alternative ways to being and the likely outcomes of this new behavior. In acting as if, the client can be reminded of this acting which, in turn, reduces defenses around change and allows the client to experience a new narrative and way of being. Watts (2003, 2013), a noted Adlerian counselor and researcher, added a reflective component to this intervention and coined it *reflecting as if (RAI)*. Watts based RAI on ideas and procedures from Adlerian therapy and constructivist and social constructionist approaches. Specifically, he viewed RAI to be relationship-focused, optimistic and anticipatory of positive change outcomes, present and future oriented, and emphasizing on existing client strengths, skills, and abilities. The process invites clients to both identify and implement new or alternate behaviors. Given that clients create the new or alternate behaviors (neither created by nor forced upon by their counselors), clients gain a greater propensity to feel ownership of the new behaviors. Thus, clients may be more likely to commit to implementing the behaviors and expect positive outcomes when enacting them. RAI comprises three phases. Phase 1 consists of brainstorming with clients. Here, clients identify new or alternative behaviors they believe would be beneficial to their life. Phase 2 of the RAI includes the creation of a list of "as if" behaviors and the evaluation of the plausibility of the behaviors. RAI phase 3 consists of three separate steps. First, clients select two or three of the easiest behaviors from the list generated in phase 2 and implement these behaviors during the upcoming week. Next, clients discuss with their counselor their experiences with enacting the "as if" behaviors. Throughout the process, as clients attempt to enact the more difficult "as if" behaviors on their list, counselors provide encouragement in their continued pursuit of change. As the behaviors become more difficult, clients may get discouraged. As the counselor focuses on the clients' strengths and abilities, differentiating between what people do and who people appear to be, they communicate affirmation regarding clients' efforts and the clients can learn to view success as forward movement.

CHOICE (REALITY) THERAPY

OVERVIEW

William Glasser's choice therapy (1965) reasons that from birth, people possess five innate basic needs; and individuals become genetically motivated to fulfill these needs in order to avoid pain. The five needs include (a) survival, (b) love and belonging, (c) power, (d) fun, and (e) freedom; and the individual revises them throughout the life span. Therefore, the inability to fulfill one of these basic needs can result in psychological problems. *Survival* represents a biological need to survive to possess the essential for life such as health, food, air, shelter, safety, and security. *Love and belonging* denotes needs tied to connecting with others, maintaining friends, and sharing an intimate relationship with others. *Power* signifies the need to be satisfied with an accomplishment or competence along with a desire for personal sense of worth. *Fun* embodies the need to pursue enjoyment, excitement, playfulness, laughter, and pleasure. *Freedom* corresponds to the human desire for autonomy and the ability to choose without restrictions. Glasser believes all five of these needs must be satisfied and that an individual will seek to fulfill these needs in personally unique ways (Glasser, 1965; Henderson & Thompson, 2011).

Reality therapy (RT), based on choice therapy, goes further to state that an individual controls how they see the environment and their behavior in this environment. Thus, counselors observe a client as needing to connect with others and meet one or more of the five basic needs. With this in mind, a counselor would suggest that a child or adolescent remain responsible for how they behave. Yet, the focus transpires not on the behavior such as criticizing, blaming, complaining, or finding fault. Instead, the counselor relies on five characteristics to help a young client understand their needs: (a) focus on choice and responsibility, (b) elimination of transference, (c) staying in the present, (d) not addressing the symptoms, and (e) challenging the common views of mental illness. In addition, counselors direct a young client to accept responsibility and identify their own role in the change process, thus satisfying their quality of life needs and behaviors (Glasser, 1965; Ziomek-Daigle, 2017).

BASIC CONCEPTS

Counselors generally use the WDEP approach to guide the counseling process. The acronym stands for (W) wants and needs, (D) doing and direction, (E) self-evaluation, and (P) planning (Wubbolding, 2000). Davis (2011) also points out the planning portion of the WDEP following its own formula. The SAMIC3/P formula dictates that the plan should be (S) simple, (A) attainable, (M) measurable, (I) immediate, (C) consistent, (C) contingent on the client's motivation to work, (C) including client commitment, and (P) implemented by the person. It becomes imperative that the young client create the plan with the help and collaboration of the counselor. The plan should be feasible in the young client's world and lead to obtaining the wants. This approach helps to ensure the connection between the counselor and the client and maintains a counseling alliance (Davis, 2011).

THEORETICAL APPLICATIONS

Davis (2011) reminds counselors of the importance of beginning RT by developing a positive relationship with the client. This requires creating a safe and accepting environment. The focus should be on the present, avoiding complaints, dealing with thoughts and action. The counselor leads the client to avoid blame, explore their perceptions, find new conditions, and focus on developing lines of developmentally appropriate communication. These ideas continue to be essential for children and adolescents. The WDEP process may be familiar to this population who use problem-solving concepts often taught in schools and homes. Adding the creative use of drawing can allow the client to be self-expressive in a healthy way when addressing their thoughts and emotions, as well as when meeting their developmental level (Davis, 2011; Leggett, 2009).

WDEP Drawing Method

The WDEP drawing method employs the wants (W), doing (D), evaluation (E), and planning (P) elements in a series of drawings. This method allows the counselor and the client to visualize each element of the process, gaining insight into the driving wants and needs of the situation (Davis, 2011). The counselor simply uses coloring pencils or crayons and paper as tools. With adolescents, a drawing journal may feel more fitting while following the same principles. Then offer the client an introduction to the WDEP concept and how this will work to help reach the goal identified. Each element of the WDEP should be described and discussed. The counselor can instruct the client that they will be creating drawings to relate to the WDEP. The client may want to use one sheet divided into four squares and identify each square with the corresponding letters, WDEP (Davis, 2011). Using a drawing journal with older clients, the page may be drawn into quarters or four pages can be used with the corresponding letters.

To get a clear understanding of what the client wants, it becomes necessary to focus on the problem. Attention should be given to understanding the situation from the perspective of the client along with an understanding of what the client *wants* to see happen or be different. It remains important for the counselor to be open to what or how the client may describe what they want. At this point, the client can draw this on the paper in the identified location. When the counselor gives the client the time to fully complete the details of their drawing, the counselor can then discuss the thoughts and feelings behind the details drawn. This will also provide an opportunity to ensure and develop realistic options (Davis, 2011). The next step would include discovering what the client is *doing* to achieve the *want* and drawing. This discussion should focus primarily on the client and their actions and behaviors. Effort must be given to stay away from what others do while around the client. This focus will help the client retain responsibility for their choices, as well as the actions in relation to the situation. This will help to avoid blaming the issues on others (Davis, 2011). The client then draws the actions in the D square or page. This drawing can be done as the client decides which could include a scene of action or a symbol of the action.

This would lead to the *evaluation* of the *what* the client did that worked or did not work to get the desired outcome they *wanted*. This portion might require the counselor to provide more guidance in determining the effectiveness of the actions. However, the *client* makes the final determination (Davis, 2011). This drawing in the E square or page might be more creative and insightful to demonstrate the outcome of the action, an illustration of the correct or incorrect outcome with the conclusion of the choice made. Openness to creativity remains helpful in allowing the client to find a way to express this image.

Finally, the counselor and client can begin the discovery and development of new ideas to meet the *wants* with different thoughts, behaviors, and actions. With this discussion, the counselor's role becomes one that listens to the client's thoughts and comments as they "speak off the top of their heads" until landing on possible options that fit the situation. It would also be fitting to include a discussion of a variety of plans to allow the client options and choices. Care should be given to narrow the new plans to those that appear realistic. The counselor follows this by focusing on a clear and measurable plan considered suitable for the situation or problem. The conversation should include the possibility of failure as an outcome to the plan (Davis, 2011). Next, the client adds the final drawing to the P square or page.

Follow-up sessions should offer a review of the drawings. Additional drawings can be created in reaction to the outcomes of the previous plan. If the original plan did not work as hoped, the counselor and the client can evaluate the outcomes while comparing these outcomes with the original one displayed in the E drawing. Next, the opportunity to create a new plan becomes available. This exchange can offer continuous evaluation and update on the original situation that brought the client in to counseling, along with the chance to observe how the client continues to deal with the issue (Davis, 2011). The concrete record the client presents of the steps taken to handle the problem or situation highlights a benefit of using the drawing method. This documentation can provide the client with a road map to meeting future challenges (Davis, 2011).

COGNITIVE BEHAVIORAL THERAPY

OVERVIEW

Cognitive behavioral therapy (CBT) appears to be the most widely known and used therapeutic approach in mental health counseling today. Counselors describe CBT as the most widely researched treatment model in the mental health field and consider it to be the first therapy identified as evidence-based (David et al., 2018). Versions of CBT, with more of a focus on the cognitive components of the therapy, began to emerge in the 1960s; but not until the 1970s did the therapies become more popular (Meichenbaum, 1977). In the 1970s, therapists organized CBTs into three different categories: (a) cognitive restructuring therapies, (b) coping skill therapies, and (c) problem-solving therapies. Cognitive restructuring targets emotional distress as the consequence of maladaptive thoughts; coping skills target the development of new adaptive skills to aid a client in various environments; and problem-solving therapies target the development of new adaptive actions and behaviors that aid a client in many different settings and situations. About 30 years ago, theorists combined cognitive and behavioral approaches as an empirically based treatment approach. Theorists consolidated behavioral approaches that emphasized desensitization and other classical conditioning approaches with cognitive approaches that focused on adapting maladaptive, or problematic, thoughts that impeded prosocial behaviors or the reinforcement of negative actions. As these two approaches evolved and merged into CBT, the treatment protocols began to take on more experiential components. As of 2017, roughly 18 different variations of cognitive behavioral approaches spanned a continuum from mainly behavioral to mainly cognitive interventions (Sperry, 2017).

BASIC CONCEPTS

All CBT therapies center on three components: (a) Cognitions impact a person's behaviors, (b) cognitions can be "monitored and altered," and (c) behavioral outcomes can be adjusted as cognitions change (Dobson & Dozios, 2010, p. 4). Therapists founded CBT on the idea that one's thinking, attitudes, and perceptions (cognitions) influence the person's understanding of an external event, which then impacts the person's emotional and behavioral responses to the event.

Importantly, clinicians should not consider cognitive therapies and behavioral therapies as stand-alone treatments. Also, these therapies should not be considered CBT. To be considered CBT, a treatment must produce both cognitive and behavioral changes for the client (Sperry, 2017). Clinicians consider CBT therapies as short term, lasting between 6 and 20 sessions. The most common and widely used CBT models include the following: rational emotive behavior therapy (REBT) by Albert Ellis, problem-solving therapy by Thomas D'Zurilla and Marvin Goldfried, cognitive therapy by Aaron Beck, schema therapy by Jeffrey Young, and acceptance and commitment therapy by Steven Hayes.

CBT, shown to be effective for children and adolescents experiencing many mental health disorders, symptoms, and problems of daily living, takes on a problem-solving approach to help this population develop a healthier worldview and corresponding cognitive behavioral skills (Knell, 1997). CBT therapists often engage in verbal dialogue and play activities including the use of toys, art, and games designed to build a therapeutic relationship; understand the child or adolescent's view of the world and behaviors; and introduce more adaptive ways of thinking and behaving in the world. Key components of treatment with this population include the integration of problem-solving skills; cognitive restructuring to reduce negative cognitions about self and others to more adaptive cognitions; emotional regulation skills; relaxation and mindfulness training; modeling of healthy, adaptive behaviors; and behavioral modification through contingency management plans (Crawley et al., 2010). In order for CBT therapies with this population to be successful, as with all of the other available therapies, a clinician must be in tune with the child's cognitive, emotional, and social developmental level.

THEORETICAL APPLICATIONS

CBTs consist of a wide range of models and interventions. Clinicians most commonly divide them into behavioral and cognitively focused interventions. More often than not, counselors center these interventions on modeling and role-playing of more healthy and adaptive ways of coping, behaving, and thinking. Role-playing, especially for children and adolescents, may be a helpful way to practice new skills and behaviors in a safe environment while obtaining ongoing feedback from the clinician. Often a client may not be comfortable role-playing or practicing a new skill. In that case, the clinician models the skill or behavior in order to provide space for the client to process before *trying on* the skill. In doing so, the client becomes able to process how the new skill will work in desired settings. The following sections present an overview of various behavioral and cognitive interventions—many of them time-efficient—available to clinicians.

Behavioral Interventions

Counselors use mindfulness and relaxation training as some of the most widely popular behavioral interventions. Mindfulness training helps clients recognize emotional cues that lead to cognitive distortions and maladaptive behaviors. Recognizing these behaviors helps clients identify the emotional responses and address them appropriately before the distortions or behaviors intensify. The cognitive behavioral cycle would then be circumvented and the client can then react to a situation in a healthier manner. Counselors use relaxation training as a technique to bring clients down from an elevated emotional state (e.g., anxiety) so that they can appropriately assess a situation and choose a behavioral response accordingly. The profession offers many relaxation-training techniques, including guided imagery and diaphragmatic breathing, to counselors. It continues to be important to note that care should be taken with any client who has experienced severe or complex trauma as some interventions such as relaxation training could intensify their emotional state (Gilman & Chard, 2015).

ABC (antecedent, behaviors, and consequences) functional analysis presents another popular behavioral intervention. ABC functional analysis allows a client to understand the causes and consequences, both positive and negative, of their behaviors. The underlying assumption of the functional analysis posits that all behavior can be influenced by the client's environment that reinforces or extinguishes behaviors, leading to increased or decreased behaviors in the future. The client begins by examining the factors, or antecedents, that lead to a maladaptive behavior. Next, the client examines the behavior following the event to determine a positive or problematic outcome. The final step in the analysis encourages the client to examine the consequences of the behavior. If the behavior seems to be problematic, the likely consequence will be negative whereas a positive behavior will likely lead to a positive consequence. Ultimately, behavior can be reinforcing or will be extinguished depending on the consequences provided.

Cognitive Interventions

Many CBT interventions fall under the concept of cognitive restructuring. Counselors design these interventions to decrease or adapt a person's cognitive distortions. Common cognitive distortions include polarized or black-and-white thinking, emotional reasoning, catastrophizing, fortune-telling or jumping to conclusions, and mind reading among many others. When engaging in cognitive restructuring interventions, the counselor may use techniques that directly dispute or challenge cognitive distortions or aid the client in recognizing the irrationality of the distortion or test the reality of the distortion. These types of interventions begin with the client learning to identify various cognitive distortions and when they engage in them leading to maladaptive thinking and behaving. Other clinicians use worksheets or activities designed to chart dysfunctional thoughts. These activities allow the client to log when the distortion or dysfunctional thought occurred, the situation in which the thought arose, the distortion or dysfunctional thought, level of emotional distress that accompanied the thought, and alternative or positive thoughts that can replace the distortion or dysfunctional thought. The use of self-statement, an intervention described as easily adaptable to working with adults, adolescents, and children, denotes another common cognitive intervention. Counselors use positive self-statements to help a client identify self-affirming statements, which enables the client to develop coping skills and positive reinforcement to complete a task or accomplish a goal.

DIALECTICAL BEHAVIOR THERAPY

OVERVIEW

Dialectical behavior therapy (DBT), created by Marsha Linehan (1993), presents a form of CBT that may be used to treat severe mental illness in women and addresses issues such as borderline personality disorder, high-risk suicidal ideation, eating disorders, and substance use disorders (Chapman, 2006). Counselors consider DBT as an evidence-based treatment for clients experiencing severe suicidality in conjunction with borderline personality disorder (Jobes et al., 2015). The treatment philosophy behind DBT originates in dialectics (Kaminstein, 1987). This philosophy and framework suggest that within all people lie opposing forces or tension. As a counselor teaches a client a new behavioral skill, it creates internal tension within the person to accept their current position rather than change. In other instances, the opposite might occur. When the counselor focuses solely on client acceptance, without change and a new behavioral skill set, it can lead to an increase in severity of symptoms.

BASIC CONCEPTS

Counselors find DBT, originally established as a treatment modality for adults, to be just as effective with adolescents between the ages of 12 and 18 who struggle with suicidality, nonsuicidal self-injury (NSSI), bipolar disorder, eating disorders, and substance use (Behavioral Tech, n.d.). DBT can often be found in treatment settings such as inpatient hospitals, intensive outpatient programs, residential facilities, and correctional facilities (MacPherson et al., 2012). The key treatment difference lies in the involvement of parents or caregivers when addressing the specific behavioral concerns in counseling. Along with individual counseling, counselors invite parents to attend family sessions and family group training sessions, where counselors teach parents the same skills as the adolescents. Most DBT interventions for adolescents last between 16 and 24 weeks.

Most DBT treatment protocols last up to 12 months for adults. The traditional format of DBT consists of weekly individual counseling centered on acceptance and barriers to change along with weekly group counseling, where the focus remains on members learning skills such as core mindfulness, emotional regulation, interpersonal effectiveness, and distress tolerance. Additional therapeutic supports include phone consultations with the counselor and the use of a consultation team consisting of the counselor and other mental health professionals. As such, Chapman (2006) considers DBT to be a treatment program rather than an intervention due to the inclusion of the various counseling modalities and resources used by the counselor and the client.

THEORETICAL APPLICATIONS

As stated earlier, clinicians originally developed DBT as a treatment model for women with borderline personality disorder. Since its inception, counselors find DBT to also be effective with clients with suicidal and self-injurious behaviors, along with those with substance use disorders, eating disorders, and depression. Dr. Marsha Linehan, the founder of Behavioral Tech, continues to distribute research regarding the effectiveness of DBT with a variety of populations and issues. To date, counselors report DBT to be effective for children as young as 7 years old. The same treatment strategies for adults may be applied to children and adolescents along with the inclusion of parents or guardians in the treatment process (Behavioral Tech, n.d.).

Acceptance and Change

The focus of DBT treatment for adults, adolescents, and older children centers on acceptance and change wherein the counselor aids the client in increasing positive skill development along with the motivation to continue to change. Counselors view validation as an integral part of the focus on acceptance and use validation within the DBT treatment protocol to understand the current implications of the client's identified concerns; acknowledge the client's thoughts, feelings, and behaviors; make sense in the face of the identified concerns; and communicate compassion and understanding for the client (Budak & Kocabas, 2019). Further, counselors use validation as the DBT element that balances acceptance for the client and the change skills being developed.

In addition to the focus on acceptance and change, DBT counselors integrate five functions of treatment, three that they consider to be client-focused and two to be counselor-focused (Chapman, 2006). The client-focused functions include (a) enhancing the client's skill and awareness capabilities, (b) generalizing these capabilities to other experiences and settings, and (c) improving the client's motivation for change leading to a reduction in maladaptive and harmful behaviors. The counselor-focused functions include enhancing counselor intervention delivery and motivation for treatment and structuring of the therapeutic environment and relationship to enhance the use of positive skill development and maintenance.

Skill Training

Ongoing skill development aids in behavioral, emotional, and cognitive change for the client. Skill development consists of mindfulness exercises, distress tolerance, emotional regulation, and interpersonal effectiveness (Budak & Kocabas, 2019). Counselors divide these skills into acceptance and change modules. Acceptance includes mindfulness and distress tolerance skills. Change includes emotional regulation and interpersonal effectiveness skills. Clients acquire these skills via weekly groups that occur in conjunction with weekly individual therapy sessions. Often these skill groups last up to 24 weeks. Group leaders may assign homework tasks to help encourage clients to practice these new skills in their day-to-day lives.

Each of the four skill areas helps enhance the client's capabilities to problem-solve concerns in different areas of functioning. Mindfulness skills help the client become more aware of themselves and the world around them while also learning to become fully present in the moment. Distress tolerance skills help the client learn to tolerate uncomfortable and difficult situations while not trying to fix or change the situation. Emotional regulation skills help the client identify various emotions and learn how to manage and control emotions preferred by the client. Interpersonal effectiveness skills help the client learn to ask for what they need or desire while maintaining self-worth and boundaries in relationships. These skills also empower a client to say "no" while maintaining healthy interpersonal relationships.

FAMILY AND FAMILY SYSTEMS

OVERVIEW

Family systems therapy, considered a revolutionary approach to therapy, made its appearance in 1940 and grew stronger in the 1950s. In the 1960s and 1970s, it became regarded as the fourth force, preceded by psychodynamic, behavioral, and humanistic approaches, which dominated the field of counseling and psychotherapy (Corey, 2017). The profession offers a variety of theories and approaches that represent family systems therapy, which all see human problems as a result of relational functions (Corey, 2017). Family counseling ascended from the observation of schizophrenia patients and involvement with their families. These observations led to findings of some communication patterns related to mental illness within families. Therefore, the seed for treating family members began and demonstrated favorable outcomes (Falke, 2009).

Family counseling works to change identified problematic, maladaptive, repetitive relationship patterns and self-defeating belief systems within a family system (Goldenberg et al., 2017). This approach considers the identified client or the family member exhibiting a problem as one who creates trouble within the family or community or system. The focus shifts to the family and the members' interactions and relations (Henderson & Thompson, 2011). This shift of focusing on the *systems* rather than the individual can be difficult for counselors. The Western perspective of autonomous individuals with the capability to make independent and free choices can often create a blind spot for understanding the systems approach. Yet, individuals come out of their families of origin bringing with them the unspoken rules, routines, and boundaries generated there (Corey, 2017). It, therefore, becomes important to understand this approach when working with children and adolescence clients. Counseling with children and adolescents involves counseling in the context of multiple systems. Two major systems impact this population—family and school (Carter & Evans, 2008). Clinical mental health counselors and professional school counselors who adopt this perspective can make an impact on the etiology and treatment for the systems of family and school (Roaten et al., 2009).

BASIC CONCEPTS

Family

Counselors identify family as a group of people who intimately share their lives with one another. Therefore, a family can include any combination of parents, siblings, extended family, and even friends and/or neighbors (Council on Foundations, 2015; Kress et al., 2019). Counselors see each family member as part of the larger family system. Hence, anything that affects one family member will impact the entire family system. Each member of the family brings different perceptions and experience into the interactions and relationships among and between the family members (Kress et al., 2019).

Identified Client

It continues to be common for one member of the family (oftentimes the child or adolescent) to be referred for counseling. The identified client comes to counseling (or someone brings them) to address a mental health concern. Regardless, the family counselor believes the root of the problem can be found within the family system. Furthermore, the counselor does not find the client to be more or less pathologic or troubled than the other members of the family. Therein lies the difference between a family counselor and other theoretical approaches that focus on the individual client (Kress et al., 2019).

Family Development

It also becomes imperative for counselors working with families to understand the family development process. This development includes the growth of both the individual and the family as a whole. As the development of an individual intersects with the family life, complexities arise (McGoldrick et al., 2016; Vernon & Schimmel, 2019). Theorists list three key components impacting this development: the family life cycle, child development, and family reconfiguration. The family life-cycle stage model describes developmental events in a family's timeline. Vernon and Schimmel (2019) identify six general stages:

- young adulthood—separating from the family of origin
- young adults forming a couple relationship
- families with young children—establishing a new nuclear family
- families with adolescents—adjusting to adolescent's increased independence outside of the nuclear family
- families in midlife—departure of children and arrival of new members as children marry
- families in later life—adjusting to retirement and old age.

Counselors do not view transitioning from one stage to another to be applicable to all individuals and families and in all cultures. It does, however, provide a normative guide for understanding the family system as it expands and contracts. These can happen at various points throughout the cycle (e.g., new members by adoption and loss of members by unexpected death or divorce). The family renegotiates their relationships with each other through each of these phases. The focus lies not on how or if a family follows the path laid out; instead, it highlights the path described as always occurring in a series of continual expansions and contractions, which impact the family system (Vernon & Schimmel, 2019).

The developmental stages of children and adolescents present significant impacts on the family, as family dynamics shift with each stage of development. The support of family and caregivers varies as a child matures and gains more independence and responsibilities. The developmental needs of the child shift, meaning that the family system then adjusts. This adjustment can create stress for families working to balance parenting along with personal and professional lives (Vernon & Schimmel, 2019). Counselors consider family reconfiguration as the realigning and renegotiating of the family system at each transition of change. These can often lead to stress on the family. This can then be manifested in an individual family member with presenting symptoms. When the individual arrives for counseling as the identified client, the family counselor looks beyond this to consider larger life patterns, thereby exploring problems in a broad and systemic framework (Vernon & Schimmel, 2019).

THEORETICAL APPLICATION

Family counselors use core counseling skills in working with clients. All family counselors incorporate several common skills and tether additional skills to the counselor's theoretical orientation and style of work. Lowenstein (2010) presents this list of common family counseling skills. *Structuring* includes creating a safe place for clients to talk about their thoughts and concerns during the initial discussion about rules in the session, intervening if conflict arises, selection of appropriate interventions for the session, and reviewing the treatment goals regularly. *Reflecting* allows the listening counselor to provide the client's words, thoughts, and feeling in an open atmosphere. This ensures that the counselor provides each family member the opportunity to express themselves openly during session. *Empathizing* demonstrates the counselor's understanding of each member of the family. An empathic response encourages family members to reveal sincere sentiments. Counselors often achieve this with a reflection of feelings and content. *Hypothesizing and formulating* takes place as the counselor ponders their thoughts about the transactions within the family. This may be from observation of the family's patterns, briefs, and behaviors in the session. These hypotheses can guide the kinds of questions the counselor may ask or issues they may raise in sessions. *Tracking* occurs when the counselor listens attentively to family stories, carefully recording the events and their sequence. This allows the family counselor to identify the sequence of events operating within the family system. This insight can help in the selection of interventions and strategies used in the session. Counselors use *reframing* to restate or reconstruct the language used by a family in discussing the problem. Other shared skills include normalizing, confronting, pacing, and providing psychoeducational information (Lowenstein, 2010). Integrating creative activities and approaches to sessions can enrich the session, eliciting insight and information. The *questions,* however, reveal clinical information, guide the clients to face issues, or enable insights. This also increases the insight of how families interconnect and operate as a system.

Children and Adolescents in Family Sessions

The challenge of working with children may present a common discomfort to family counselors. Clinicians highlight a number of reasons not to include children in a family session. Some counselors may decide that the child needs to be protected from the information shared or that the information may hurt the child. Some counselors may encounter difficulty connecting with the adults and the child at the same time. In addition, the theoretical orientation may not be appropriate for young client interaction or that the problem and solution fall within the parental subset (Sayger & Horne, 2007). Parent consultation models, as done by professional school counselors, may be a consideration for working with children and parents separately. The following becomes the focus of parent consultation: (a) educating parents on improving communications between parent and child and (b) explaining the process and goal of counseling (Boswell, 2017, p. 256). This process begins with the initial contact with the family and continues through the counseling relationship. These consultation sessions with parents should engage them in cooperation with explanation and understanding of the counseling process. Furthermore, the counselor should explore with the parent ways for them to engage in the counseling process. Models of consultation consist of parent education, solution development, and parent trainings (Boswell, 2017).

Young Children in Family Sessions

There can also be anxiety around involving children in the family session because they can sometimes be noncommunicative or disruptive to the session. Lowenstein (2010) suggests integrating engaging and developmentally appropriate techniques into the session that will involve the children and prevent disruptive behavior (p. xxx). Counselors who feel uncomfortable in their ability to communicate with children can use simplified language, while being careful not to be patronizing. Feeling posters can be helpful for identifying and referring to emotions. Puppets, finger puppets, and dolls, as well as figurines, can be used as tools to communicate with children. Other key elements needed for child-focused family counseling consist of art- and play-based techniques with creative and playful approaches (Lowenstein, 2010).

Horton et al. (2017) point out *directive filial therapy* as a therapeutic model for very young children aged zero to six. This intervention engages parents as the therapeutic agents with their own children. This includes (a) infant/child's parent in the therapeutic process; (b) goals of improving various aspects of parent–child relationship, child outcome, and parent functioning; and (c) elements of direct instruction or coaching from the counselor. Counselors use regularly three evidence-based models with this approach area: Attachment and Biobehavioral Catch-up, Child–Parent Psychotherapy (CPP), and Parent–Child Interaction Therapy (PCIT) (Horton et al., 2017, p. 186).

Adolescents in Family Sessions

Teens and adolescents commonly present as aggressive or hostile and moody during family counseling. If the adolescent presents with a reluctance to participate in the session, it may be best to avoid direct questions about how they feel or make direct eye contact. Furthermore, teaching, lecturing, and giving advice should also be avoided. It may be helpful to ask the teen client to observe the session and provide written feedback of key moments in the session (Lowenstein, 2010). Utilizing a creative or expressive approach may be a valuable process. While a teen may not like being approached directly in a family session, they may be more comfortable allowing their parents to listen to music meaningful to them. This strategy and other creative or expressive modes to work with adolescents in a family session may allow the family members to access modes of communications not always available through language (Hudspeth et al., 2018).

GESTALT THERAPY

OVERVIEW

Born in 1893 in Berlin, Germany, Frederick ("Fritz") Perls and his wife Laura Perls originally developed Gestalt therapy in the 1940s. Perls studied with many of the psychoanalytic greats such as Karen Horney and Wilhelm Reich. During World War II, Perls and his wife moved from Germany to the United States in the 1940s, where Perls finalized his theory of personality. Psychoanalysis, psychodrama, humanistic theories, phenomenology, and existentialism influenced Gestalt therapy (Oaklander, n.d.). At its core, Gestalt therapy may be considered to be a process-oriented therapy centered on a healthy, integrated functioning of the entire organism or person (Perls et al., 1951). Self-regulation remains the fundamental tenet of Gestalt therapy. Via self-regulation, a person becomes able to get their psychological needs met, which leads to an increase in healthy functioning, learning, and potential. Healthy functioning includes an integration of the senses, body, emotions, and mind (Oaklander, n.d.). This healthy functioning leads a person to change via an awareness of "what they are doing, how they are doing it, and how they can change themselves" (Oaklander, n.d., para. 2). What a person experiences and perceives appears to be valued more than explanations and rationalizations for behavior.

BASIC CONCEPTS

Gestalt therapy consists of many important concepts and components that a clinician must understand in order for the theory to be both useful and effective. First and foremost for needed change, Gestalt therapy presents four conditions. These include (a) both the client and counselor being fully present and engaged in the therapeutic work together, (b) the client displays a desire or want to change, (c) the client appears open to recognizing boundary problems that cause a disturbance while remaining open to change and feedback, and (d) the client displays a nondefensive attitude.

VIEW OF PEOPLE

Perls believed all people to be fully functioning organisms at birth. Each person's interactions with the environment, or field, serve as a means to get their needs met, and the person begins to find various ways to address and satisfy these personal needs and wants. As a person seeks to interact with the environment in order to get personal needs met, contact boundaries emerge leading to an understanding of an individualized self. These contact boundaries differentiate self from others. Perls noted that the I-boundary develops through safe, nurturing environments. Unhealthy environments represent boundaries that come across as rigid and inflexible or those that seem permeable and open lead to a sense of discomfort, an unhealthy sense of self, rejection, and abandonment (Carroll, 2009). For children specifically, they "do not have the cognitive or emotional maturity to discriminate what fits from what does not fit for them or the situation, and they therefore tend to accept everything they hear, or imagine they hear, about themselves" (Carroll & Oaklander, 1997, p. 187). The more a client, specifically a child, hears negative messages about themselves, the more the person feels a sense of disconnect and loss of self, leading to fragmentation.

WHOLENESS AND POLARITIES

Perls believed that all people could enact personal change providing exposure to a positive, nurturing, and corrective environment. This includes a person being willing to connect with their senses and emotions, to be in the here and now, and to be authentic to their true self (Perls, 1969). Perls determined that being connected with one's self and in contact with the world meant embracing a willingness to explore all experiences and senses, including those considered both positive and negative or painful. Counselors establish the goal of treatment to provide a safe environment that allows a person to restore healthy self-regulation, begin to experience self in relation to others and the environment, and use the person's internal resources as a means to get their needs and wants met.

THEORETICAL APPLICATION

Today, many Gestalt institutes worldwide provide research, literature, and best practices for clinicians interested in concepts and techniques grounded in Gestalt theory. Violet Oaklander and her institute, the Violet Solomon Oaklander Foundation, brought many Gestalt concepts to clinicians working with children and adolescents. She and other Gestalt clinicians and researchers published many articles and texts illustrating the use of Gestalt play therapy techniques and activities.

Two-Chair Method

Gestalt therapy offers another common strategy the two-chair method (originally called the empty chair technique). Counselors consider this to be a common intervention in which a client holds a conversation, or dialogue, with an aspect of themselves or a significant person in the client's life. The client imagines an aspect of the self or significant person to be sitting across from the client. As the client dialogues with the imagined aspect of self, the counselor encourages the client to sit in each chair and take on the role of the different aspect or the significant person. In this method, the client develops greater awareness of their needs through self-dialogue as the counselor encourages the client to play out different pieces of oneself. Additionally, the two-chair method aids the therapeutic process in allowing unfinished business within the client or with a significant person to be understood and resolved. This process helps the client view the conflict from various angles and gain insight into why they feel and behave in a certain way. When working with clients, including children and adolescents, the use of this technique can aid in resolving neglect and abandonment issues along with issues such as guilt, abuse, and trauma (Elliott et al., 2004; Trijayanti et al., 2019). It remains important to note that careful attention should be given to clients with a risk or retraumatization or suicidality as this technique may not be appropriate.

Awareness

Gestalt clinicians use a variety of strategies that aid in developing greater awareness of a person's genuine self and needs. These strategies can be simple awareness statements such as "What are you aware of now?" and the use of "I" statements versus "you" statements to better understand the needs the person wants met. The counselor may emphasize awareness through repetition of a behavior or exaggeration that leads to an overawareness. At times, the counselor may also want to focus on an awareness of self and others by asking the client to become the other person by taking on the person's behaviors and affect to enhance awareness of feelings of what seems important to each person.

Unfinished Business

Perls considered one major concept, the idea of unfinished business or unresolved conflicts, to be at the root of many human problems. Being authentic to oneself and working through unfinished business leads a person to make independent and thoughtful choices regarding how and when to act in various situations versus living a more reactionary life. When working with a client, one must spend time developing a safe and trusting relationship. Once developed, the counselor aids the client in understanding the true, authentic self, reviews unfinished business, and learns skills to better self-regulate during times of crisis and stress (Wheeler & Axelsson, 2014). Gestalt counselors, whether working with adults, adolescents, or teens, integrate techniques such as the two-chair and other expressive modalities including creative arts, play, movement, sand tray, and others to help clients facilitate greater awareness during counseling sessions.

NARRATIVE THERAPY

The counseling field considers Michael White and David Epston to be common names associated with narrative therapy. Narrative therapy, a postmodern social constructionist narrative approach, presents a collaborative approach with special attention to respectful listening to the client's story. Counselors use questions to engage and facilitate clients in their exploration of their story. This story shapes client reality with regard to the social and cultural framework. This approach provides the power to create and rewrite one's own story. The process can give the client the chance to discover where their story might not be accurate or real as well as changed (Rice, 2015). The counselor approaches this work collaboratively with clients. The focus involves assisting clients in reauthoring their own story. No interpretation of life events occurs; rather, an interest in helping the client find new meaning within the events becomes the focus. The counselor provides the opportunity for clients to tell and retell their story from various angles. This method permits clients to increase the descriptions and details of the events as they move through the telling and retelling. This approach also helps to externalize client problems, revealing that the problem does not define them. Counselors consider *the problem* itself to be the problem

(McHenry & McHenry, 2015). Furthermore, these stories can uncover the dominant cultural influences that the client may not perceive to be present. Narrative therapy can shed light on the issue of power, knowledge, and dominance that may be a part of a client's society and family (Haskins & Mingo, 2017).

This approach allows children and adolescents to create an identity that separates them from society, their family, or any oppressive dominant presence. The counselor welcomes clients by listening to them with an open mind, encouraging them to share their story, maintaining a curious respectful stance, and helping the client to see that the problem does not define them. *The problem* continues to be the problem (White 1995 as cited in Haskins & Mingo, 2017). Kottman and Meany-Walen (2015) point out narrative therapy can be useful with clients who may choose to speak little or not speak at all, especially younger clients. The counselor would observe the capturing of a story that goes along with the client's drawing or selection of toys.

BASIC CONCEPTS

Taylor de Faoite (2011) provides recommendations when using this approach with children and adolescents. The goal should not be to replace the client's story with the counselor's; rather, the goal should be to empower the client to participate in the collaborative process for creating and renovating the meaning of their story. With this population, it becomes important that the counselor takes time to first expand their knowledge about the client's social and cultural history as well as other stories they carry with them. This creates a safe place for the client to open up as the counselor listens to them tell their story. In this safe place, a relationship can develop that will allow the counselor and the client to coconstruct a new or alternative story and self. There are four elements that are incorporated.

1. *The ambiguity of stories.* The counselor is uncertain about where the story may go or lead to. There is also the uncertainty about what alternative stories might arise.
2. *The coconstruction of the narrative.* With intentional and skillful listening as well as questioning, the counselor can assist in the construction of a new narrative.
3. *The story is a purposeful act.* The configuration of a story has a beginning, middle, and end that engage in the purposeful act of retelling the stories.
4. The counselor goes further to acknowledge and explore any existence of cultural elements or components (Taylor de Faoite, 2011).

THEORETICAL APPLICATION

The application of this approach does not include specific techniques. However, counselors employ three considerations: questions, externalization, and deconstruction and creating alternative stories (Ziomek-Daigle, 2017), which they intertwine through the six-stage process of narrative therapy to generate collaboration between the counselor and the client. This allows the client to describe their experience in a new and fresh language. Counselors use *questions* to collect the experience of the client rather than just information. The counselor's approach appears to be a stance of not knowing, curious, and openness, thereby encouraging the client to explore different perspectives of their life experiences while dismantling problem-saturated stories. Counselors view *externalization* as imperative in that it separates the client from identifying with the problem. Before *creating the new story,* the previous story must be *deconstructed. Possibility questions* help the client to see a new future and explore what it might be like when things take a different perspective in the new story. To complete the process, the counselor helps the client find an audience that will validate this new story (Ziomek-Daigle, 2017).

Externalizing the Problem: Sculpture and Processing

Narrative therapy can be used with various art and creative forms. Clark's (2018) distinctive approach includes the use of clay, Play-Doh, Model Magic, or any sculpting medium in place of paper and pencil. This approach focuses on externalizing the problem, naming the problem, and beginning the process of restorying. Clark considers this approach to be suitable for both children and adolescents.

The counselor first begins by providing the sculpture medium to the client and asks them to create an image of the problem that brought them in today. Time will be needed for the client to create their sculpture. Sometimes a client may be hesitant to begin. Encouragement may be needed along with assurances that the outcome of the creation will not be evaluated or judged. The counselor must provide a safe place for this creation. Next, when the client completes the sculpture, the counselor should allow the client time to name it, to name their problem. From this point forward, the name given to the sculpture should be used (Clark, 2018). Then the counselor should discuss how the client felt while creating the sculpture. Time should be given to discuss the story of the sculpture, the creations of it, the naming, and its meaningfulness to them. Counselors view reflections of feelings, empathy, along with curiosity and not knowing stance as appropriate interventions during this exploratory storying step and progress toward the deconstruction of the story (Clark, 2018).

Subsequently, beginning the steps of externalizing the problem at this time will include allowing the client to describe how it feels to know the problem and to see the problem outside of themselves. The counselor follows this with the coconstruction of the new story: life without the problem. This purposeful action and new story should be wrapped with questions of inquisitiveness that pull together the beginning, middle, and end that support the new narrative (Clark, 2018). As the session comes to an end, the counselor should provide the client with choices about their sculpture. They may want to keep it to be a reminder of a problem that they overcame, a story of their past. Others may wish to simply return it to the original shape and container. It would not be unexpected that some might consider throwing it in the trash. Keep in mind that the name given to the sculpture should be used throughout this time. Within the last moments of the session, the counselor should provide a conclusion of the events, summarize the session, and include questions about the possibility of doing anything differently assessing how this information might be used going forward (Clark, 2018).

PLAY THERAPY

OVERVIEW

The United Nations High Commission for Human Rights considers play an integral aspect of children's development and a right of all children (Ginsberg, 2007). Play therapy methods help children explore the world around them and express their thoughts and feelings in a safe environment. The Association for Play Therapy defined play therapy as "the systematic use of a theoretical model to establish interpersonal processes wherein trained play therapists use the therapeutic powers of play to help clients prevent or resolve psychosocial difficulties and achieve optimal growth and development" (n.d., para. 2). Credentialed clinicians practicing as play therapists receive special training that allows them to assist children in exploring their feelings, increasing positive interactions with others, and developing appropriate social skills using play, their natural form of communication (Kottman & Meany-Walen, 2015; Landreth, 2012).

Bratton and Ray (2000) conducted a meta-analysis of play therapy research completed since 1942 and found over 100 case studies that concluded that play therapy proved to be effective in improving many different presenting issues. Further, Bratton and Ray concluded that 82 experimentally designed studies demonstrated effectiveness with various client issues. In a more recent meta-analysis of play therapy research, Bratton et al. (2005) identified that play therapy treatment methods revealed a larger treatment effect when compared to methods that did not utilize play therapy tenets. They completed a meta-analytic review of 93 research articles, both published (n = 43) and unpublished (n = 50), about play therapy, filial therapy, family play therapy, therapeutic play, and play in therapy to determine the effectiveness of these treatments.

NONDIRECTIVE PLAY APPROACHES

Play therapy historically encompassed two different approaches—nondirective and directive. Nondirective play therapy approaches focused on Virginia Axline's (1947) specific tenets and beliefs about therapy with children. Axline stressed that nondirective play therapy can be used to help children better understand their feelings and inner struggles through their natural form of communication—play. She also noted a child–counselor relationship should be built on trust, acceptance, and the belief that the child's inner drive toward healthy functioning will lead to increased growth and emotional maturity.

Play therapy, specifically nondirective, child-centered play therapy, connotes a "dynamic interpersonal relationship between a child and a therapist trained in play therapy procedures who provides selected play materials and a safe, therapeutic environment in which the child becomes able to explore and fully express himself or herself" (Landreth, 2012, p. 16). Clinicians commonly view play as a child's natural form of communication and assist the counselor to help the child grow and develop to their full potential (Kottman & Meany-Walen, 2015; Landreth, 2012). Landreth (2012) encouraged counselors and play therapists to recognize play as a child's language and toys as the child's words.

DIRECTIVE PLAY APPROACHES

Directive play approaches allow the counselor to work with their client at their appropriate developmental level. This addresses any verbal or developmental inability to express feelings. The counselor can then assume the responsibility to communicate effectively with clients of all ages and offers the client the opportunity to respond, bridging the gap between experiences, thoughts, and feelings. The approach allows the client to express these in concrete forms (Leggett, 2009; Leggett et al., 2016). Directive play tenets speak to an integrative approach that combines a counseling theory with the use of toys to address the needs of the client. Other names for this approach include structured, prescriptive, focused, and nonhumanistic. The focus includes the use of games, toys, metaphors, or make-believe to elicit responses from the client. The counselor guides and interprets the play interaction (Leggett & Boswell, 2017).

BASIC CONCEPTS OF DIRECTIVE PLAY THERAPY

A counselor uses directive play therapy to focus attention, stimulate further activity, gain information, interpret, or set limits. The counselor selects purposeful activities structured to elicit responses from the client. The counselor remains responsible for the guidance and interpretation of the play interactions. Thought and intentionality must go into the selection of toys and materials to match the circumstance and presenting problem the client might be facing. Jones et al. (2003) offer some recommendations for planning and selecting toys and materials. These recommendations emanate from three stages of the structured play model: (a) opening, (b) working, and (c) termination (Knell, 1997). An added level of consideration concerns the determination of the level of intensity for each session. These levels include (a) evoking anxiety, (b) challenging to self-disclose, (c) increasing awareness, (d) focusing on feelings, (e) focusing on the here and now, and (f) focusing on the threatening issues. With these elements in mind, the counselor plans for each session to determine the level of intensity needed and then weighs the direction of the session, activities, and materials or toys (Jones et al., 2003; Leggett & Boswell, 2017). These elements and key concepts become threaded together with the core theory of operation. Some examples of these include post-Jungian, solution-focused, humanistic sand tray therapy; eye movement desensitization and reprocessing and play; bibliotherapy; trauma-focused CBT; and the list grows. The counselor seeks to obtain a deeper understanding of the therapeutic power of play based on their understanding of the therapeutic remedies (Schaefer & Drewes, 2016).

RATIONAL EMOTIVE BEHAVIOR THERAPY

OVERVIEW

REBT ranks as one of the most researched and identifiable CBTs (Corey, 2013; Haskins & Mingo, 2017). REBT shares some characteristics with other cognitive behavioral theories. REBT encompasses (a) cognitive change to create a new feeling and behavior; (b) counselor directedness; (c) collaboration in the counselor–client relationship; (d) an understanding of how cognitive distortions and dysfunction create psychological distress; (e) time limitation; and (f) interventions that target the identified or presenting problem (Corey, 2013; Haskins & Mingo, 2017). Counselors who choose REBT agree that thoughts impact emotions and behaviors. The awareness of thoughts and the decision to change those thoughts lead to change. Albert Ellis (1962), the originator of this theoretical approach, rationalized that human tendencies could be understood as inclinations to want, to need, and to criticize themselves, others, and the world when faced with immediate unmet needs. This results in absolute and unrealistic goals, desires, and absolute and unrealistic preferences often identified as *shoulds*, *oughts*, and *musts*. This system of rigid thoughts that formulate into patterns can lead to emotional problems for children and adolescents. Helping children and adolescents to think and behave in a more satisfying personal way that allows them to realize that they can choose between self-defeating rigid thoughts and behaviors or efficient, enriching, and positive behaviors become the goal of REBT. Doing so allows children and adolescents to take responsibility for their own logical thinking and the natural consequences and behaviors that follow it (Henderson & Thompson, 2011).

BASIC CONCEPTS

REBT utilizes the *ABCDE* model, which illustrates the basic constructs of the theory. The *A* stands for the activating event, which can be positive or negative, real or perceived, and in the past or present or future. While some children and adolescents might believe this event causes their emotional and behavioral reaction, the belief about the event, *B*, leads to these reactions. The *C*, the consequence, results in the emotional and/or behavioral demonstration. The *D* for this model denotes the disputation of the thoughts. This process can be challenging for children and adolescents. Concrete, psychoeducational, as well as, creative and expressive techniques help with this change. The *E* represents the effective new thought, feeling, and behavior (Henderson & Thompson, 2011). Corey et al. (2018) expanded this model by adding *F* creating a new model, *ABCDEF*. The *F* represents the new feeling the client experiences under effective disputing. Therefore, when *D* appears successful, the counselor evaluates the effect (*E*) with the client. In this process, the evaluation will reveal changed feelings and actions due to the altered belief (Erford, 2020).

Vernon and Schimmel (2019) took REBT further with the development of a model primarily aimed at working with children and adolescents—*C.A.T.* The *C* stands for connect. This integral component involves listening, providing unconditional positive regard, honesty, patience, respect, and genuine interest in clients. The *A* represents assessing the activation event, the emotional and behavioral consequence, and rational and irrational beliefs. A developmentally appropriate format and intervention should include creative and expressive components along with concrete strategies, which will allow the child or adolescent to assess and understand the process. Finally, the *T* represents teaching and treating. When disputing the irrational belief, it continues to be important to help a client identify a new and effective way to think, feel, and behave (Vernon & Schimmel, 2019).

THEORETICAL APPLICATIONS

Ellis (1996) determined that a child's psychological problems may be due to rigid beliefs and that children hold the possibility for rational thinking when they stop blaming self and others. Children often fall into three groups of thoughts.

- *I must do to win approval. . .or I'm no good.*
- *Other people must treat me well. . .if they don't, they are no good.*
- *I must get what I want. . .if I don't, life is no good.*

REBT allows counselors to understand the thoughts, feelings, and behaviors of children and adolescents. Counselors begin with identifying the client's irrational belief and then move to an intervention to demonstrate to the client the means to dispute the belief and substitute a more rational belief. Finally, the counselor discusses the evaluation of the effect of disputing the irrational belief (Ziomek-Daigle, 2017).

ABCDEF MODEL

Rational Emotive Imagery

Maultsby developed the technique of rational emotive imagery (REI) to establish patterns of emotional adaptation. This format allows the client to visualize their thinking, feeling, and behaving as they would hope it to be every day. The primary goal focuses on allowing the client to change emotions from unhealthy to healthy through this process (Erford, 2020; Seligman & Reichenberg, 2013). Initially, the client must identify the irrational belief and then collaboratively the counselor and client can begin the following seven-step process (Seligman & Reichenberg, 2013).

VISUALIZE AN UNPLEASANT ACTIVATING EVENT

The counselor encourages the client to visualize the details of the event that holds the irrational belief. For young clients, it may be helpful to use story squares (see Figure 5.1). The client can create a sequence of drawings that reveal the events. This will create a vivid element while allowing the client a chance to gain a full perspective. The number of squares needed may be determined by the story and the client's choice. The client needs time to complete the drawing of the story to ensure the inclusion of rich details.

EXPERIENCE THE UNHEALTHY NEGATIVE EMOTIONS

The client must identify the feelings that surface during this event and spend several moments sitting with these feelings. The story squares will help the client to more clearly identify when the emotions occurred.

CHANGE THE EMOTION

Once the client experiences the unhealthy emotions, they will need to spend time considering the feeling and determining the appropriate response. With the story squares, the client can visualize themselves responding with healthy emotions to this event. Counselors call this healthy response positive imagery.

EXAMINE THE PROCESS

At this point, the counselor can help the client understand the impact of changing their belief system (B) and how it will affect the activating event (A) and the resulting emotional consequence (C). Furthermore, it remains imperative that the client understands how their self-talk changes from the old belief to bring about the new more rational belief.

To make the change more concrete, it may be helpful to create a new individual story square. The client can draw a new picture in this square that reflects the new

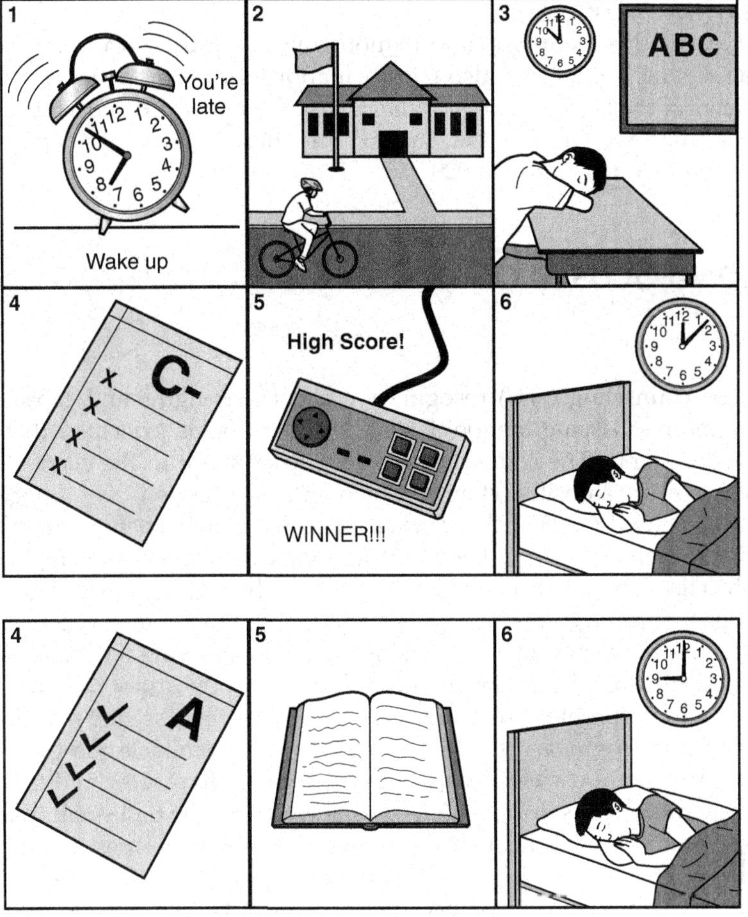

FIGURE 5.1 Story squares.

healthy response and place it over the previous story square that reflected the unhealthy inappropriate feeling. A small piece of tape will allow the new square to cover the former square. This will also allow the new square to be flipped up to allow a visual review of the change: a glimpse of before and after.

REPETITION AND PRACTICE

Best practices require the client to repeat steps 1 to 3 at least 10 minutes every day until they no longer experience the unhealthy feelings in response to the activating event.

REINFORCING THE GOAL

With some time, usually several weeks, the client should be able to experience a healthy, appropriate emotion while experiencing little, or none, of the previously experienced inappropriate feelings when they faced the activating event. A review of the story squares with the changes made to the new square will reinforce the accomplished goal.

GENERALIZATION OF SKILLS

As the client learns this technique and demonstrates comfort with it, they can then use it for other activating events that also trigger inappropriate emotional responses. Again, consider reviewing the story squares of the original event and discuss how other events appear to be similar and/or different. Include attention to the client's choices to change their self-talk and feelings (Erford, 2020).

SOLUTION-FOCUSED COUNSELING

OVERVIEW

Solution-focused counseling (SFC) recognizes a client's strengths and capacities to access and develop a more satisfying life (de Shazer, 1985) and holds principles that advocate for children and adolescents. The counselor maintains confidence in the client's ability to use inner resources to make a positive change (Corcoran & Stephenson, 2000; Leggett, 2017). The signature questions used in SFC help the client to focus on how change can take place. This allows the client to tell their story. The client formulates questions allowing connections to be made as the client shares ideas and key thoughts. Through this exchange, collaboration between the client and the counselor crafts a new or alternative meaning or approach to a situation. Furthermore, the new ideas and thoughts lead to pathways for change and solutions. The time-limited focus on the problem still provides an opportunity for the counselor to reorient the client to the problem, seek out clues as to how others see the situation, and notice changes (Gillen, 2011). This moves the focus to a clear goal. The miracle question "...if a miracle happened tonight while you were asleep and you woke up tomorrow and the problem that brought you here today was solved by magic, what would be the first small thing you would notice that told you this miracle happened?" allows the client to look past the present and into the future. The client can open their imagination to a time when experiences seemed better and the problem did not exist. Hope becomes increased. Clarity evolves from the miracle by noticing what seems to be different and who notices these differences. Recognizing and identifying exceptions stand out as another key theoretical component—those moments in the past when some of the miracles happened or when the problem did not occur. Murphy (1994) points out five methods that assist a client in noting exceptions: (a) eliciting times when the problem did not exist; (b) elaborating the details and circumstance of these times; (c) expanding the exception to other contexts; (d) evaluating exception in sight of the goals and details of the miracle; and (e) empowering the client to intentionally continue this change over time.

Scaling questions provide a concrete notation of achievements measuring the client's success as well as the proximity to the goal. The client can point out their impressions on a scale from 1 to 10 with 1 meaning *the problem controls the client* or *no success*, and 10 meaning *the client controls the problem* or *success*. The counselor can gain insights into the client's hopefulness, motivation, and confidence. The final step often includes three basic parts including complements to the client's strengths, a bridge to connect these identified strengths and successes to the task or suggestion, as well as to the goal, and the suggestion or task given to move the client into the future and closer to their goal (Leggett, 2017).

BASIC CONCEPTS

These SFC concepts provide counselors with the freedom to expand their work and begin to creatively integrate around these SFC concepts to meet the needs of children and adolescents. Expanding the basic model opens the client to verbal and nonverbal tools of expression. Developmentally appropriate adjustments can be easily made for the client. Finally, communication between the counselor and the client increases, all while facilitating the relationship (Leggett, 2009, 2017). The counselor includes experiential activities to serve as the means for the SFC dialogue. These could be a selection of books and literature, drawings, selected toys, puppets, and sand tray. The counselor can use these tools to help the client establish groundwork for new thinking and coconstruct new and alternative meanings of situations as well as provide a means to change and solutions (Leggett, 2017).

THEORETICAL APPLICATIONS

Describing the Problem and Establishing the Goals

The initial prompt, "What brings you here today"?, allows the client to describe their story and the chance to identify what they want different or to change. This exchange can lead to establishing a goal. The goal for this population should (a) fit the client's needs; (b) be relevant, meaningful, and individualized to the situation; and (c) be concrete, behavioral, and measurable. The use of books, drawings, and selected toys can help children and adolescents express or communicate the situation or problem they face. They can also help to normalize what the client experiences and assist in helping the client externalize the problem (Leggett, 2017).

Miracle Question

This question, designed to allow the client to look beyond their situation or problem into the future, lets the client see how life will be when things appear different, mainly when the client achieves the goal. For children and adolescents, this may be too abstract a visualization without help. Books and drawings can help to facilitate this stage.

The profession provides various picture books that describe a *perfect day*. Beginning this conversation with a selected book will provide a foundation for understanding the concept of a day or time without a problem. These books can be simple picture books or ones with more content and depth. The selection should match the client's development level. While it may seem awkward to some adolescents when an adult reads a book to them using this technique, they will generally accept and participate in the strategy with some explanation. The books help the client grasp the abstract idea of the miracle question. This begins by reading the book to the client followed by the discussion of the features described by the main character's perfect day. Exploring the character's perfect day opens the client's imagination to the possibilities of their own perfect or miracle day. This leads the session into the client's own description and exploration of the details that construct their own miracle (Leggett, 2017).

Exploring for Exceptions

The search for moments when the problem ceases, or happens not as often, can also be an abstract idea for this population. Rather than searching for several exceptions, it may be best for this age group to concentrate on only one exception no matter how small it may be. The use of drawings can allow the client to carefully examine even the tiniest exception to their situation. Allowing the client to draw this moment can give the client opportunity to concentrate on the event and the details, to identify random or deliberate behaviors, and to determine how to repeat this happening. This activity, as with so many, must allow time for the client to draw the exception with related details and descriptions (Leggett, 2017).

Scaling Questions

The scaling question permits the client to evaluate their own progress. A visual representation of a scale makes this concrete as well. The question should be altered to fit the selection of the visual scaling question. Nims (2007) presents drawing and physical responses as examples that can be used. Counselors describe a physical response as a unique format arranged on the floor with designated locations for the number line marking from 0 through 5 or 10. Then, the client can decide where to stand to represent their place on the scale. Follow-up questions would create opportunity to investigate what drew the client to the selected number and what needs to be different to move a half or whole number closer to the goal, 10. Keep in mind to stay with small increments to encourage small changes, which counselors consider to be signature to SFC (Leggett, 2017).

CASE STUDY 5.1: CASE STUDY WITH RATIONAL EMOTIVE BEHAVIOR THERAPY/ABCDEF MODEL AND STORY SQUARES

Daniel is a middle school student who identifies as male. He does not demonstrate any cognitive or learning issues. Also, he has not previously had any reports of behavior issues. His teacher notes he has been arriving late to school and sometimes falls asleep. The teacher is worried about Daniel and has referred him to the counselor on campus. Mr. Martinez, the counselor, arranges to meet with Daniel to get a better idea of his situation, needs, and how he might be able to help Daniel.

After building a counseling relationship with Daniel, Mr. Martinez decided to spend three or four additional sessions with Daniel. As a counselor, Mr. Martinez uses REBT to guide his counseling sessions and interventions. Furthermore, he has expanded his use of the ABCDE model to the ABCDEF model, which allows him to include an evaluation of the changed feelings or behaviors. To be more effective in his work with Daniel, Mr. Martinez has selected REI, more specifically the use of story squares to help Daniel. This will allow Daniel to (a) visualize what is happening, (b) recognize any unhealthy negative emotions or behaviors, (c) make a change, (d) process this change, (e) practice the change, and finally (f) reinforce the goal and (g) generalize skills.

Mr. Martinez begins by offering Daniel a story squares template and asks him to draw out the events that are taking place currently. After spending some time drawing out the events, Daniel shared the following comments.

(*continued*)

CASE STUDY 5.1 (*continued*)

> *I know I need to do something so that I am not so tired in the morning before school. It is hard to wake up because I'm playing my game so late at night. When I sleep through my alarm, I end up being late for the bus. My mom has to take me to school and then she is late for work. Even when I am at school, I end up falling asleep or forgetting homework. It sucks! I know I need to do better, but I hate missing out on playing the game with my friends.*

Mr. Martinez and Daniel spend more time exploring what might change to help Daniel reach his goal. Looking at the story squares, Daniel decides squares 4, 5, and 6 could be different. Mr. Martinez and Daniel process how these changes could impact things for Daniel, at home and at school. Daniel believes if he changes his actions and behaviors here, things will be different. He draws new pictures of how things could be different.

> *I do not want to stop playing my game. I enjoy it. I get to hang out with my friends and we have a lot of fun. Maybe if I stop playing earlier in the evening. . .say 10 or 11 p.m. instead of after midnight, then it will be easier for me to wake up and get to school on time. It might also help me keep from falling asleep in class.*

Daniel makes new drawings for squares 4, 5, and 6. He tapes these new images onto the story squares. In the final sessions with Daniel, Mr. Martinez explores how Daniel has implemented the changes. Furthermore, they explore changes in Daniel's feelings as well as the impact of these. In addition, Mr. Martinez took some time to ask Daniel where else he might want to make similar changes. This added exchange allowed Daniel to see where else he might be able to make a change that would lead to better outcomes.

CHAPTER SUMMARY

Counselors must consider how to approach the struggles, fears, and vulnerabilities young clients face in schools and communities and how to help them make sense of their world (Vernon & Schimmel, 2019). Counselors must understand their own level of self-awareness, cultural knowledge, theory of orientation, and commitment to counseling this population. Roaten (2011) and Landreth (2012) point out that counselors cannot treat these clients as *mini-adults*. Instead, they must utilize effective techniques and strategies that meet their developmental and cultural needs. Children and adolescents must gain a sense of control through counseling and feel respected and valued. Counselors identify the use of counseling theories listed in this chapter along with creative strategies and expressive approaches (e.g., drawings, music, toys, and books) as best practices for working with young clients (Leggett & Boswell, 2017; Roaten, 2011).

POINTS TO REMEMBER

- Be grounded in your theory of orientation.
- Be attuned to the difference of working with children and adolescents.
- Be aware of the varying amount of time a young client might need to progress through the session.
- Be prepared if deciding to integrate purposeful activities and interventions (e.g., games, books, drawings, and toys).
- Be comfortable providing time and space to explore and process insights gained in the activities.
- Be mindful that only one or two steps may be accomplished during one session.

OTHER HELPFUL INFORMATION FOR CONSIDERATION

The professional organizations and conferences listed in the following provide efficacious continued education to learn current trends and best practices in the mental health profession (Leggett et al., 2009).

- American Counseling Association: www.counseling.org
- Association for Child & Adolescent Counseling: acachild.org
- Association for Creativity in Counseling: www.creativecounselor.org
- Association for Play Therapy: www.a4pt.org
- Beck Institute for Cognitive Behavior Therapy: beckinstitute.org
- Behavioral Tech: A Linehan Institute Training Company: behavioraltech.org
- Glasser Institute for Choice Theory: wglasser.com
- North American Society for Individual Psychology: www.alfredadler.org
- Solution Focused Brief Therapy Association: www.sfbta.org
- Violet Solomon Oaklander Foundation: vsof.org

QUESTIONS FOR FURTHER DISCUSSION

- In what ways might counselors go about selecting their foundational theory?
- How do counselors decide which creative or expressive activity would work best with their client?
- In what ways are activities best integrated into a session?
- What may be the most difficult element of integrating with the theory?

- How will a counselor know when the theory and the activity worked or did not work well in the session?
- How will a counselor know the efficacy of the theory and the activity used with the client?

KEY REFERENCES

Only key references appear in the print edition. The full reference list appears in the digital product on Springer Publishing Connect: connect.springerpub.com/content/book/978-0-8261-4764-6/part/part02/chapter/ch05

Adler, A. (1956). Social interest. In H. Ansbacher & R. Ansbacher (Eds.), *The individual psychology of Alfred Adler* (pp. 127–132). Basic Books.

Axline, V. M. (1947). *Play therapy* (rev. ed.). Ballantine Books.

Behavioral Tech. (n.d.). DBT helps adolescents. https://behavioraltech.org/wp-content/uploads/2018/09/Adolescents.pdf

Boswell, J. N. (2017). Directive approaches when working with parents. In E. S. Leggett & J. N. Boswell (Eds.), *Directive play therapy: Theory, technique, & treatment* (pp. 255–273). Springer Publishing Company.

Carroll, F. (2009). Gestalt play therapy. In K. J. O'Conner & L. D. Braverman (Eds.), *Play therapy theory and practice: Comparing theories and techniques* (2nd ed.). John Wiley & Sons.

Goldenberg, I., Stanton, M., & Goldenberg, H. (2017). *Family therapy: An overview* (9th ed.). Brooks/Cole Publishing Co.

Knell, S. M. (1997). Cognitive-behavioral play therapy. In K. J. O'Connor & L. M. Braverman (Eds.), *Play therapy theory and practice: A comparative presentation* (pp. 79–99). John Wiley & Sons.

Kottman, T., & Meany-Walen, K. (2015). *Partners in play: An Adlerian approach to play therapy* (3rd ed.). American Counseling Association.

Leggett, E. S. (2017). Solution focused play therapy. In E. S. Leggett & J. N. Boswell (Eds.), *Directive play therapy: Theories and techniques* (pp. 59–80). Springer Publishing Company.

Leggett, E. S., & Boswell, J. (2017). Directive play therapy. In E. S. Leggett & J. N. Boswell (Eds.), *Directive play therapy: Theory, technique, and treatment* (pp. 1–16). Springer Publishing Company.

Wubbolding, R. E. (2000). *Reality therapy for the 21st century*. Brunner-Routledge.

CHAPTER 6

Theoretical Approaches and Modalities Used With Children and Adolescents

Priscilla Rose Prasath, J. Claire Gregory, Mahsa Maghsoudi, Stacy Speedlin Gonzalez, and Crystal Morris

LEARNING OBJECTIVES

After completing this chapter, the reader should be able to:

- Identify theoretical approaches and modalities for working with children and adolescents.
- Explain how developmental, systemic, relational, and multicultural concepts intersect with each approach or modality.
- Employ developmentally appropriate creative strategies in counseling children and adolescents.

CACREP STANDARDS FOR THIS CHAPTER

- CACREP 2016: 2.F.1.f.; 5.a,b,j; 3.i.; 5.b.f.g.; School Counseling: 5.G.2.l.; 3.d.e.f.h.; Clinical Mental Health Counseling: 5.C.1.b.; 2.a.j.k.; 3.b.
- CACREP 2009: II.G.1.f.; 2.d; 3.b.d.h.; 5.b.c.d.e.; School Counseling: 3C.1; Clinical Mental Health Counseling: 3C.8; E.3.

INTRODUCTION

Working with children and adolescents, whether in a school or clinical mental health setting, calls for intentional practices. Professional school counselors and clinical mental health counselors work with clients from developmental, systemic, relational, and multicultural perspectives that inform theoretical lens to better conceptualize the needs of young clients. In this chapter, we describe various perspectives of child and adolescent client needs using theoretical approaches and modalities. Here, the authors discuss the following approaches: strengths-based approaches, experiential-based learning (EBL), social-emotional learning (SEL), relational approaches, systemic approaches, multidisciplinary approaches, group counseling, trauma-informed counseling (TIC), neurofeedback, and motivational interviewing (MI). Additionally, the authors discuss systemic contexts, the use of creativity, relational context, and multiculturalism to illuminate how intersectionality occurs with the perspective of each approach.

STRENGTHS-BASED APPROACHES

Literature examining strength concepts extends beyond an individual's inherent talent. Strength promotes energy when individuals experience successful performances and foster motivation to engage and remain productive. The strength perspective provides a positive paradigm that allows counselors to see the glass as half full rather than half empty. In such strengths-based approaches, counselors place emphasis on clients' assets rather than their deficits or problems (Burt et al., 1998). Strengths-based approaches present a dramatic paradigm shift in psychotherapy, from the medical model (which focused on pathology) to a model that stresses on developing assets (Seligman, 2011; Walsh, 2004). Focusing on strengths does not mean ignoring challenges or spinning struggles into strengths. Rather, a strength focus allows the counselor to place emphasis on health and well-being. This positive, strengths-based approach aids in empowering children and adolescents to learn, grow, and succeed in and out of school.

Well-known traditional counseling theories currently highlight strengths-based perspectives. *The Adlerian theory* uses the term encouragement and describes the process of developing a child's inner resources with the courage to make positive choices (Adler & Porter, 1931). Within the *behavioral theories,* principles of positive reinforcements provide practical steps toward behavior modification and shaping of desired outcomes within children and adolescents. Furthermore, Frankl's (1963) *logotherapy,* which may be used with some adolescents, forms a cornerstone for strengths-based counseling, with its emphasis on the search to find meaning out of adverse life circumstances. *Cognitive behavioral therapy* recognizes that clients need to restructure their negative thoughts to facilitate change in their behavior. The key concepts of *relational-cultural theory (RCT),* such as growth-fostering relationships, relational resilience, zest, authenticity, and mutual empathy, underscore the strengths-based positive orientation of human nature (Duffey & Somody, 2011). Therapists with social constructivist and postmodern assumptions may engage in solution-building conversations with their clients (de Shazer, 1985, 1994) through *solution-focused brief therapy (SFBT),* resulting in optimism and confidence (de Shazer, 1988). Additionally, they may use narrative strategies so that clients can retell their life stories and portray themselves as survivors rather than victims within the *narrative therapy* framework.

STRENGTHS-BASED APPROACHES FROM A DEVELOPMENTAL PERSPECTIVE

Strengths-based interventions need to be developmentally appropriate. Strengths-based counseling provides a theoretical and practice framework designed to engage counseling professionals in capacity and asset building across a person's life span (Benson et al., 1995). Early in age, "children need to develop and use as many of their strengths of character as possible" (Peterson, 2006, p. 157). Character strengths, defined as "pre-existing qualities that arise naturally, feel authentic (and) are intrinsically motivation to use" (Brdar & Kashdan, 2010, p. 151), subsist as the foundation of lifelong healthy development. Character strengths serve as protective factors and aid in mitigating psychopathology and enabling flourishing qualities (Park & Peterson, 2008). Members of the counseling profession consider Peterson and Seligman's (2004) Values In Action (VIA) classification system of virtues and character strengths as an empirically measurable guiding framework for a strengths-based approach. The system comprises six virtues divided into 24 subordinate character strengths (visit www.viacharacter.org to see the detailed description of the framework and to take the free online test). Clinicians use two age-appropriate assessments to measure character strengths: (a) VIA Youth Survey (for ages 10–17) and (b) VIA Adult Survey (for ages 18+). Character strength categories provide the necessary help that enables counselors to identify a client's positive attributes, focus on what appears to be going right in a person's life, and place such strengths within an overall framework of the client's psychological and social functioning (Peterson & Seligman, 2004).

RELATIONAL CONSIDERATION IN STRENGTHS-BASED APPROACHES

Building meaningful relationships and activities grounded firmly in the strengths of individuals and communities remains the primary focus of strengths-based approaches in counseling children and adolescents. This focus appears to be juxtaposed to connecting with others from a perspective of "what is wrong." Contrarily, a strengths-based framework supports the starting point of "what is right with people" (Seligman, 2011). Positive change occurs in the context of authentic relationships, which begins the journey of transformation to a place "unknown" from a familiar place of confidence and comfort. By facilitating a mutually empathic and supportive relationship, clients can know someone cares and will be there unconditionally for them. Clients then take risks, drawing upon their resources of motivation and hope, and create sustainable change through experiential growth.

STRENGTHS-BASED APPROACHES USING SYSTEMIC PERSPECTIVES

Strengths-based approaches value the capacity, skills, knowledge, connections, and potential in not just individuals but also communities (Pattoni, 2012). In incorporating a strengths-based framework, counselors need to take the whole system of family, school, and close peer relationships into consideration.

Family System

While working with young kids, strengths-based parent education may appear ubiquitous. When strengths-based approaches appear in parent education, parents tend to display improved effect, make more positive statements about their child, and also exhibit more physical affection toward their children (Steiner, 2011). In working from a strengths-based perspective, counselors help parents positively conceptualize their children's behavior. For example, professionals may coach parents of children with autism in identifying positive characteristics of their children and their relationship. This appears particularly beneficial because the stressors associated with the disability develop into chronic stressors, which may become difficult to master (Gray, 2006). Thus, engaging in a strengths-based approach necessitates viewing the positive aspects of a child's behavior, highlighting areas of competence and identifying areas that facilitate development.

Peer System

Strengths-based approaches not only involve family but peer relationships. Positive Peer Culture (PPC) emerged as one of the programs developed to counteract negative peer groups, which form within educational and social settings (Commonwealth, 2007). The goal of the program grew to one which teaches students how to help one another when challenges arise. Students assist in creating a climate where positivity flourishes and they can reflect on their decisions and actions toward others (Commonwealth, 2007). PPC groups help students to overcome the influences of negative peer interaction and promote positive change between their peers.

School System

In addition to developing academic excellence, schools stand as ideal institutions for teaching and building students' strengths and psychological well-being (Benninga et al., 2006; Peterson, 2006). Without a doubt, ameliorating suffering and negative experiences such as bullying, substance abuse, and other unhealthy behaviors remains a goal for schools. However, when schools put in place practices that systematically build character and well-being, they move from being a "police department" to "the good school" (Peterson, 2006, p. 284). With the American School Counselor Association recognizing the limitations of the traditional deficit-reduction emphasis in school counseling, Akos and Galassi (2008) proposed the Strengths-Based School Counseling model (SBSC) displays and indicates that "it is difficult to imagine school counselors impacting development for all students without operating from a strengths-based perspective" (p. 66). This paradigm shift involves a movement away from a primary emphasis on pathology and deficits that impede development in a small percentage of students, to a primary focus on personal strengths and environments that facilitate positive development for all students (Akos & Galassi, 2008). Counselors direct strengths-based positive psychological interventions at the individual and institutional levels. With the rapid growth of applying concepts such as the "positive education" (Oades et al., 2011), the "enabling institutions," and "the good school" (Peterson, 2006, p. 284), strengths-based interventions in educational institutions appear to be progressively gaining momentum at fostering academic excellence.

STRENGTHS-BASED APPROACHES FROM A MULTICULTURAL PERSPECTIVE

Every individual possesses strengths. They need to be recognized, celebrated, edified, and used. The goal of positive youth development (PYD) should not be merely surviving in the face of adversity but flourishing and thriving. Measures of problems, deficits, and weaknesses remain plentiful within education and mental health, whereas positive development practices appear to be missing. Identifying and understanding each individual's character strength profile provides essential bases for individually tailored interventions for children from diverse backgrounds. School counselors who adopt a strengths-based approach can "relanguage" their counseling practice by expanding their vocabulary to highlight student strengths. For example, while working with students with a history of disability or low achievement (if the focus remains on their "signature strengths"), the counselor brings out the client's optimism, hope, and confidence. In doing so, they frame problems from a strengths-based perspective as well as help students to see potential strengths in their weaknesses (White & Waters, 2015).

INFUSING CREATIVITY IN STRENGTHS-BASED APPROACHES

The strengths-based paradigms of *positive psychology* (Seligman, 2002) offer new approaches for bolstering psychological resilience and promoting mental health. Counselors offer creative ways of incorporating positive psychological interventions within intake, assessment, and evaluation phases by asking for positive introductions, identifying signature strengths, writing gratitude journals, savoring assignments, composing a family tree of strengths, and putting strengths in action plan (Gladding, 2016; Rashid, 2015).

TIME-EFFICIENT METHODS AND STRENGTHS-BASED APPROACHES

Counselors characterize strengths-based approaches as goal-oriented. They measure individuals' strengths and mobilize them to continuously move forward toward goal-setting. The goal orientation principle in SFBT and MI, for example, invites clients to explore their best selves in a defined time frame. The use of an appreciative inquiry framework enables the development of affirmative skills to identify strengths and provide support.

EXPERIENTIAL-BASED LEARNING

Based on the principles of interdisciplinary and constructivist learning, EBL embodies learner experiences through reflecting, reconstructing, and evaluating (Andresen et al., 2000). EBL supports a participative learner-centered approach with a focus on engagement, holistic learning, social and cultural applications, relatable applications, and prior experiences. In the experiential learning environment, learners analyze their experiences and construct their reality and meaning, either individually or in groups. EBL applies to informal education around the world, and it promotes student self-awareness with multicultural and ethical implications of learning and teaching (Andresen et al., 2000).

EBL theories provide various learning models, among which the Kolb's development of Lewinian experiential learning cycle applies. Kolb's model posits that knowledge results from grasping and transforming experiences. Kolb describes learning as the combined product of concrete experiences, abstract conceptualizations, and reflective observations. Such an approach to EBL emphasizes how experiences, including cognition, environmental factors, and emotions, influence the learning process.

EXPERIENTIAL-BASED LEARNING FROM A DEVELOPMENTAL PERSPECTIVE

EBL stands as a vital resource in the developmental process of children and adolescents. According to the study by Newman et al. (2017), experiential learning through groups and teams revealed a positive relationship in the youth's development. Teams that participated in adventure therapy and outdoor education resulted in increased positive development in prosocial character as well as in life skill development (Newman et al., 2017). Furthermore, developmentally appropriate teaching and active learning strategies consist of service learning, field investigations, group projects, and interactive classroom sessions along with active learning styles in education, which enhance students' attitudes, behaviors, and overall knowledge (Alexandar & Poyyamoli, 2014).

EXPERIENTIAL-BASED LEARNING FROM RELATIONAL CONSIDERATIONS

Virginia Satir pioneered a relational approach using experiential-based educational processes (Woods & Martin, 1984), a connection that remains vital when providing EBL (Pasco et al., 2012). Studies show that individuals who participated in experiential exercises and role-play practice demonstrated increased self-efficacy, communication, and relationship-building skills (Pasco et al., 2012).

EXPERIENTIAL-BASED LEARNING FROM SYSTEMIC APPROACHES

A systemic approach to education encompasses a case-based classroom experiential learning environment (Georgiou et al., 2008). Experiential learning consists of reflective observations, real experiences, and experiments with abstract conceptualizations (Georgiou et al., 2008). Systemic instruction promotes learning via general and theoretical principles that offer experiential influence.

Family System

Families play a vital role in children and adolescent learning. Through the support of experiential learning, students can foster growth within their family systems. Students with strong family support achieve higher academic success (Jeynes, 2005). Parental involvement in homework, school activities, and social events showed a positive effect on students' academic achievements (Jeynes, 2005). Thus, families who directly support children and adolescents produce higher levels of academic achievement in students.

Peer System

EBL regards peer interactions as a crucial part in the success of students. A Michigan school in the Montcalm Outdoor Challenge Program tailors student learning to peer support by providing project-based activities with peer groups (Commonwealth, 2007). In this program, students participate in service, experiential, and electives (SEE). SEE activities involve student-to-student groups, the enhancement of interpersonal relationships, and the fostering of leadership skills. Student activities include primitive fire building skills, ground-based group building initiatives, water navigation skills, orienteering skills, earth shelter construction, art projects, creative writing activities, earth oven cooking, and music (Commonwealth, 2007).

School System

Encouraging a "whole-school" connectedness allows students to experience a sense of belonging in their school environment. According to Rowe and Stewart (2009), child and adolescent health, social well-being, and education stand as essential components for experiential student learning. Taking a comprehensive whole-school approach to promote school connectedness involves family, school personnel, and the community (Rowe & Stewart, 2009). The Health Promoting School (HPS) model, used in school settings to promote connectedness, addresses the school holistically. It assesses the curriculum, teaching, school policies, procedures, organization, physical and social environment, as well as families, community, health services, and community agencies (Rowe & Stewart, 2009). In their research study, Rowe and Stewart (2009) conduct interviews and focus groups that reveal how social cohesion and social capital coexist as essential parts of school connectedness among students.

EXPERIENTIAL-BASED LEARNING FROM A MULTICULTURAL PERSPECTIVE

Experiential learning can take place in blended environments that facilitate multicultural competency (Roux et al., 2018). While serving culturally diverse clients, it is important to consider their cultural values and beliefs, as cultural sensitivity aids in communication and lack thereof poses significant barriers (Logan et al., 2014).

Multicultural counseling shifted from the monocultural perspective to a more humanistic view, becoming more aware and knowledgeable along with the implementation of an experiential-based curriculum (Hill, 2003). With a paradigm shift beyond the monocultural view to multiculturalism, counseling educators may aim to incorporate multicultural counseling competency development among students and counselors-in-training through reflective and experiential teaching and learning practices (Sue et al., 2019). Therefore, EBL effectively helps in meeting differences in students' communication, learning styles, and problem-solving as well as provides a culturally relevant, student-oriented, curriculum-based intervention (Hill, 2003; Sue et al., 2019).

Integrating a cultural worldview perspective within the curricula of practicum/internship courses promotes experiential learning (Hill, 2003).

INFUSING CREATIVITY USING EXPERIENTIAL-BASED LEARNING

Lewis and Williams (1994) highlight two types of EBL: (a) field-based experiences and (b) classroom-based learning. They promote creative examples of ways to incorporate these approaches when counseling children and adolescents through field-based experiences (e.g., internships, practicums, cooperative education, shadowing, peer coaching, mentoring, apprenticeships, student teaching, and service learning). Other creative classroom EBL approaches include role-playing, games, case studies, simulations, and various types of group work (Lewis & Williams, 1994). Additionally, Jackson (1992) includes panel, debate, buzz groups, screened speech, small/large group collaboration, autobiographies, visual maps, in-depth inquiry, file card feedback, reflective journals, letters to prospective students, student-developed criteria, student-select evaluators, and developed individualized plans as viable EBL techniques. This also includes art, which can be easily integrated with a variety of theoretical approaches, including solution-focused, person-centered, and cognitive behavioral therapy (CBT). An example would be asking students to draw a picture of their family or neighborhood. Also, prop interventions allow students to engage in dialogue by holding a prop.

TIME-EFFICIENT METHODS USING EXPERIENTIAL-BASED LEARNING

Children and adolescents can participate in EBL interventions such as solution-focused brief activities that encourage internal schemas to assist in problem-solving and social issues (Dansereau et al., 2013). Adventure-based counseling (ABC), an intervention that can be implemented in school settings, includes group juggling, team tasks, or a blind maze, where one student leader guides other students through a maze (Dansereau et al., 2013). Interventions facilitated by professional school counselors with their students continue to be necessary for positive growth-fostering relationships (Dansereau et al., 2013).

SOCIAL-EMOTIONAL LEARNING

SEL provides an avenue for multidimensional growth for children and adolescents. Rooted in Bandura's Social Cognitive Learning Theory (1997), SEL assists individuals with tools for developing behavior patterns adequate to cope with personal and environmental stressors.

SOCIAL-EMOTIONAL LEARNING FROM A DEVELOPMENTAL PERSPECTIVE

Ee and Ong (2014) define SEL as "the process of developing knowledge and skills in understanding and managing emotions, empathizing, and caring for others, building and maintaining positive relationships, making responsible decisions as well as dealing with challenging issues in an effective manner" (p. 26). Hence, SEL remains an appropriate theory for providing personal, social, and emotional maturity with children and adolescents.

A SEL framework offers the following measures: self-awareness, social awareness, self-management, relationship management, and responsible decision-making. Self-awareness involves how accurately an individual appraises their strengths and weaknesses, identifies their emotions, and their ability to understand their own values and attitudes (Ee & Ong, 2014). Social awareness describes a person's ability to empathize and understand the needs of others and to appreciate diversity.

SOCIAL-EMOTIONAL LEARNING FROM A RELATIONAL APPROACH

The literature defines self-management as a person's capability of managing their own reactions and emotions in a disciplined manner (Ee & Ong, 2014). Relationship management involves the ability to resolve conflict, listen effectively, and build and maintain relationships (Ee & Ong, 2014). Lastly, Taylor and Kilgus (2014) define responsible decision-making as the means by which an individual effectively identifies and analyzes life problems. Decision-making can be viewed as *responsible* based on whether a person can weigh the pros and cons of a decision, consider their own strengths and areas for growth, and determine how the solution can affect future outcomes in relation to others.

SYSTEMIC APPROACHES

A myriad of issues can arise when children and adolescents lack social-emotional skills, including with family, peers, and school. Failure to develop these vital skills can result in frequent peer conflicts, underdeveloped relational strategies, long-standing familial strain, and impaired academic performance (Taylor & Kilgus, 2014). Children and adolescents with social-emotional skill deficits exhibit a higher utilization of referrals, increased dropout rates in school settings, poor discipline in school and home, and increased problematic behaviors (Taylor & Kilgus, 2014). In contrast, children and adolescents with higher capabilities in their SEL show improved outcomes within family, peer, and educational systems (Dugas, 2017).

Family System

In the most ideal situation, family systems positively reinforce SEL. Typically, continuous systemic disruptions (e.g., poverty, trauma, lack of parental skills, and mental health concerns) inhibit this type of learning (Taylor & Kilgus, 2014). Youth who grow up with such disruptions will exhibit a lack of self-control and poor concentration. Counselors who work with children and adolescents should meet with family members to help reinforce SEL skills at home.

Peer System

Peers provide an avenue for growth and development of social learning tools. Contemporary literature describes the value of peers regarding social learning (Taylor & Kilgus, 2014). Unhealthy peer relations, often seen as correlational with poor familial relations and subpar academic performance, should also be conceptualized when working with this population. Counselors should consider how peer relation formation assists their clients in the development of social and emotional skills.

School System

Morgan (2014) describes the possible benefits of implementing SEL within the context of the classroom to include improving student engagement, helping them to do their best work, and increasing success potential. Research describes SEL as the missing piece in educational settings (Bridgeland et al., 2013). Since SEL posits a redirection toward a differentiated approach, this can improve skills, which make students increasingly ready for life as opposed to more content-based curricula focused on course knowledge. Despite a large number (93%) of teachers and counselors who reported their belief of SEL to be vital to their students' growth and development, only 28% of high school teachers surveyed reported the use of SEL programming in their schools (Dugas, 2017). This also holds true in counseling. SEL now emerges as a strong modality in the counseling field.

INFUSING CREATIVITY USING SOCIAL-EMOTIONAL LEARNING

The counseling profession defines *creativity* as "a broad term for practices that typically include a variety of therapeutic approaches used in a creative way" (Rosen & Atkins, 2014, p. 292). Therefore, counselors working with students and clients infuse creativity with various learning styles or developmental stages. To infuse creativity with SEL, teachers, professional school counselors, and clinical mental health counselors may need to think beyond the scope of their own pedagogic training in order to implement strategies. This may require synthesis with structured modalities along with impromptu activities.

Contemporary literature recommends differentiated instruction as strategies for teachers to meet students, where they guide them in their educational path more effectively (Birnie, 2015; Dugas, 2017; Levy, 2008). Further, Wallin and Durr (2002) recommend the following techniques: students writing short stories about self-control; artwork about anger control issues/consequences of responsible behavior; music and poetry for teaching students how to avoid problem behaviors; and peer-facilitated feedback about character enhancing and problem-solving. Students can also play games and discuss methods for achieving academic success. These techniques can be modified based on the developmental stage or chronologic age of the students.

TIME-EFFICIENT METHODS

The counseling profession recommends and encourages the use of effective methods; therefore, replication of such processes could prove to be time-efficient. The Collaborative for Academic, Social, and Emotional Learning (CASEL; 2020) website (www.casel.org) provides five recommended actions for implementing SEL within school settings. These five actions include the following: (a) communicate the value of SEL and the school's commitment to social-emotional competencies to staff and families; (b) develop an action plan collaboratively with stakeholders for adoption, implementation, and evaluation of systematic needs; (c) commit time and monetary support toward professional development for educators; (d) ensure that the school make dedicated resources available for adoption and implementation processes; and (e) create intentional processes to avoid SEL being taken away from important academic instruction.

RELATIONAL APPROACHES

RCT emerged from the belief that traditional psychotherapeutic frameworks excluded the relational experiences of women and other cultural groups (Comstock et al., 2008).

To be more inclusive, RCT provided a model across the life span that continues a focus on relational development (Comstock et al., 2008). More specifically, RCT emphasizes the value and impact of mutual empathy to promote healing in growth-fostering relationships (Comstock et al., 2008).

RELATIONAL APPROACHES FROM A DEVELOPMENTAL PERSPECTIVE

RCT focuses on individual growth and development through growth-fostering relationships (Jordan, 2000). Jordan (2000) discussed how individuals learn, throughout the life span, to move toward mutuality and stay away from separation. To be more exact, mutual empathy and mutual empowerment continue to be key to the healthy development of individuals at any given time (Jordan, 2000). Therefore, development cannot exist outside of the context of the relationship and in return, development serves as the final aim to foster mutually empathic and empowering relationships (Miller & Stiver, 1997).

RELATIONAL CONSIDERATIONS

As Jordan (2000) emphasized, RCT consists of seven core tenets (see Figure 6.1):

1. Individuals grow throughout the life span toward and through relationships.
2. Individuals become mature and functioning through mutuality, not separation.
3. Psychological growth means being able to participate in diverse relational networks.
4. Individuals involved in a relationship must show not only mutual empathy, but also mutual empowerment, so that the relationship continues to be growth-fostering.
5. Individuals must be authentic in order to demonstrate real engagement in growth-fostering relationships.
6. As a result of participating in and contributing to growth-fostering relationships, individuals grow in that development process.
7. Individuals ought to realize their increased relational competence over the life span and through their growth-fostering relationships.

SYSTEMIC APPROACHES

Counselors who practice RCT emphasize the importance of growth-fostering relationships within family, peer, and school systems. RCT offers a guideline in working with various systems. As Jordan (2004) specified, a healthy system assists individuals to move from holding *control over* each other to sharing a supported vulnerability; to showing mutual empathy and support for all members of the system moving away from one-way support; and to creating meaning in an expansive relational manner rather than in a self-centered way. In this perspective and approach, members of the system become more resilient and more relationally competent. This relational competence stimulates depth and meaning in relationships.

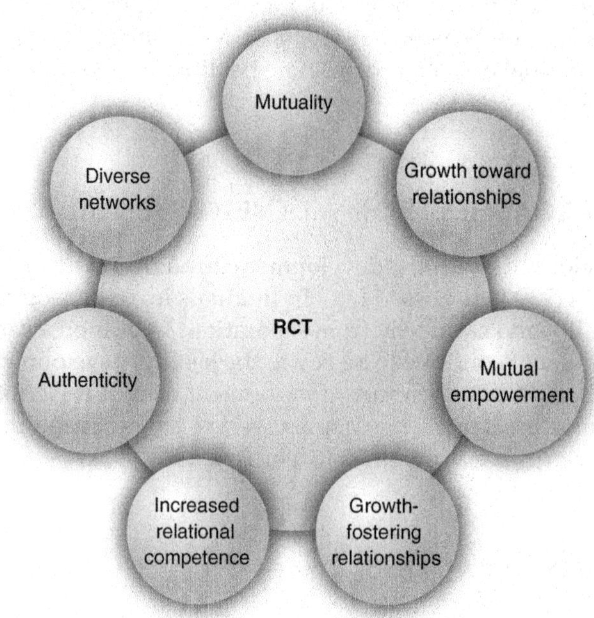

FIGURE 6.1 Relational-cultural theory principles.

RCT, relational-cultural theory.

Source: Jordan, J. V. (2018). *Relational-cultural therapy* (2nd ed.). American Psychological Association.

Family System

According to Jordan (2010), growth of any individual depends on the individual's growth-fostering connections. Therefore, family systems and relationships within this system become an integral part of individuals' identity and growth process. As Miller (1986) highlighted, every healthy connection consists of several characteristics to include a sense of zest, which refers to a sense of well-being stemming from growth-fostering relationships; empowered individuals with motivation to take action; an understanding of one's self and others in the context of a relationships; an understanding of one's thoughts and feelings; and finally, a strong system that promotes action.

Peer and School System

RCT emphasizes the development of growth-fostering relationships crucial for adolescents who struggle with a sense of belonging in a group (Akos, 2005). In early adolescence, individuals strive to understand their identity as independent individuals. During this time, peer groups become an inseparable part of their lives. This becomes the time when adolescents experience challenges in uncovering their own authentic selves, connection with their peers, and forming their desired relationships. Therefore, it remains imperative for professional school counselors and clinical mental health counselors to use RCT as a means to assist adolescents in navigating through this confusing time of their lives. As a part of that confusion, adolescents experience rapid developmental changes, so counselors must possess a culture of connection rather than disconnection. This will provide a safe environment for students to engage in growth-fostering relationships, through which they can learn about themselves and others (Robb, 2006).

MULTICULTURAL PERSPECTIVE

Sole acquisition of multicultural knowledge does not guarantee culturally sensitive practices and attitudes (Alberta & Wood, 2009; Arredondo & Toporek, 2004). RCT can play an important role in connecting with individuals and assisting them in developing mutual empathy and mutual empowerment, which can result in the development of growth-fostering relationships. Furthermore, counselors sometimes fail to consider the contextual factors of clients' stories when helping them navigate through mainstream culture. Duffey and Somody (2011) suggested that this dismissal may result in disconnection in the counseling session, ultimately causing clients to feel misunderstood. Therefore, it becomes significantly important for counselors to increase their skills and competence in understanding and reflecting upon contextual factors.

INFUSING CREATIVITY USING RELATIONAL APPROACHES

Jordan (2010) based RCT on changing attitudes, rather than techniques; however, RCT does not prohibit the use of creative techniques that do not contrast with the relational-based nature of this theory. Some of the creative techniques include music, art, and expressive writing. Mainly, RCT utilizes therapeutic authenticity and mutual empathy to meet the therapeutic goals.

TIME-EFFICIENT METHODS

Clinicians do not consider RCT to be a short-term counseling approach. RCT focuses on deepening relational connections that, in nature, require time to establish. However, some practitioners utilized RCT in short-term services. Even in using RCT as a short-term counseling approach, the counselor still places emphasis on raising awareness about relational patterns and images and building skills for healthier connections. Clinicians consider the lack of counselor emphasis on termination to be the difference between short-term and long-term RCT.

GROUP COUNSELING

Counselors view group counseling, an essential element for providing a sense of connectedness with others, to be copiously beneficial for individuals across their life span. The literature highlights various authors in the development of group counseling concepts (e.g., Moreno, Yalom, Prat, and others). The profession recognizes Bruce Tuckman, a well-known psychologist, for his group counseling terms "forming, storming, norming, and performing" (1965, p. 396). This four-stage group process depicts how groups span from the initial stage of a first group session, working through conflict concerns, reaching cohesion, and ending with flexibility and functionality (Tuckman, 1965). Knowing these group stages can aid the counselor in awareness about how groups form. In relating this to children and adolescents, group counseling offers numerous advantages. Children and adolescents face similar struggles as adults and experience feelings of disconnection with others. By participating in group counseling, children and adolescents could enhance feelings of relatedness to others in a phenomenon known as universality. Universality happens when group members grasp the notion that others experience similar experiences (Fineran et al., 2016).

Yalom (2008), another primary-source author popular in group counseling literature, posits along with Tuckman (1965) that the salient outcomes of group counseling consist of feelings of universality, development of social skills, emotional regulation, and group cohesiveness. Further, group counseling offers a safe environment for children and adolescents to process their feelings, gain peer acceptance and support, and receive the opportunity to help support peers through their struggles (Fineran et al., 2016).

GROUP COUNSELING FROM A DEVELOPMENTAL PERSPECTIVE

When planning and organizing a group, group leaders will want to consider the group's goals, and pay specific attention to the developmental stages of the children and adolescents (Fineran et al., 2016). Considering the notion that all children develop uniquely, group leaders could benefit from acknowledging that some children fit better in individual counseling. Also, it remains vital for group leaders to consider incorporating inclusion and exclusion criteria for the group. At times, group leaders may make every attempt to create a template for an exceptional group, and feel a sense of frustration if the group does not turn out as planned (e.g., when one child becomes disruptive). Even with proper planning, groups ebb and flow, and predicting the outcome may be difficult. Children and adolescents develop with unique ways of responding to counseling interventions. After the group leadership experience, group leaders can assess the level of achievement of their goals and objectives and adjust accordingly.

Also, when creating a group, group leaders will want to remain cognizant that chronologic age does not always coincide with developmental level. Some group leaders may choose to incorporate varying levels of development while others may not, which appears to be contingent on the group's goals. However, children and adolescents who possess a developmental delay frequently lack feelings of inclusion and social interactions (Grunblatt, 2016).

RELATIONAL CONSIDERATIONS FOR GROUP COUNSELING

A considerable number of children and adolescents' concerns derive from disruptions in relationships. Children and adolescents come to group counseling with an array of abusive experiences (e.g., neglect, sexual, emotional) and relationship concerns with parents, teachers, peers, or siblings (Grunblatt, 2016). However, a group leader, after establishing an awareness of these relational dynamics, can observe group member behaviors and tailor the sessions to help build relational connections. The children and adolescents in the group may reside in family situations lacking healthy, relational connections. If this appears to be true, the group leader can model a healthy and safe authority figure.

SYSTEMIC APPROACHES TO CONSIDER DURING GROUP COUNSELING

Children and adolescents, just as adults, live in a world with numerous rich contexts. Having the group leader experience a child or adolescent's inner world and how they relate during sessions provides benefits in group counseling. Group counseling, in a sense, can be seen as a little society on its own. The group members bring to the group their viewpoints of caretakers, siblings, school, sports, and other areas. How they relate to the group members allows the group leader to see into their world.

Family System

Every child and adolescent commences group counseling with experience from at least one group—their family system. This may or may not be a growth-fostering system for the child or adolescent. Their family structure may be working through addiction, family conflicts, siblings leaving for college, divorce, and numerous other family system issues (Grunblatt, 2016). These experiences could lead the child to feeling isolated, disconnected and unwanted. Despite the group being in a private practice, school, or inpatient setting, group leaders will want to glean information about the members' family systems. To best understand a child, or an adult, group leaders need to consider the contextual factors of a family system.

Peer System

Learning to relate to their fellow peers, children and adolescents could develop essential social skills and prosocial behaviors (Hoorn et al., 2016). Both social acceptance and approval coexist as important elements for child and adolescent development. Children grow into adolescence, and their peers' opinions increase in importance. A crucial aspect of Bandura's (1986) Social Learning Theory (as discussed in Chapter 1) examines how peer influence leads to social change. According to this theory, adolescents view and learn social behaviors from their peers, especially if their peers reinforce their behavior. For example, a child may see his best friend playing baseball, they learn how to throw and catch the ball, and the best friend cheers when the child catches the ball. Hence, a group setting could be ideal for fostering positive change for children or adolescents' behavior. In addition, peer acceptance often becomes a good motivator for a child to change their behavior (Grunblatt, 2016). A group leader could guide the group to achieve certain tasks together to promote social learning, and ideally, prosocial tendencies will then result in desired outcomes.

School System

The school system continues to be an integral part of children and adolescent's development. During their time in school, students experience their own specific school culture and its associated nuances. Several groups that students may encounter in school may involve teachers, parents/caregivers, other students, and the like. With all these varying groups already in place, group leaders will want to be aware of the school culture and climate.

Professional school counselors reside in school settings and serve as vital supports for helping children and adolescents navigate their developmental growth. They help students in areas of academic achievement, social/emotional development, and career development. School counselors facilitate different groups with a few core groups presented in psychoeducational and task group formats.

MULTICULTURAL PERSPECTIVE DURING GROUP COUNSELING

Group counselors should envision culture from a broad viewpoint. Every group consists of a unique blend of members who bring with them their own worldviews of family, friends, culture, race, and an emergence of defined ideas about genders and sexual orientation, for example. It remains imperative that group leaders continuously seek additional training about multicultural topics.

INFUSING CREATIVITY IN GROUP COUNSELING

Children and adolescents develop through and with creative endeavors. Incorporating creativity in group counseling remains a long-standing practice for counselors as they must continually engage group members with creative ideas, tasks, games, or processes (Gladding, 2016). According to Duffey et al. (2016), school-age children and socially young children often stay in tune with their creativity. Their creative experiences and imaginations make children and adolescents curious about life and excellent at problem-solving. Unfortunately, as youths grow into adulthood, they become socialized and lose touch with their creative selves (Duffey et al., 2016). Group counselors can tap into their once (or current) creative mind-sets and use this energy to create cohesion and optimal functioning within the group.

TIME-EFFICIENT METHODS FOR GROUP COUNSELING

Sometimes school and inpatient settings require brief group sessions with time limitations. This may result in group counselor mindfulness of asking group members to process at deep levels. Processing trauma or grief at deeper levels, for example, may open a child or adolescent to a vulnerable state. A time restraint may then limit group members from adequately working through their presenting concern.

ADDITIONAL APPROACHES AND MODALITIES

TRAUMA-INFORMED COUNSELING

TIC and best practices continue to evolve, and counselors must understand the current literature and effectively apply sensory process treatment and cognitive treatments (Steele & Malchiodi, 2012). Counselors should steer away from solely using cognitive-based theories with children and adolescents since the trauma may not be primarily cognitive. Counselors should seek additional training for TIC skills and use their creativity to connect children and adolescents to their trauma, while also respecting their space to grieve, be scared, or feel withdrawn. More information on TIC will be addressed in Chapter 12.

NEUROFEEDBACK

Clinicians define biofeedback modalities as specific interventions that can help children and adolescents learn about their mind–body connection and how to develop self-regulation skills (Marzbani et al., 2016). Marzbani et al. (2016) view neurofeedback as a division of biofeedback that uses quantitative electroencephalogram (qEEG) technology and operant conditioning to encourage change in brain wave activity. From this perspective, mental health concerns present as variations in brain wave frequencies. Neurofeedback protocols provide clients with audio and visual feedback for when their brain waves maintain a certain frequency band (Marzbani et al., 2016). Therefore, the client learns how to self-regulate their brain waves. Self-regulation of brain waves with neurofeedback training produces promising results for treatment of anxiety and trauma (Jones & Hitsman, 2018; van der Kolk et al., 2016), sleep disorders (Cheon et al., 2015), and attention deficit hyperactivity disorder (ADHD; Van Doren et al., 2019). Currently, neurofeedback appears to be increasingly researched (Marzbani et al., 2016). This research aids professionals with knowledge about neuroscience-infused treatments.

Different helping professions and clinicians treat mental health concerns with varying protocols, theories behind neurofeedback, and equipment. However, the basic structure of a neurofeedback session remains the same. For example, clients presented with an audio feedback protocol will hear the music clearly when they come into the desired threshold for the brain waves. Though, if the client maintains a certain undesirable brain wave frequency, the music will lower in volume and make it difficult to hear. The practitioner presets the thresholds for the neurofeedback protocols. The practitioner recognizes these as set thresholds on the computer software and determines this by the qEEG, symptoms, or standardized protocols. See Figure 6.2 for the neurofeedback demonstration.

Neurofeedback appears to present promising outcomes for children and adolescents. For example, EEG brain wave data show variations in certain areas of the brain connected with development (e.g., prefrontal cortex) and attention (Edwards, 2016). Edwards further states that neurofeedback aids children and adolescents in controlling their behavioral concerns. If children and adolescents learn how to self-regulate their behaviors, their peer and school relationships grow. From a developmental perspective, children and adolescents' brain chemistry will vary from genetics and experiences. To date, the majority of children and adolescent neurofeedback consists of using neurofeedback protocols for treating ADHD and improving attention. Whether receiving biofeedback or neurofeedback, counselors will want to consider a child or adolescents' culture and understanding of the brain (Harvey et al., 2015). For example, there are ranges of cultural norms surrounding substance abuse, modesty, and educational level when discussing biofeedback treatments (Harvey et al., 2015).

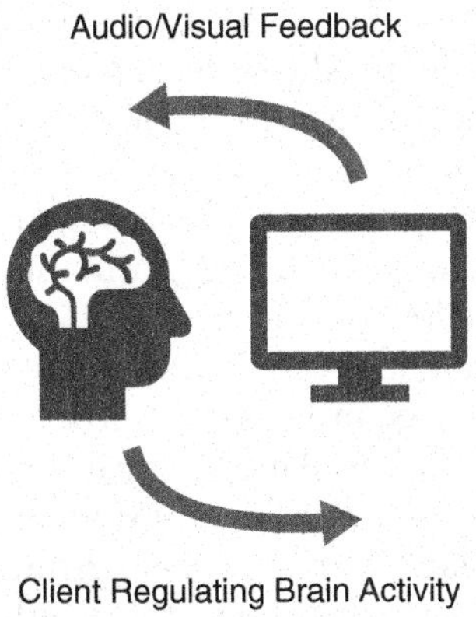

FIGURE 6.2 Neurofeedback demonstrations.

MINDFULNESS

Mindfulness originated from Eastern mind-sets, which require a person's full attention to the present moment without passing judgment on their self (Kabat-Zinn, 1990). In addition, mindfulness asks for a person to remain aware and open to their experience while remaining nonreactive (Testa & Sangganjanavanich, 2016). This skill can greatly benefit people at any age as it could offset anxiety and judgment toward self, to take a breath; and calm and recenter the self after an argument, high anxiety, a terrible test, and so forth. With a counselor's help, children and adolescents using mindfulness skills may develop greater levels of mental clarity and less anxiety or judgment toward themselves. Mindful yoga can be used as a mind–body skill, which focuses on breathing, holding postures, and movement. Other mind–body and mindfulness skills include meditation, tai chi, creative outlets (e.g., art, dance, music), guided imagery, and deep breathing (National Center for Complementary and Alternative Medicine, n.d.). Relationally and systemically, mindfulness fosters a sense of awareness with self and others. When the child or adolescent tunes into their breathing with their peers, fellow classmates, teachers, and family, they achieve a nonverbal, empathic connection. This may produce a ripple effect of empathy and compassion for varying levels within a system. Teachers can implement mindfulness skills before class begins or during the class as needed. Also, research suggests that professional school counselors hold a prime position to conduct mindfulness small-group sessions (Su & Swank, 2019). Brief mindfulness exercises appear to be successful at teaching attention (Su & Swank, 2019) and other skills. Because of this, teachers, counselors, and parents can integrate a brief mindful drawing exercise, meditation, or mindful movement to a morning or bedtime routine.

MOTIVATIONAL INTERVIEWING

MI, an effective framework that propels people to act, focuses on "arranging conversations so that people talk themselves into change, based on their own values and interests" (Miller & Rollnick, 2013, p. 4). MI can be beneficial for children and adolescents. Professional school counselors and counselors working in different environments may find MI to be efficacious when helping a child or adolescent walk through the change process. This involves different communication styles and the counselor knowing when to use them. The *directing style*, for example, refers to a counselor providing advice or instruction (Miller & Rollnick, 2013). Next, the *following style*, considered as the opposite of the directing style, can be illustrated in counseling when a child listens to a caretaker without talking back. Miller and Rollnick (2013) believe a middle style, *guiding communication style*, falls between the follower and the director. According to Miller and Rollnick (2013), most counselors use this style during their sessions.

Using MI, counselors also recognize the attention to ambivalence to be important during individual and group counseling sessions. A normality of the human experience seems to be a desire to change, yet the client experiences ambivalence to change at the same time (Miller & Rollnick, 2013). Ambivalence occurs when a person becomes slightly closer to the change marker versus the nonchange mind-set. Children and adolescents may be ambivalent about their identity and/or gender. Ambivalence about school work, peers, sports, or other activities and choices remains salient in children and adolescents' lives. To illustrate this concept, a child may find themself in an unsafe group of friends and bullying occurs. The child appears scared of losing their friend group and does not want to leave, but also knows the bullying can be hurtful. The child sees the school counselor, and the counselor works with them about their ambivalence toward losing friends versus being mistreated. Counselors using MI remain steadfast in not becoming fearful of the ambivalence present with a developing mind-set; instead, they use supportive skills and techniques. Therefore, a start of change for a person could be first moving to an ambivalent viewpoint.

INTEGRATED BEHAVIORAL HEALTH

Counselors view integrated behavioral healthcare (IBHC) as a fast-growing approach in the counseling profession. The Institute of Medicine (2001) designates the main goal of this approach to be increasing both the physical and mental health of patients from a holistic framework. Using an IBHC approach, primary care and behavioral health providers work together as a team to help patients and their families. Behavioral health consultants (BHCs) provide consultation to primary care physicians in order to provide patient-centered care by utilizing a systemic approach. This type of care considers behavioral and mental health factors that impact chronic illness and physical symptoms. Offering behavioral health services on primary care sites increases the likelihood of patients following through with their appointments, as they can visit not only their primary care physician but also their BHC all within one appointment.

CREATIVITY IN COUNSELING APPROACHES

Creativity can be a developmental, relational, and mutually growth-promoting quality when shared with others. Developmentally speaking, children communicate primarily through play (Kottman, 2014). Young children demonstrate play, by making art, making music, using humor, creating games, and using their imaginations (Duffey et al., 2016). Counselors working with creativity in counseling (CIC) promote growth within clients through innovative and relational means. Social connections and relationships support children's creativity. Counselors place emphasis on supporting the internal and therapeutic processes of creativity and expression among children and adolescents rather than primarily focusing on the analysis of the product. Counselors identify play therapy, art therapy, music therapy, dance/movement therapy (DMT), animal/pet-assisted therapy, expressive writing, and bibliotherapy as some of the most popular modalities of creative interventions among children and adolescents. See Table 6.1 for a detailed list of research-based creative interventive modalities utilized among children and adolescents. Often, creative interventions serve as a communication tool between therapists and children (Kottman, 2014). Using creative interventions like child play in counseling allows children to gain more information about their own lives, culture, and problems in a safe and accepting climate without judgment. CIC provides an appropriate environment for a child's reflection to develop cognitive skills and improve behavioral patterns, thus going beyond information gathering and assisting the youth in gaining optimal levels of insight. Furthermore, creativity within the counseling environment increases adaptive and relational skills of mutual empathy and openness (Lawrence et al., 2015). Also, by using creative problem-solving skills, counselors can foster growth within educational programs. Exhibit 6.1 provides a list of counseling organizations and conferences where counselors may seek opportunities for professional growth.

CHAPTER SUMMARY

The authors recommend theories for working with children and adolescents as a lens to further understand the needs of this population. Using various approaches and modalities, counselors in school and community settings can develop a more comprehensive understanding of the needs of clients and their families. Further, approaches and modalities can help counselors better understand the systems surrounding the client and how to develop a more effective support system. The authors provide at the end of this chapter a list of research-based, best-practice expressive arts interventions as well as a list of professional organizations and conferences where more information on expressive arts techniques may be obtained.

POINTS TO REMEMBER

- The profession encourages counselors who work with children and to stay cognizant of contextual, multicultural, and developmental factors.
- Counselors describe creativity as a salient tool for incorporating into all counseling theories for children and adolescents.
- Counseling theories highlight different aspects about child and adolescent development; however, all theories agree that counselors remain aware of individual variations during development.
- Counselors begin with a theoretical lens and during sessions they add tenets from other theories, approaches, or modalities, or tailor their current theory to meet their client's needs.
- Children and adolescents do not always express concerns verbally; hence, counselors infuse art, music, videos, or other creative modalities to enhance their communication.

OTHER HELPFUL INFORMATION FOR CONSIDERATION

See Table 6.1 for a comprehensive summary list of research-based, creative intervention studies done among children and adolescents and Exhibit 6.1 for a list of professional growth organizations and conferences for counselors.

- See Figure 6.1 to understand RCT.
- See Figure 6.2 to understand neurofeedback demonstration.
- Need for and Steps Toward a Clinical Guideline for the Telemental Healthcare of Children and Adolescents | *Journal of Child and Adolescent Psychopharmacology.*
- Review of Experimental Social Behavioral Interventions for Preschool Children: An Evidenced-Based Synthesis, Tonya Hall, 2020.

- Mindfulness- and Compassion-Based Interventions in Relational Contexts.
- Motivational Interviewing as Evidence-Based Practice? An Example from Sexual Risk Reduction Interventions Targeting Adolescents and Young Adults.
- Making Positive Changes Counseling (MPCC) Program: A Creative Adaptation of Motivational Interviewing for Use with Children in School Settings.
- Evidence-Based Psychosocial Treatments of Conduct Problems in Children and Adolescents: An Overview.
- Children and Adolescents Mental Health: A Systematic Review of Interaction-Based Interventions in Schools and Communities.
- Evidenced-Based Practices.
- Predictors of Use of Evidence-Based Practices for Children and Adolescents in Usual Care.
- Mindfulness Based Interventions for Youth.
- Evidence-Based Treatments for Children and Adolescents: Issues and Commentary.
- Investigating Adherence Promoters in Evidence-Based Mental Health Interventions with Children and Adolescents.
- Systematic Review and Meta-Analysis of Parent and Family-Based Interventions for Children and Adolescents with Chronic Medical Conditions.
- Mindfulness-Based Approaches with Children and Adolescents: A Preliminary Review of Current Research in an Emergent Field.
- A Systematic Review and Evaluation of Video Modeling, Role-Play and Computer-Based Instruction as Social Skills Interventions for Children and Adolescents with High-Functioning Autism.
- Practitioner Review: Cognitive Bias Modification for Mental Health Problems in Children and Adolescents: A Meta-Analysis.
- A Systematic Review of Strengths and Resilience Outcome Literature Relevant to Children and Adolescents.
- Effect of a Music Therapy Social Skills Training Program on Improving Social Competence in Children and Adolescents with Social Skills Deficits.
- Family-Based Interventions for Child and Adolescent Disorders.
- Attachment-Based Clinical Work with Children and Adolescents.
- Meta-Analysis of Trauma-Focused CBT for Treating posttraumatic stress disorder (PTSD) and Co-Occurring Depression Among Children and Adolescents.
- Ed Jacobs creative counseling interventions, books, and workshops: impacttherapy.com/

CASE STUDY 6.1

Blake, a straight-A, 14-year-old student, currently lives with his mother, grandmother, and two younger sisters. His high school recommended him for community-based counseling after a teacher found him in the library curled up in a fetal position under a desk. Historically, Blake demonstrated a good relationship with the school counselor, and always expressed a willingness to talk with her when he felt sad or anxious. However, when the school counselor met with him, Blake refused to talk. The school counselor called his mother, shared her concerns, and recommended a counselor in their area.

Blake met with the counselor and did not make eye contact due to his shyness and discomfort about talking with adults. He further self-reported a diagnosis of panic disorder with agoraphobia, generalized anxiety, and depression. He informed the counselor about his current medication but reported he does not believe the medicine to be effective. The counselor asked him what makes him feel comfortable; he said, "I like music. It helps me." After the first session, Blake's mother asked to speak with the counselor. She informed the counselor that Blake had struggled with anxiety since childhood. Blake's mother told the counselor that she recently left an abusive relationship. She informed the counselor that her ex-fiancé controlled, hit, and screamed at her in front of Blake. She regretted that Blake went through all of this, but stated it took a while to leave because of her limited support.

Presently, Blake and his mother and siblings live with their grandmother. His mother reported how Blake loves his grandmother and feels closest to one of his uncles who comes over frequently. His mother also reported Blake can become so anxious that he experiences panic attacks and can even pass out. She reported this to the school and asked for accommodations for him, but they told her anxiety did not constitute a diagnosis appropriate for an admission, review, and dismissal (ARD) meeting. She wants her son to succeed and appears afraid that his grades will be affected if he does not get help.

Activity 6.1: Questions for Further Discussion

- Based on the case vignette, identify Blake and his family's current needs.
- As a counselor, what type of approach or modality would you utilize when working with him?
- In what ways do you see the need to advocate for this client?
- How do multicultural, systemic, relational, and developmental perspectives shape your view of Blake?
- What strengths does Blake display that can support his progress in counseling?
- What type of creative strategies would you suggest for working with Blake to reduce his anxiety in and out of counseling sessions?

TABLE 6.1 CREATIVITY: RESEARCH-BASED EXPRESSIVE ARTS INTERVENTIONS

Study Citation and Hyperlink	Issue/Population Addressed	Creative Intervention Used	Outcome
1. Akesson, B., D'Amico, M., Denov, M., Khan, F., Linds, W., & Mitchell, C. A. (2014). "Stepping back" as researchers: Addressing ethics in arts-based approaches to working with war-affected children in school and community settings. *Educational Research for Social Change (ERSC), 3*(1), 75–89. https://ssrn.com/abstract=2476379	Ethical issues of art-based therapy with children are affected by global adversity, including children affected by war.	The study implemented the use of participatory arts-based methods such as photo voice, drama, and drawing.	Participatory arts-based methods help children affected by war to tell their stories.
2. Armstrong, S. N., & Richard, R. J. (2016). Integrating rap music into counseling with adolescents in disciplinary alternative education program. *Journal of Creativity in Mental Health, 11*(3–4), 423–435. https://doi.org/10.1080/15401383.2016.1214656	Coping response regulation is used with minority at-risk adolescent.	Incorporating rap music into counseling practices as listed in the following: Activity 1: Catching Feelings and Expressing Emotions • Teaches students to identify emotions and use effective coping skills. Activity 2: Dollars & Dreams • Encourages students to identify and differentiate values and goals; create goals based on values.	Creative techniques that incorporate music help adolescents understand and regulate coping responses to difficult and emotionally sensitive situations.

(*continued*)

TABLE 6.1 CREATIVITY: RESEARCH-BASED EXPRESSIVE ARTS INTERVENTIONS (*CONTINUED*)

Study Citation and Hyperlink	Issue/Population Addressed	Creative Intervention Used	Outcome
3. Bazargan, Y., & Pakdaman, S. (2016). The effectiveness of art therapy in reducing internalizing and externalizing problems of female adolescents. *Archives of Iranian Medicine (AIM), 19*(1). https://pdfs.semanticscholar.org/58a9/3df7fe10298857ce99f637a79dc40c732fb4.pdf	Issues addressed are reducing internalizing/externalizing problems in adolescent girls 14–18 years old.	Art therapy intervention is used with six painting sessions. Experimental. Groups and art therapy theories are used as interventions.	Counselors use art therapy to effectively reduce internal issues. More sessions are needed for external issues.
4. Beauregard, C. (2014). Effects of classroom-based creative expression programmes on children's well-being. *The Arts in Psychotherapy, 41*(3), 269–277. https://doi.org/10.1016/j.aip.2014.04.003	Children (5–17 years old) in school settings are the population. Exploring the effects of classroom-based creative expression interventions on children's mental health is addressed.	Art, drama group therapy, visual arts, music, dance/movements, sand trays in classroom setting at school are interventions used.	Improvement was found in hope, coping and resiliency, prosocial behaviors, self-esteem, impairment, emotional and behavioral problems. Reduced posttraumatic and depressive symptoms were displayed.
5. Bungay, H., & Vella-Burrow, T. (2013). The effects of participating in creative activities on the health and well-being of children and young people: A rapid review of the literature. *Perspectives in Public Health, 133*(1), 44–52. https://doi.org/10.1177/1757913912466946	Culturally appropriate health promoting strategies are presented in children 11–18 years old.	Music, dance, singing, drama, and visual arts are interventions used.	Creative activities can have a positive effect on behavioral changes, self-confidence, self-esteem, levels of knowledge, and physical activity.

6. Cortina, M. A., & Fazel, M. (2015). The Art Room: An evaluation of a targeted school-based group intervention for students with emotional and behavioral difficulties. *The Arts in Psychotherapy, 42*, 35–40. https://doi.org/10.1016/j.aip.2014.12.003	Students with emotional, behavioral difficulties and psychological difficulties that impede students' school experience are discussed.	Interventions used are a story, an object, and a work of art. The Art Room structured weekly interventions in a calm environment within the school for 1–2 sessions over a 10-week period. Questionnaires on psychological functioning were administered and teachers completed the SDQ and children completed the sMFQ.	Students showed a significant reduction in emotional and behavioral problems. Students report reduction in depressive symptoms and improvements of positive "prosocial" behavior.
7. Davis, E. S., Pereira, J. K., & Dixon, A. (2015). Introducing reality play therapy: Reactions and perceptions from elementary school counselors. *Journal of Creativity in Mental Health, 10*(4), 402–422. https://doi.org/10.1080/15401383.2015.1093984	Elementary school students are investigated by school counselors' perceptions of the introduction of reality play therapy through a series of trainings and its potential.	Reality therapy and play therapy (sand trays, puppets, and drawing) are interventions used based on the concepts of choice theory.	School counselors state reality play therapy is an option for working with upper-grade elementary students.
8. Davis, K. M. (2010). Music and the expressive arts with children experiencing trauma. *Journal of Creativity in Mental Health, 5*(2), 125–133. https://doi.org/10.1080/15401383.2010.485078	Case studies of Caucasian and Latinx backgrounds are studied in rural areas with children and adolescents in grades 3–5. Self-awareness and self-understanding including materials, facilitation, and processing of musical activities in group format are discussed.	Feelings Ensemble and Symphony interventions are applied with students composing and performing their own compositions regarding personal feelings.	Students were able to process their emotions better with their families.

(continued)

TABLE 6.1 CREATIVITY: RESEARCH-BASED EXPRESSIVE ARTS INTERVENTIONS (*CONTINUED*)

Study Citation and Hyperlink	Issue/Population Addressed	Creative Intervention Used	Outcome
9. Dilawari, K., & Tripathi, N. (2014). Art therapy: A creative and expressive process. *Indian Journal of Positive Psychology, 5*(1), 81. https://search.proquest.com/docview/1614312498?accountid=7122	Children and youth learn to deal with traumatic events, develop coping skills, reduce stress and anxiety, promote health, and increase self-esteem.	Interventions used are guided imagery, journaling, collages with magazines, mandala, art therapy (drawing, painting, and sculpting).	Children and youth were able to better cope with traumatic experiences and manage stress levels.
10. Dos Santos, A., & Wagner, C. (2018). Musical elicitation methods: Insights from a study with becoming-adolescents referred to group therapy for aggression. *International Journal of Qualitative Methods, 17*(1), 1609406918797427. https://doi.org/10.1177/1609406918797427	Six adolescent participants with aggression were studied.	Poststructuralist paradigm, musical elicitation methods such as drumming, creating images during music listening, song writing, and group musical therapy were applied.	Group musical therapy provided ease to adolescents experiencing aggression, thus creating meaning, purposeful relationships and kindness within.
11. Edgar-Bailey, M., & Kress, V. E. (2010). Resolving child and adolescent traumatic grief: Creative techniques and interventions. *Journal of Creativity in Mental Health, 5*(2), 158–176. https://doi.org/10.1080/15401383.2010.485090	Resolution of traumatic grief in children and adolescents was discussed.	Writing and drawing trauma, narratives, epitaphs, and acrostic poems are used for interventions.	Promoted a strengthened internal locus of control and enhanced the child's perception that they can cope with grief and loss. Allowed children to expose themselves to the traumatic aspects of their loss through the lens of personal ownership of their work.

12. Fairchild, R., & McFerran, K. S. (2019). "Music is everything": Using collaborative group songwriting as an arts-based method with children experiencing homelessness and family violence. *Nordic Journal of Music Therapy, 28*(2), 88–107. https://doi.org/10.1080/08098131.2018.1509106	15 children and adolescents aged 8–14 years who experience homelessness and family violence are presented.	Interventions such as music-based focus groups that involved writing (two) songs about what music meant to them are applied.	Music song writing provided a way to escape from the realities of current issues and provide hope.
13. Ferreira, R., Eloff, I., Kukard, C., & Kriegler, S. (2014). Using sandplay therapy to bridge a language barrier in emotionally supporting a young vulnerable child. *The Arts in Psychotherapy, 41*(1), 107–114. https://doi.org/10.1016/j.aip.2013.11.009	3.5-year-old HIV positive Sotho-speaking orphans are studied and the use of sand play therapy to bridge the language barrier was explored.	Sand play therapy. 18 sessions of sand play therapy. Psychoanalytical developmental model, an object relation, and a Gestalt therapy perspective are applied as interventions.	The orphan's emotional, social, and communicative functioning improved. Sand play therapy may be useful for vulnerable children with preverbal trauma.
14. Goicoechea, J., Wagner, K., Yahalom, J., & Medina, T. (2014). Group counseling for at-risk African American youth: A collaboration between therapists and artists. *Journal of Creativity in Mental Health, 9*(1), 69–82. https://doi.org/10.1080/15401383.2013.864961	Facilitating self-expression, self-confidence, emotion regulation, coping and communication. Communication skills that enhance personal resilience and a sense of connection with one's community are discussed.	Children's Art and Talk (CHAAT) program met weekly for 8 weeks, 2-hour sessions after school in a community center located in the heart of an urban African American neighborhood.	Children were able to open up and talk about family and personal obstacles they faced and to problem-solve challenges.
15. Gorbel, J. E. (2017). Examining adolescent student photography and revealed processes to inform day treatment school curricula and behavior interventions. https://scholarworks.waldenu.edu/dissertations/3991/	Seven adolescent participants (students) with psychiatric disorders such as cognitive limitations, maladaptive behaviors, and social functioning deficits are presented.	Interventions used in the qualitative study with semiotics as a conceptual framework are applied, and a photography program in day treatment school uses photographs taken by adolescent day treatment school students.	Photography activities are motivating and provide interest and perspective in effective academic and behavioral interventions in educational settings.

(*continued*)

TABLE 6.1 CREATIVITY: RESEARCH-BASED EXPRESSIVE ARTS INTERVENTIONS (*CONTINUED*)

Study Citation and Hyperlink	Issue/Population Addressed	Creative Intervention Used	Outcome
16. Hibbin, R. (2016). The psychosocial benefits of oral storytelling in school: Developing identity and empathy through narrative. *Pastoral Care in Education, 34*(4), 218–231. https://doi-org.libweb.lib.utsa.edu/10.1080/02643944.2016.1225315	Helping psychosocial emotional development effects and benefits of school-age children are discussed.	Oral storytelling that uses self-expression, identification, empathic understanding of self and others, and bidirectional communication is applied.	Oral storytelling strongly reinforces the idea that "social skills are not taught, but rather absorbed" and "learned through relationship."
17. Kim, S., & Ki, J. (2014). A case study on the effects of the creative art therapy with stretching and walking meditation—Focusing on the improvement of emotional expression and alleviation of somatization symptoms in a neurasthenic adolescent. *The Arts in Psychotherapy, 41*(1), 71–78. https://doi.org/10.1016/j.aip.2013.11.002	A single case study of a neurasthenic adolescent, investigating how the creative art therapy with stretching and walking meditation can improve the emotional expression of a neurasthenic adolescent and alleviate her somatization symptoms.	Stretching and walking meditation are applied.	Improvement of emotional expression ability and alleviation of the somatization symptoms helped the neurasthenic adolescent.
18. Kennedy, H., Reed, K., & Wamboldt, M. Z. (2014). Staff perceptions of complementary and alternative therapy integration into a child and adolescent psychiatry program. *The Arts in Psychotherapy, 41*(1), 21–26. https://doi.org/10.1016/j.aip.2013.10.007	Children with psychiatric illnesses are investigated with various forms of alternative therapies.	Art, music, dance/movements, and yoga therapies provide coping skills, relaxation, and stress relief to patients.	Complementary and alternative therapies benefit youth in psychiatric hospital programs.

19. Kuban, C. (2015). Healing trauma through art. *Reclaiming Children and Youth, 24*(2), 18. https://search.proquest.com/docview/1705355391?accountid=7122	Children with trauma are treated using interventions such as drawing. Art provides youth with a medium to express and explore images of self that are strengths-based and resilience-focused.	Through drawing, children can portray the depth of their terror and loss, externalizing the implicit messages and meanings of traumatic experiences.	Art therapy provided the youth the healing of traumatic images and experiences.
20. Kuo, N. C., & Plavnick, J. B. (2015). Using an antecedent art intervention to improve the behavior of a child with autism. *Art Therapy, 32(*2), 54–59. https://doi.org/10.1080/07421656.2015.1028312	A case study of autistic children applying coping skills to reduce off-task behavior is investigated.	Interventions applied are art therapy, crafting with beads, animal figurines, direction following games, storytelling, and movie watching in groups.	An antecedent art intervention can be an effective procedure to reduce off-task behavior of a child with autism.
21. Lindsey, L., Robertson, P., & Lindsey, B. (2018). Expressive arts and mindfulness: Aiding adolescents in understanding and managing their stress. *Journal of Creativity in Mental Health, 13*(3), 2288–2297. https://doi.org/10.1080/15401383.2018.1427167	Students from grades 6–8 manage stress with expressive arts and mindfulness.	Interventions applied were mindfulness, mask making in 12-hour groups over 6 weeks, which measure self-efficacy, depression, anxiety, and stress.	Significant self-reported reductions of anxiety and stress at the 3-week follow-up revealed a positive outcome for adolescents.
22. Marino, R. C., Thorton, M. D., & Lange, T. (2015). Professional school counselors address grief and loss: A creative group counseling intervention. *VISTAS Online, Article, 66*, 1–12. https://www.counseling.org/docs/default-source/vistas/article_66965a22f16116603abcacff0000bee5e7.pdf?sfvrsn=84c422c_4	Children and adolescents address grief and loss with creative group counseling.	An intervention using Marge Heegaard's book *When Someone Very Special Dies:* Children *Can Learn to Cope With Grief* is applied in 11 group counseling sessions such as art therapy, drawing, painting, visual, literary, and performing art.	The grief/ loss group teaches beneficial ways to utilize healthy coping skills and gain positive social support systems to aid in their healthy grieving process.

(continued)

TABLE 6.1 CREATIVITY: RESEARCH-BASED EXPRESSIVE ARTS INTERVENTIONS (*CONTINUED*)

Study Citation and Hyperlink	Issue/Population Addressed	Creative Intervention Used	Outcome
23. McDermott, P., Falk-Ross, F., & Medow, S. (2017). Using the visual and performing arts to complement young adolescents "close reading" of texts. *Middle School Journal, 48*(1), 27–33. https://doi.org/10.1080/00940771.2017.1243925	The challenges of reading literacy of young adolescents are explored.	Visual (paintings) and performing arts (music videos) are used as interventions.	Students are engaged and motivated to read.
24. Nsonwu, M. B., Dennison, S., & Long, J. (2015). Foster care chronicles: Use of the arts for teens aging out of the foster care system. *Journal of Creativity in Mental Health, 10*(1), 18–33. https://doi.org/10.1080/15401383.2014.935546	Teens in foster care engage and assist vulnerable youth to address developing aspects of self-image, self-healing, self-efficacy, and lessons learned.	Narrative and drama therapies as creative therapeutic interventions are applied in group setting by building on youths' individual and collective strengths in writing, speaking, and acting.	Teens talked at length about how meeting at a college campus gave them confidence that they could set and reach goals. Art therapy helped them heal around issues of abandonment and loss.
25. Otting, T. L., & Prosek, E. A. (2016). Integrating feminist therapy and expressive arts with adolescent clients. *Journal of Creativity in Mental Health, 11*(1), 78–89. https://doi.org/10.1080/15401383.2015.1019167	Feminist therapy is integrated with adolescent clients to provide a voice to the silent experiences, intuitions of adolescents and promote identity development of the holistic self through increased self-awareness and other awareness, known as connectedness.	Feminist therapy and expressive arts are integrated to support biopsychosocial/spiritual–existential axes of personal power. Spiritual interventions using plant and garden are applied.	Expressive arts can be integrated to foster identity development and alleviate symptoms of distress in adolescents.

26. Ovsyannilova, O. A. (2017). Social adaptation of teenagers with deviant behavior through art. *Paradigmata poznáni, 2*(1), 88–91. https://doi.org/10.24045/pp.2017.1.18	Adolescents/teenagers with behavioral problems such as defiant behavior and social adaptation are explored.	Phototherapy and video therapy art interventions are applied.	Art therapy via phototherapy and video therapy helped with the emotional, social interactions and personality of adolescents in expressing feelings, thoughts, and moods.
27. Perryman, K. L., Moss, R., & Cochran, K. (2015). Child-centered expressive arts and play therapy: School groups for at-risk adolescent girls. *International Journal of Play Therapy, 24*(4), 205–220. https://doi.org/10.1037/a0039764	At-risk adolescent female insecurities, self-awareness, stress relief, relationships, families, and expression of feelings are investigated.	Artist of color, counselors, African dance and music, mask making, and storytelling.	Adolescents exhibited an awareness of a transference of skills learned in the group, in outside relationships.
28. Quinlan, R., Schweitzer, R. D., Khawaja, N., & Griffin, J. (2016). Evaluation of a school-based creative arts therapy program for adolescents from refugee backgrounds. *The Arts in Psychotherapy, 47*, 72–78. https://doi.org/10.1016/j.aip.2015.09.006	Refugee adolescents 15 years of age are presented.	Intervention comprising creative arts therapy over the course of a school term.	School-based creative art therapy programs are valuable with young people from refugee backgrounds. A significant reduction in emotional symptoms was found for the treatment group.
29. Reed, K., Kennedy, H., & Wamboldt, M. Z. (2015). Art for Life: A community arts mentorship program for chronically ill children. *Arts & Health, 7*(1), 14–26. https://doi.org/10.1080/17533015.2014.926279	Addresses chronically ill children, adolescents 12–18 years old.	Mentorship program such as Art for Life, along with interventions like art, music and dance/ movement, and relational were applied.	Common themes include the perceived importance of mentorship and relationships. An increase in students' self-esteem, enhanced family bonds, and development of new coping skills were reported.

(continued)

TABLE 6.1 CREATIVITY: RESEARCH-BASED EXPRESSIVE ARTS INTERVENTIONS (*CONTINUED*)

Study Citation and Hyperlink	Issue/Population Addressed	Creative Intervention Used	Outcome
30. Sawyer, C. B., & Willis, J. M. (2011). Introducing digital storytelling to influence the behavior of children and adolescents. *Journal of Creativity in Mental Health, 6*(4), 274–283. https://doi.org/10.1080/15401383.2011.630308	Changes in social behaviors of children and adolescents are reviewed.	Digital storytelling. Combined with narrative therapy, drama, music, and visual imagery were the interventions applied.	Pilot study to help elementary students with social behavioral skills by using digital narratives was helpful.
31. Slyter, M. (2012). Creative counseling interventions for grieving adolescents. *Journal of Creativity in Mental Health, 7*(1), 17–34. https://doi.org/10.1080/15401383.2012.657593	Grieving adolescents and their developmental issues are explored.	Music, visual arts, bibliotherapy, drama, and cinematherapy are the interventions used.	Creating developmentally appropriate counseling to match adolescent grieving helps in their grieving process.
32. Thanasiu, P. L., & Pizza, N. (2019). Constructing culturally sensitive creative interventions for use with grieving children and adolescents. *Journal of Creativity in Mental Health, 14*(3), 270–279. https://doi.org/10.1080/15401383.2019.1589402	Exploring cultural sensitivity when counseling children and adolescents who are navigating the grieving process.	Play therapy, drawing, creating with clay, writing poetry and stories, and the use of sand tray are presented in two case studies.	When counselors are culturally competent, they can meet developmental and coping needs of diverse students.

33. Tyrer, R. A., & Fazel, M. (2014). School and community-based interventions for refugee and asylum-seeking children: *A systemic review. PloS One, 9*(2). https://doi:10.1371/journal.pone.0089359	Refugee children. See progress of refugee children in school settings.	Exposure through writing. Creative expression. Interventions: supportive therapy and creative arts—music therapy, creative play, drama, and drawing.	Findings suggest that interventions delivered within the school setting can be successful in helping children overcome problems.
34. Vela, J. C., Smith, W. D., Rodriguez, K., & Hinojosa, Y. (2019). Exploring the impact of a positive psychology and creative journal arts intervention with Latina/o adolescents. *Journal of Creativity in Mental Health, 14*(3), 280–291. https://doi.org/10.1080/15401383.2019.1610535	Studying reducing depression symptoms, building resiliency, and improving attitude in Latinx adolescents.	PPIs such as gratitude, forgiveness, strengths, meaning-oriented, and creative journal arts therapy are interventions applied over 7 weeks of group counseling.	Findings suggest higher levels of life satisfaction and positive affect after using PPIs.
35. Vivaldi, R. A., Jolley, R. P., & Rose, S. E. (2020). From mind to picture: A systemic review on children's and adolescents' understanding of the link between artists and picture. *Developmental Review, 55*, 100895. https://doi.org/10.1016/j.dr.2020.100895	Systematic analysis of children's and adolescents' understanding of the relation between artists and pictures.	Freeman's intentional network theory, PRISMA flow diagram, pictorial understanding of symbolic development, pictures (drawings), and paintings are applied.	Revealed a developmental pattern in preadults' understanding of the A–P link that children first acknowledge intention and later become more aware of how artist's attributes are communicated.

(*continued*)

TABLE 6.1 CREATIVITY: RESEARCH-BASED EXPRESSIVE ARTS INTERVENTIONS (*CONTINUED*)

Study Citation and Hyperlink	Issue/Population Addressed	Creative Intervention Used	Outcome
36. Heck, N. (2015). The potential to promote resilience: Piloting a minority stress-informed, GSA-based, mental health promotion program for LGBTQ youth. *Psychology of Sexual Orientation and Gender Diversity, 2*(3), 225–231. https://doi.org/10.1037/sgd0000110	10 participants in the Gay–Straight Alliance address minority stressors among LGBTQ youth.	**Handouts—Yes** **Instructions—No** A mental health promotion program is used to address minority stressors and promote coping skills among LGBTQ youth.	The use of community-based and school-based programs has shown to increase resilience in LGBTQ youth.
37. Carsley, D., Health, N. L., & Fajnerova, S. (2015). Effectiveness of a classroom mindfulness coloring activity for test anxiety in children. *Journal of Applied School Psychology, 31*(3), 239–255. https://doi.org/10.1080/15377903.2015.1056925	52 children participated and were evaluated for test anxiety before and after coloring before a spelling test.	**Handouts—Yes** https://www.therapistaid.com/therapy-worksheet/mandalas https://read.amazon.com/kp/embed?asin=B004Z8W1F0&preview=newtab&linkCode=kpe&ref_=cm_sw_r_kb_dp_BPjyEb8YHKHZJ **Instructions—Yes** Intervention used is mindfulness-based structured versus unstructured coloring.	Males reported a greater anxiety reduction in the free coloring and females with mandala condition.

38. Cho, A. S. (2016). *Suicide and non-suicidal self-injury: Art therapy and mindfulness techniques in a school setting to help decrease levels of anxiety, depression, and stress in adolescents* (Doctoral dissertation, The Chicago School of Professional Psychology). https://libweb.lib.utsa.edu/login?url=https://search.proquest.com/docview/1811634427?accountid=7122	Prevention and awareness of suicidal ideation and nonsuicidal self-injury for ninth to 12th grade girls are explored.	**Handouts—Yes** **Instructions—Yes** https://www.therapistaid.com/therapy-worksheet/dbt-emotion-regulation-skills https://www.therapistaid.com/therapy-worksheet/what-is-mindfulness https://www.amazon.com/dp/1572246022/ref=cm_sw_em_r_mt_dp_U_i1jyEbJH3YY4Y Interventions used are art therapy, emotion regulation (DBT), and mindfulness.	Mindfulness-based art therapy manual shown to be helpful when working with nonsuicidal self-injury.
39. Brown, E. C., & Gibbons, M. M. (2018). Addressing needs of children of incarcerated parents with child-centered play therapy. *Journal of Child and Adolescent Counseling, 4*(2), 134–145. https://doi.org/10.1080/23727810.2017.1381931	Children whose parents are incarcerated, who experience relational detachment, stigma, shame, and instability.	**Handouts—No** **Instructions—Yes** Child-centered play therapy	Researchers found child-centered play therapy to be culturally and developmentally appropriate intervention with positive outcomes.
40. Parisian, K. (2015). Identity formation: Art therapy and an adolescent's search for self and belonging. *Art Therapy, 32*(3), 130–135. https://doi.org/10.1080/07421656.2015.1061257	A Filipino adolescent who struggled with identity formation, social and adjustment difficulties is investigated.	**Handouts—No** **Instructions—Yes** A case study examining the application of four art therapy sessions and family art therapy.	The adolescent began to interact and gain acceptance with peers at school.

(continued)

TABLE 6.1 CREATIVITY: RESEARCH-BASED EXPRESSIVE ARTS INTERVENTIONS (*CONTINUED*)

Study Citation and Hyperlink	Issue/Population Addressed	Creative Intervention Used	Outcome
41. Allen, S. N. (2015). Adolescents, social media, and the use of self-portraiture in identity formation. https://digitalcommons.lmu.edu/cgi/viewcontent.cgi?article=1159&context=etd	Explores the tension between self-doubt and the desire to be seen of adolescent high school students.	**Handouts—No** **Instructions—Yes** Selfie in art therapy, photography, and self-portraiture are interventions applied.	Self-portraiture and selfies online can be therapeutic acts.
42. Alati, C. S. (2019). A theoretical exploration of feminist perspectives and art therapy for body image issues in adolescent females. https://spectrum.library.concordia.ca/985281/	Adolescent females with body image issues are explored.	**Handouts—No** **Instructions—Yes** Feminist approaches in the prevention and treatment of body image issues and art therapy are the interventions applied.	Feminist perspectives reduce stigma in school settings and increase social support in adolescent females.
43. Wood, D. M. (2015). Beauty or brains? The impact of popular culture on the development of adolescent rural gifted girls' identity and subsequent talent development. https://ro.uow.edu.au/cgi/viewcontent.cgi?article=5529&context=theses	Rural adolescent gifted girls dealing with identity issues.	**Handouts—No** **Instructions—No** Differentiated Model of Giftedness and Talent. Social media photography, selfies.	Popular culture was found to support talent development.

44. Sosin, L. S., & Rockinson-Szapkiw, A. J. (2016). Creative exposure intervention as part of clinical treatment for adolescents exposed to bullying and experiencing posttraumatic stress disorder symptoms. *Journal of Creativity in Mental Health, 11*(3–4), 391–408. https://doi.org/10.1080/15401383.2016.1251370	Children and adolescents who are bullied and develop PTSD.	**Handouts—Yes** **Instructions—Yes** CBT-(in vivo imagery or imagery rescripting), mindfulness techniques, and art therapy techniques.	A case illustration revealed that the creative interventions helped the adolescents with PTSD from bullying.
45. Laffier, J. (2016). Empowering bullying victims through artistic expression (L'autonomisation des victims d'intimidation par l"expression artistique). *Canadian Art Therapy Association Journal, 29*(1), 12–20. https://doi.org/10.1080/08322473.2016.1171987	Children in elementary school who were victims of bullying use artistic expressions.	**Handouts—No** **Instructions—Yes** A 14-week art therapy program is used with children.	Artistic expression in art therapy provided participants with opportunities to develop PE and develop emotional and cognitive changes such as increased self-efficacy, competence, influence, control, motivation, and self-esteem.
46. Hickey, M. (2018). "We all come together to learn about music": A qualitative analysis of a 5-year music program in a juvenile detention facility. *International Journal of Offender Therapy and Comparative Criminology, 62*(13), 4046–4066. https://doi.org/10.1177/0306624X18765367	Adolescent male and female residents in a large detention center in Chicago participate in a music program.	**Handouts—No** **Instructions—No** 700 youth in a PYD in a music composition program over a period of 5 years created primarily rap music compositions.	Participants enjoyed the program and built competence and positive feelings.

(continued)

TABLE 6.1 CREATIVITY: RESEARCH-BASED EXPRESSIVE ARTS INTERVENTIONS (*CONTINUED*)

Study Citation and Hyperlink	Issue/Population Addressed	Creative Intervention Used	Outcome
47. Lee, S. Y. (2015). Flow indicators in art therapy: Artistic engagement of immigrant children with acculturation gaps. *Art Therapy, 32*(3), 120–129. https://doi.org/10.1080/07421656.2015.1060836	Art therapy for three Korean boys (ages 7–11) from immigrant families who migrated to the United States.	**Tables—Yes** **Instructions—Yes** Two or three art therapy sessions that were videotaped or audiotaped explored their daily lives, with parent interviews and evaluation of children artwork. Semistructured interviews and postsession interviews were conducted.	Art therapy helps with children coping with acculturation challenges.
48. Linesch, D., Aceves, H. C., Queada, P., Troche, M., & Zuniga, E. (2012). An art therapy exploration of immigration with Latino families. *Art Therapy, 29*(3), 120–126. https://doi.org/10.1080/07421656.2012.701603	Examining anxieties, stressors, traditional values, and bi-cultural agents of acculturation among eight Latinx families that immigrated to the United States	**Tables—Yes** **Instructions—Yes** Three focus groups using family drawings and verbal communication were applied.	Art therapy can facilitate communication about the complex nature of acculturation through family drawings and research.
49. Tepper-Lewis, C. (2019). Description and evaluation of a dance/movement therapy programme with incarcerated adolescent males. Body, *Movement and Dance in Psychotherapy, 14*(3), 159–176. https://doi.org/10.1080/17432979.2019.1631885	Three adolescent males incarcerated in NSPs participated in a DMT program to improve self-restraint skills and a predictive factor of recidivism while incarcerated.	**Tables—Yes** **Instructions—Yes** The researcher created a movement observation sheet to complement the WAI-SF, based on Laban Movement Analysis and Chacian DMT theory, and recorded observations after every session.	The DMT program appeared partially successful in its goal of improving participants' self-restraint.

A–P, artist–picture; DBT, dialectical behavior therapy; DMT, dance/movement therapy; NSP, needle and syringe program; PE, psychological empowerment; PPI, positive psychology intervention; PRISMA, Preferred Reporting Items for Systematic Reviews and Meta-Analyses; PTSD, posttraumatic stress disorder; PYD, positive youth development; SDQ, Strengths and Difficulties Questionnaire; sMFQ, Short Mood and Feelings Questionnaire; TF-CBT, trauma-informed congnitive behavioral therapy; WAI-SF, Working Alliance Inventory-Short Form.

EXHIBIT 6.1

Professional Growth Organizations and Conferences for Counselors

Professional Organizations and Conferences for Counselors Related to Child and Adolescent Counseling

Child- and Adolescent-Focused Professional Organizations

American Counseling Association (ACA): https://www.counseling.org/about-us/about-aca

Divisions
Association for Specialists in Group Work (ASGW)
Association for Counselor Education and Supervision (ACES)
Association for Creativity in Counseling (ACC)
Association for Child and Adolescent Counseling (ACAC)

Branches
Alabama Counseling Association (ALCA)
Alaska Counseling Association (AKCA)
Arizona Counselors Association (AzCA)
Arkansas Counseling Association (ARCA)
California Counseling Association (CCA)
Colorado Counseling Association (CCA)
Connecticut Counseling Association (CCA)
District of Columbia Counseling Association (DCCA)
Florida Counseling Association (FCA)
American Counseling Association of Georgia (ACA of Georgia)
Hawaii Counselors Association (HCA)
Idaho Counseling Association (ICA)
Illinois Counseling Association (ICA)
Indiana Counseling Association (ICA)
American Counseling Association of Iowa (ACA of IOWA)
Kansas Counseling Association (KCA)
Kentucky Counseling Association (KCA)
Louisiana Counseling Association (LCA)
Maine Counseling Association (MECA)
Maryland Counseling Association (MCA)
Michigan Counseling Association (MCA)
Minnesota Counseling Association (MnCA)
Mississippi Counseling Association (MCA)
Missouri American Counseling Association of Missouri (ACAM)
Nebraska Counseling Association (NCA)
Nevada Counseling Association (NCA)
New Jersey Counseling Association (NJCA)
The New Mexico Counseling Association (NMCA)
The American Counseling Association of New York (ACA of New York)

(*continued*)

EXHIBIT 6.1

North Carolina Counseling Association (NCCA)
North Dakota Counseling Association (NDCA)
Ohio Counseling Association (OCA)
Oklahoma Counseling Association (OCA)
Oregon Counseling Association (ORCA)
Pennsylvania Counseling Association (PCA)
Puerto Rico Asociacion Puertorriquena Consejeria Profesional
South Carolina Counseling Association (SCCA)
South Dakota Counseling Association (SDCA)
Tennessee Counseling Association (TCA)
Texas Counseling Association (TCA)
Utah Counseling Association (UCA)
Virginia Counselors Association (VCA)
American Counseling Association of the Virgin Islands (ACA of the VI)
West Virginia Counseling Association (WVCA)
Wisconsin Counseling Association (WCA)
Wyoming Counseling Association (WCA)

Regions
The Midwest Region of the American Counseling Association
The North Atlantic of the American Counseling Association
The Southern Region of the American Counseling Association
The Western Region of the American Counseling Association

American Mental Health Counselors Association (AMHCA): https://www.amhca.org/home
AMHCA Affiliated Chapters

Midwest Region
Illinois—Illinois Mental Health Counselors (IMHCA)
    Illinois School Counselor Association (ISCA)
Indiana—Indiana Mental Health Counselors Association (IMHCA)
    Indiana School Counselor Association (ISCA)
Iowa—Iowa Mental Health Counselors Association (IMHCA)
    Iowa School Counselor Association (ISCA)
Michigan—Michigan Mental Health Counselors Association (MMHCA)
    Michigan School Counselor Association (MSCA)
Missouri—Missouri Mental Health Counselors Association (MMHCA)
    Missouri School Counselor Association (MSCA)
North Dakota—North Dakota Mental Health Counselors Association (NDMHCA)
    North Dakota School Counselor Association (NDSCA)
Ohio—Ohio Mental Health Counselors Association (OMHCA)
    Ohio School Counselor Association (OSCA)
Oklahoma—Oklahoma Mental Health Counselors Association (OKMHCA)
    Oklahoma School Counselor Association (OSCA)

(*continued*)

EXHIBIT 6.1

South Dakota—South Dakota Mental Health Counselors Association (SDMHCA)
South Dakota Association of Counselor Educators & Supervisors (SDACES)
South Dakota School Counselors (SDSCA)

North Atlantic Region
Connecticut—Connecticut Mental Health Counselors Association (CMHCA)
Connecticut Career Counseling and Development Association (CCCDA)
Connecticut Association for Counselor Education and Supervision (CACES)
Connecticut School Counselor Association (CSCA)
District of Columbia—District of Columbia Mental Health Counselors Association (DCMHCA)
District of Columbia School Counselor Association (DCSCA)
Maine—Maine Mental Health Counselors Association (MEMHCA)
Maine School Counselor Association (MESCA)
Maryland—Licensed Clinical Professional Counselors of Maryland (LCPCM)
Maryland School Counselors Association (MSCA)
Massachusetts—Massachusetts Mental Health Counselors Association Inc. (MaMHCA)
Massachusetts School Counselor Association (MSCA)
New Hampshire—New Hampshire Mental Health Counselors Association (NHMHCA)
New Hampshire School Counselor Association (NHSCA)
New Jersey—New Jersey Mental Health Counselors Association (NJMHCA)
New Jersey School Counselor Association (NJSCA)
NJ Association of Creativity in Counseling (NJACC)
NJ Association of Multicultural Counseling (NJAMC)
NJ Career Development Association (NJCDA)
NJ Association for Child & Adolescent Counseling (NJACAC)
NJ Association for Counselor Education & Supervision (NJACES)
NJ Association for Specialists in Group Work (NJASGW)
New York—New York Mental Health Counselors Association (NYMHCA)
New York State School Counselor Association (NYSSCA)
Pennsylvania—Mental Health Association in Pennsylvania (MHAPA)
Pennsylvania School Counselor Association (PSCA)
Rhode Island—Rhode Island Mental Health Counselors Association (RIMHCA)
Rhode Island School Counselor Association (RISCA)

Southern Region
Alabama—Alabama Mental Health Association (ALMHA)
Alabama School Counselor Association (ALSCA)
Arkansas—Arkansas Mental Health Counselors Association (ArMHCA)
Arkansas School Counselors Association (ArSCA)
Florida—Florida Mental Health Counselors Association (FMHCA)
Florida School Counselor Association (FSCA)
Georgia—Licensed Professional Counselors Association of Georgia (LPCA)
Georgia School Counselor Association (GSCA)
Louisiana—Louisiana Mental Health Counselors Association (LMHCA)
Louisiana School Counselor Association (LSCA)

(*continued*)

EXHIBIT 6.1

Mississippi—Mississippi Licensed Professional Counselors Association (MLPCA)
Mississippi School Counselor Association (MSCA)
North Carolina—Licensed Professional Counselors Association of North Carolina (LPCANC)
North Carolina School Counselor Association (NCSCA)
South Carolina—South Carolina Association of Licensed Professional Counselors (SCALPC)
South Carolina School Counselor Association (SCSCA)
Tennessee—Tennessee Mental Health Counselors Association (TMHCA)
Tennessee School Counselor Association (TSCA)
Texas—Texas Mental Health Counselor Association (TMHCA)
Texas School Counselor Association (TSCA)
Virginia—Virginia Association of Clinical Counselors (VACC)
Virginia School Counselor Association (VSCA)
West Virginia—West Virginia Licensed Professional Counselors Association (WVLPCA)

Western Region
Idaho—Idaho Mental Health Counselors Association (IMHCA)
Idaho School Counselor Association (ISCA)
Montana—Mental Health America of Montana (MHA of MT)
Montana School Counselor Association (MSCA)
New Mexico—The New Mexico Counseling Association (NMMHCA)
New Mexico School Counselor Association (NMSCA)
Utah—Utah Mental Health Counselors Association (UMHCA)
Utah School Counselor Association (USCA)
Washington—Washington Mental Health Counselors Association (WMHCA)
Washington School Counselor Association (WSCA)

American School Counselor Association (ASCA): https://schoolcounselor.org/

American Psychological Association: https://www.apa.org/about/

Divisions
School Psychology
Society for Child and Family Policy and Practice
Society for Couple and Family Psychology
Developmental Psychology
Society of Clinical Child and Adolescent Psychology

Mental Health America (MHA): https://www.mhanational.org/

National Alliance on Mental Illness (NAMI): https://www.nami.org/Home

National Board for Certified Counselors (NBCC): https://www.nbcc.org/

National Center for School Mental Health (NCSMH): http://www.schoolmentalhealth.org/

National Institute of Mental Health (NIMH): https://www.nimh.nih.gov/index.shtml

(*continued*)

EXHIBIT 6.1

Texas Counseling Association (TCA): https://pgc.txca.org/

Divisions
Texas Mental Health Counselors (TMHC)
Texas Association for Counselor Education and Supervision (TACES)
Texas Association of Marriage and Family Counselors (TAMFC)
Texas School Counselor Association (TSCA)

Conferences for Counselors

American Counseling Association Conference
ALCA Annual Conference
American Mental Health Counselors Association Annual Virtual Conference
All Ohio Counselors Conference (AOCC)
ARCA Conference
ASGW
American School Counselor Association Conference
MHA Annual Conference
CCA—California
CCA—Colorado Mental Health Professional Online Conference
CCA—Connecticut Annual Conference Counseling Connections
FCA—Annual Florida Counseling Association Convention
Georgia ACA
ICA & ISCA
Illinois—ICA Annual Conference
Indiana—ICA Annual Conference
Iowa—ACA of IOWA Break through Conference
Kanas KCA/KSCA Counseling Conference
Kentucky KCA Conference
LCA 2020 Conference
MECA Annual Conference
MCA Virtual Conference
MnCA Spring Conference
Mississippi—MCA Conference
Missouri ACAM Annual Conference
National Alliance on Mental Illness Child and Adolescent Mental Health Conference
NCA Spring & Fall Conference
National Center for School Mental Health Conference
NCCA Annual Conference
NDCA Annual Conference
NJCA Annual Conference
NMCA Annual Conference
OCA Spring Conference
Oklahoma OCA Summer Leadership Retreat & Annual Conference

(*continued*)

EXHIBIT 6.1

ORCA Conference
PCA Virtual Conference
SCCA Annual Conference
SDCA Conference
Tennessee Annual TCA Conference
Texas Counseling Association Annual Professional Growth Conference
VCA Convention
WCA Annual Conference online
Wyoming WCA Annual Conference
WVCA Fall Conference

KEY REFERENCES

Only key references appear in the print edition. The full reference list appears in the digital product on Springer Publishing Connect: connect.springerpub.com/content/book/978-0-8261-4764-6/part/part02/chapter/ch06

Duffey, T., & Somody, C. (2011). The role of relational-cultural theory in mental health counseling. *Journal of Mental Health Counseling, 33*(3), 223–242. https://doi.org/10.17744/mehc.33.3.c10410226u275647

Gladding, S. (2016). *The Creative Arts in Counseling.* American Counseling Association.

Harvey, R., Lin, I., & Booiman, A. (2015). Multicultural and diversity training considerations for biofeedback practitioners. *Biofeedback (Online), 43*(4), 163–167. https://doi.org/10.5298/1081-5937-43.4.05

Jordan, J. V. (2000). The role of mutual empathy in relational/cultural therapy. *Journal of Clinical Psychology, 56*, 1005–1016. https://doi.org/10.1002/1097-4679(200008)56:8<1005::AID-JCLP2>3.0.CO;2-L

Kottman, T. (2014). *Play therapy: Basics and beyond.* John Wiley & Sons.

Marzbani, H., Marateb, H., & Mansourian, M. (2016). Neurofeedback: A comprehensive review on system design, methodology and clinical applications. *Basic and Clinical Neuroscience, 7*(2), 143–158. https://doi.org/10.15412/J.BCN.03070208

Miller, W., & Rollnick, S. (2013). *Motivational interviewing helping people change* (3rd ed.). Guilford Publications.

Taylor, C. N., & Kilgus, S. P. (2014). Social-emotional learning: It's easy to forget the importance of social-emotional learning when the emphasis on academic learning is so intense, but it's counterproductive to do so. *Principal Leadership*, 15, 12–16.

Yalom, I. (2008). *Theory and practice of group psychotherapy* (5th ed.). Basic Books.

CHAPTER 7

Counseling Sessions Involving Children and Adolescents

Christopher Leeth

LEARNING OBJECTIVES

After completing this chapter, the reader should be able to:

- Describe the purpose of the counseling session.
- Identify necessary skills used to conduct a counseling session.
- Plan a basic outline for a counseling session.

CACREP STANDARDS FOR THIS CHAPTER

- CACREP 2016: 2.f.5.b.c.; 3.e.; 5.a.b.c; School Counseling: 5.G.1.a; 3.d.f.h.; Clinical Mental Health Counseling: 5.C.2.a.l.;3.a.
- CACREP 2009: II.G.3.e.; 5.b.c.; School Counseling: A.3; C.3.5; D.5.; K.1.; Clinical Mental Health Counseling: III.A.3.,C.8; E.3.

INTRODUCTION

The counseling session remains the focus of what most counselors-in-training (CITs) think of when they reflect on the type of work that they will be undertaking. It appears, perhaps, to be the culmination of all the training and education that CITs go through. Questions to new counselors, such as "What happens in the counseling session?," usually evoke a likely response, "Well, we talk. We establish rapport and discuss the client's issue." However, when pressed for additional details about what occurs in the counseling session, new counselors may struggle to describe more specific responses. Consequently, this type of ambivalence inspires the focus of this chapter, the stages of a counseling session.

COUNSELING IN MULTIDISCIPLINARY SETTINGS

Counselors work in a variety of settings. These settings include private practice, community-based agencies, government programs, and school settings. Counselors appear quite adept at working with clients from diverse backgrounds throughout the life span. After leaving graduate school, counselors possess the fundamental knowledge, awareness, and skills to work with diverse populations and client issues. Of the different settings that counselors work in, the most notable two happen to be in schools and community agencies (clinical mental health centers).

CLINICAL MENTAL HEALTH COUNSELING

Clinical mental health counselors and professional school counselors focus on alleviating client distress, and clients learn techniques that they may use outside of counseling. The goals for clinical mental health counselors include helping clients reach personal fulfillment, alleviating symptoms (when present), and helping clients reach their potential (Bruce, 1984).

Clinical mental health counselors (or professional counselors) work in community agencies to provide mental healthcare for any number of issues. A few examples of these agencies include postsecondary counseling centers, veteran centers, hospitals, and eating disorder clinics. Clinical mental health counselors work with a diverse clientele, on diverse issues ranging from clinical diagnoses to career counseling.

SCHOOLS

Professional school counselors serve as critical staff members in pre-K–12 schools and remain well versed in counseling theory. They work with children and adolescents and stay current with federal and state laws and guidelines. Professional school counselors work with a variety of issues that children and adolescents face. This includes bullying, academic achievement, career and college readiness, phase of life concerns, and family problems.

School counseling serves as an early intervention to help alleviate and prevent problems that youth might face. Ensuring that children remain engaged at school (i.e., working toward their education) becomes a primary goal for professional school counselors. Pre-K–12 students face many different issues, and professional school counselors offer ways to help identify students at risk and help develop a plan that keeps students safe.

CLINICAL AND COUNSELING PSYCHOLOGY

Magyar-Moe et al. (2015) highlight two types of psychologists who practice mental health counseling—clinical psychologists and counseling psychologists. Clinical psychologists hold advanced training in assessment and diagnosis (Magyar-Moe et al., 2015). They focus heavily on the role of brain function and dysfunction. Counseling psychologists possess similar training, with more attention given to how nonclinical issues impact a client (Magyar-Moe et al., 2015). Both types of psychologists view client functioning from a medical model. A medical model categorizes human functioning as either healthy or unhealthy. Additionally, there appears to be an emphasis on the neurobiological aspects of what the client seems to be experiencing.

PSYCHIATRY

Psychiatry refers to a branch of medicine that focuses on mental health (Baruch & Treacher, 2018). As trained physicians, psychiatrists focus on symptom reduction and medication management. They also practice mental health counseling. Like psychologists, psychiatrists work from a medical model and emphasize a distinction between normal and abnormal behavior. Table 7.1 shows a comparison of the types of providers described earlier.

CLINICAL SOCIAL WORK

Clinical social workers, psychologists (clinical and counseling), and psychiatrists all provide counseling sessions in addition to professional counselors. The differences lie in

TABLE 7.1 COMPARISONS OF MENTAL HEALTH PROFESSIONS

Profession	Focus With Client	Training	Emphasis
Clinical mental health	Goal attainment	Wellness model: ACA	Wellness and development
School counseling	Growth and development	Wellness model: ACA and ASCA	Wellness and development
Clinical psychology	Diagnosis and assessment	Medical model: APA	Symptom management/ reduction
Counseling psychology	Assessment	Medical model: APA	Symptom management/ reduction
Social work	Gaining resources	Varies: ASWA	Case management
Psychiatry	Medication use	Medical model: AMA	Medication management

ACA, American Counseling Association; AMA, American Medical Association; APA, American Psychological Association; ASCA, American School Counselor Association; ASWA, American Social Work Association.

the content of the session. While each professional can utilize theory, create treatment plans, and diagnose, significant variations in the process and focus of the session exist.

For clinical social workers (Parker, 2017), tremendous attention revolves around case management and the utilization of community resources. Clinical social workers can provide mental health counseling, though their education and training heavily emphasize advocacy, resource acquisition, and client assistance toward sustainable living.

FOCUS ON WELLNESS AND PREVENTION

Counseling sessions for professional counselors focus on wellness and prevention (American Counseling Association, 2014; Young, 2017). Professional counselors consider all aspects of the client's life. *The whole becomes greater than the sum of the parts.* Counselors inquire about client background information (e.g., the client's family, heritage, environment, age, and cultural factors) with developmental, systemic, multicultural, and relational considerations. Each of these aspects, in addition to the uniqueness of the individual, contributes to the client's experience and how the counselor goes about working with the client (i.e., treatment planning).

Clinical mental health counselors represent a group of clinicians who focus on client wellness (Young, 2017). Although professional counselors receive similar training to psychologists (e.g., counseling theory, diagnosis, and assessment) and can provide nearly identical services, there lies a distinction in how they view and explain client issues. Professional counseling certainly acknowledges the role of neuroscience and the brain but greatly emphasizes culture and development. Professional counselors work from a wellness model (as opposed to a medical model), where they view the client *as a whole.* What may be considered a clinical symptom from a medical perspective can be explained by a number of different points that appear more accurate than a diagnosis.

Counselors also focus on prevention (American Counseling Association, 2014; Young, 2017). This seems especially true when counselors work in a school or other youth settings. The goals for counseling become not just the amelioration of the client's concerns, but also the prevention of resurgence later on. This includes preventing the development of additional problems. Clients should leave the counseling process, and counseling sessions, with new tools and strategies that they can utilize to stymie future problems.

TECHNOLOGY IN COUNSELING

Advancements in the counseling profession include the utilization of technology (American Counseling Association, 2014; Kupczynski et al., 2017). Currently, technology use in counseling appears less of a possibility, and more of a probability. In fact, some would say that the use of technology should now be expected. As with so many other fields, the field of counseling appears to be changing along with the technological landscape.

Kupczynski et al. (2017) present online counseling as one way in which counselors utilize technology. They offer online counseling as a method to deliver services via a computer, phone, or other digital devices. Naturally, this carries certain ethical considerations—such as privacy and confidentiality concerns, licensure portability (e.g., a counselor living in a different state than the client), and changes in communication—with the practice, which counselors addressed at the national level (i.e., American Counseling Association Code of Ethics [2014]). As a result, counselors now shift their attention to the effectiveness and best practices for online counseling with a developmental, systemic, relational, and multicultural focus.

Kupczynski et al. (2017) identify accessibility as one of the major benefits of online counseling. Receiving counseling services via an online platform makes counseling much more possible for many people. Clients may elect online counseling for several reasons: One such reason involves accessibility; there may not be a counselor within accessible, physical distance of the client. In other words, the nearest counselor (or nearest counselor who specializes in a particular client concern) may be too far away. However, with the advent of secure Health Insurance Portability and Accountability Act (HIPAA) compliant platforms, clients who otherwise would be unable to attend counseling can now receive a wide range of options.

Some clients may be reticent to seek counseling because the symptoms of their problems keep them from traveling or being face to face with a counselor. Take for example, agoraphobia; a client may be so fearful or uncomfortable leaving their home that they cannot even leave the house to seek help. However, with online counseling, a client may be more comfortable sitting behind their keyboard instead of in front of a professional.

Chapin (2016) offers neurofeedback, a great tool that helps both the client and the counselor understand how different behaviors affect the body, as another way that counselors utilize technology. Neurofeedback teaches clients how to regulate their body (e.g., mindful breathing, thoughts, and feelings) so that they can feel more in control. Not only do counselors provide many resources that support the efficacy of neurofeedback, it also appears that many people genuinely want to understand how the brain works.

Additionally, technology can be used as a method of intervention (Barnett & Johnson, 2015), which, for example, allows clients to call or text under certain conditions. A couple of decades ago, this would not be feasible. Now, clinicians dedicate this modality as the best way to communicate with clients so that their information remains protected and the client feels as though the counselor continues to be accessible outside of session.

Counselors also utilize technology in an administrative capacity. Although many clinicians still use paper files to record clinical notes, it appears much more common for professional counselors to use electronic medical records (EMRs). These EMRs assist counselors to provide a secure and confidential place to store clinical notes; make appointments with clients; communicate securely with clients; and keep track of schedules. As technology expands and improves, it will also become more refined in the ways that it enhances the counseling session.

OPENING A COUNSELING SESSION

As with nearly any relationship, the opening remains a critical step (Brammer, 1973; DeSole et al., 2006; Sommers-Flanagan & Sommers-Flanagan, 2015). This phase literally establishes the first step in creating the collaborative, working relationship that defines the counseling relationship. As with any first-time encounter, the CIT will need to make a good impression and set the stage for the counseling process. This includes establishing rapport; discussing confidentiality; explaining the role of the counselor; beginning to conceptualize the problem; and establishing goals with the client.

ESTABLISHING RAPPORT

Effective counseling correlates highly with good relational factors with clients. Rapport building with clients establishes the level of connection between a counselor and the client; and offers one, if not the most, crucial element in the counseling relationship (DeSole et al., 2006; Sommers-Flanagan & Sommers-Flanagan, 2015). With good rapport, clients feel more able to express themselves and divulge more personal information. Clients also appear more likely to be open to receive help from the counselor. In the absence of rapport, clients may only share surface-level details about themselves or their lives; they will not feel comfortable discussing and sharing substantive details; consequently, the importance of rapport cannot be understated.

The process of establishing rapport begins at first contact with the client (DeSole et al., 2006; Sommers-Flanagan & Sommers-Flanagan, 2015). During the initial encounter, the client may experience some trepidation. Therefore, laying the groundwork for building rapport becomes incumbent on the counselor. This includes several simple tasks that the counselor can carry out, such as mirroring the client's body posture and tone; maintaining appropriate eye contact; demonstrating active listening; and taking a nonjudgmental stance with what the client discloses.

Body language (influenced by systems and culture) can greatly enhance or inhibit rapport with clients (Ivey et al., 2017). Even the physical space between a counselor and the client can affect rapport (Ivey et al., 2017). If a client sees a counselor who sits with a more defensive posture (e.g., sitting back, arms folded), the client may not feel comfortable and may, in fact, feel that there appears to be antagonism in the session. Conversely, sitting in an overly casual manner (e.g., legs placed on a desk and appearing bored), the client might think that the counselor seems uninterested about what the client wants to share. The same can be said about eye contact: too much (i.e., staring) can make some clients feel uncomfortable, and too little eye contact can be offending. Although counselors should be comfortable during the counseling session, they must also be aware of how culturally responsive behaviors (e.g., body posture/language and eye contact) communicate, and that this can greatly impact the counseling session.

Counselors use active listening as a skill to keep track of client–counselor disclosures in the counseling session. Specifically, active listening enables counselors to hear, retain, and understand what the client says (Ackerman & Hilsenroth, 2003; Desole et al., 2006). At its most basic level, active listening enhances the counselor's ability to fully hear and remember what the client discloses (both earlier in a session, and throughout multiple sessions). Finally, active listening helps the client to comprehend the counseling process. Counselors can demonstrate active listening by using nonverbal cues, such as nodding, facial expressions, and leaning toward or away from the client (as appropriate), and using minimal verbal encouragers, such as "I see," "Ok," and "mm-hmm." These cues can signal to the client the counselor's level of engagement.

Counselors can build and enhance rapport developmentally, systemically, relationally, and multiculturally by adopting a nonjudgmental stance with their clients (Ivey et al., 2019; Rogers, 1957). Many times, clients worry that they may be judged for their behaviors, thoughts, or feelings. Working from a nonjudgmental stance, counselors express that they accept the client without deeming them bad, faulty, or otherwise. Counselors express that they stand on the client's side and do this both through nonverbal actions such as maintaining positive or neutral body language, as well as overtly by stating to the client "I am here with you, to help you, not judge or condemn you."

CONFIDENTIALITY

Aside from introductions, an explanation of confidentiality and its limits appears to be one of the first topics that a counselor should initiate with a new client (American

Counseling Association, 2014). Alternatively, when working with minors, the counselor should also explain privacy to the (minor) client and their guardians. The profession holds counselors ethically and legally responsible for explaining confidentiality, which sets a tone of safety for the client and serves as the foundation for a productive counseling experience.

Confidentiality denotes a legal term used to explain how clients' information will be kept private. It presents the guarantee (with the exception of a few limitations) that counselors will not disclose any of the clients' information without permission. The counselor will not identify the client as a recipient of counseling to others; will not discuss client concerns in an identifiable way with other people; and will protect any records containing client information (e.g., notes and billing information). With this information, the client can more confidently decide how to proceed with sharing personal information. This remains a necessary part of the informed consent process.

While explaining confidentiality, the counselor must also make the client aware of limitations. A limitation of confidentiality can be seen in a situation in which the counselor may disclose information about the client to a third party. Situations that may lead to this type of disclosure include the client appearing to be an imminent threat to self (i.e., suicide) or others; suspicion of child or older adult abuse; or consultation with other treatment providers.

In situations where a client expresses suicidal ideation, the counselor will follow the applicable state laws to help the client. Many times, this involves calling authorities or emergency personnel to help get the client into a setting where suicide becomes less likely. This usually means getting the client to an ED or a crisis center. Counselors may also call an emergency contact that the client previously listed in the intake paperwork. It remains vital that counselors inform clients of the ethical (and legal) responsibility of reporting imminent danger, *at the beginning of the counseling process.* When clients seriously consider suicide, it can be incredibly detrimental to inform them and then—for the *first* time—that the counselor may need to break confidentiality.

Child and older adult abuse represent two additional situations in which a counselor can break confidentiality. Like suicide and threat to others, legal and ethical requirements prevail, and counselors must abide by them in the case of suspected abuse. Regarding child abuse, counselors should inform parents or other guardians about the reporting requirement. It remains important for new counselors to understand that they do not need to *confirm*. Rather, if counselors even *suspect* abuse, they must report this to the state's child protective services department. That department then takes responsibility to investigate the claim. Today, many youths live with adult caretakers. Similarly, when counselors suspect abuse of an older person or a vulnerable adult (e.g., an adult with intellectual disability disorder and severe autism spectrum disorder), the counselor must report this to the state's adult protective services department. As with child abuse, that department will investigate the claim; counselors need not confirm the suspected abuse. For both types of abuse, the counselor should disclose the reporting requirement to everyone involved with the counseling process. This includes the client *and* the client's guardians.

Counselors may disclose client information to other treatment providers *who simultaneously work with the same client.* Additionally, the information that the counselor discloses should be limited to pertinent information only. For example, a counselor may want to consult with a client's physician to discuss medication management for depression. The counselor may share the symptoms, and severity of those symptoms with the physician, but should not disclose details that appear unrelated to depression (e.g., details such as family secrets).

Finally, counselors may need to disclose information if the client shares that a previous counselor acted unethically. This can be a complex situation, which appears beyond the scope of this chapter. Suffice it to say that if a previous counselor engaged in egregious, unethical behavior with a client, the current counselor should report this to the state licensure board. An example would be if a client shares involvement in a sexual relationship with a prior counselor.

When working with minors, counselors cannot guarantee the same level of confidentiality that they would with an adult client (Glosoff & Pate, 2002). Professional school counselors abide by Family Educational Rights and Privacy Act (FERPA), which is covered in greater detail in Chapter 14. Counselors may discuss the role of *privacy* with minors and their guardians. Minors cannot *consent* to counseling; and they cannot make legal decisions for themselves. Minors can only *assent* to counseling; meaning, they can agree to go to counseling. Not having confidentiality means that a guardian can ask the counselor for information about the counseling sessions/process, and the counselor would be compelled to share that information. However, during the beginning of the session, counselors can remind both the minor and the guardians that privacy can be a meaningful element in the counseling process. Although guardians can request information at any time, the counselor can conduct a family/group session and ask the guardians to respect the privacy of the minor, by not compelling the counselor to disclose session details. While it remains important for the counselor to make and explain the distinction between privacy and confidentiality, ultimately, that decision remains with the guardian to allow the minor privacy.

COUNSELOR AND CLIENT ROLES

Many clients will enter the counseling process with only a basic understanding of the counseling process. Clients may gain the understanding that they (the clients) own the problem, and that the counselor speaks with them about it. However, this appears to be an oversimplification of the counseling process; the counselor should provide additional details about the role and expectations of the counselor, as well as the role and expectations of the client.

The counselor's role appears quite robust. Counselors serve as a sounding board for clients as well as confidants. On the one hand, counselors make use of theory and techniques that enable clients to solve problems and achieve personal growth. Conversely, the profession does not expect counselors to serve as "professional advice-givers." Counselors should explain that they do not hold expertise on the client's life and do not possess the ability to solve problems that the client might be experiencing.

Clients, on the other hand, become the recipient of the counselor's education, training, and experience. Counselors explain that the *client* serves as the expert on the client's life, and that while the counselor possesses a great deal of knowledge about mental health, the client possesses a tremendous amount of knowledge about the situation. Clients need to participate in an active role in the counseling session and should voice their ideas and concerns to the counselor.

Professional school counselors and the students they work with each take on and carry out specific roles as well. A professional school counselor's ability to work with students in a way that helps develop the students' abilities (American School Counseling Association, 2016; Bowers & Hatch, 2005) includes the students' academic abilities, professional capabilities, personal growth, and social connection. While in school, students move from grade level to grade level, ultimately leading to graduation. Professional school counselors, uniquely positioned to evaluate and work with students so that they can achieve academic success, carry out a role that involves monitoring students' grades and performances and remaining aware of difficulties that students might experience. Professional school counselors also work with students to develop professional interests and career goals (American School Counseling Association, 2016; Bowers & Hatch, 2005; Gysbers & Henderson, 2013; Texas Education Agency, 2018). These counselors help students to foster interests and potential career ambitions. School counselors do this partly by working with individual students, and partly by using various career counseling techniques and assessments. Professional school counselors may also help students to understand how to obtain a job (e.g., interviewing techniques, job opportunities, networking opportunities).

Helping students with their personal growth becomes an imperative task for professional school counselors. These counselors remain in a unique position to see students within their peer groups, the classroom, and in the counselor's office. With so many opportunities to get to know students, professional school counselors stay positioned to help guide and enhance student growth (American School Counseling Association, 2016; Bowers & Hatch, 2005). Additionally, professional school counselors can witness barriers to growth such as bullying, developmental delays, and systemic issues, to name a few. Professional school counselors make use of the same counseling theories that clinical mental health counselors use, and they use these theories to help students achieve self-actualization.

Professional school counselors serve the faculty, staff, and administration of schools (American School Counseling Association, 2016; Bowers & Hatch, 2005; Gysbers & Henderson, 2013). They consult with teachers and administrators on a number of student issues, including bullying prevention/remediation, individualized education plans, and outreach to families. These counselors communicate with other mental health professionals, such as licensed specialists in school psychology, special education teachers, and off-campus mental healthcare providers. Professional school counselors can provide guidance, support, and effective referrals to the parents or guardians of students.

CONCEPTUALIZATION

During the start of the counseling process (including during the informed consent portion), the counselor explains their theoretical orientation and the way in which the counselor views client issues. Counselors should conceptualize the counseling process with clients using developmental, systemic, relational, and multicultural lens. This includes sharing the counselor's techniques, ideas about human behavior, the purpose of counseling, and how it may help the current client. The opposite of this would be the client coming to counseling, sharing their experiences and concerns, and the counselor working from within a "locked box." In this situation, the client must uncritically trust the counselor, which may not be helpful for the rapport between the two individuals. As counselors listen to the client, they piece together an idea of presenting client concerns. The counselor utilizes theory, training, and experience to help narrow down what the client needs or stands to gain from counseling. This seems to be a process that counselors continuously revise over time, as new information and insight become available. As the counselor becomes more aware of the client's story and concerns, the counselor can then start to formulate an idea. When shared with the client, the counselor can further refine this idea. Conceptualizing the client issue remains one of the earliest steps in helping a client achieve goals. It serves as a road map for creating a treatment plan and incorporating appropriate interventions and techniques.

SETTING GOALS FOR THE COUNSELING SESSION

Like conceptualization, goal setting becomes a collaborative process between the counselor and the client (Mackrill, 2011). Setting overarching and session goals should be done early in the counseling process, tentatively by the end of the first session. Overarching goals help the client and counselor work toward a long-term outcome, such as achieving recovery from substance use; eliminating self-harmful behavior; or learning to live life after a traumatic event. To reach those overarching goals, the client and the counselor work together in each session and work toward a session goal for each meeting. Session goals include practicing new skills; incorporating interventions; or discussing life events. Goals establish a means for the counselor and client to work toward. Goals clarify what the client wants to achieve by the end of their work with the counselor. Goal setting takes both the counselor's and the client's perspective of the problem (Mackrill, 2011). Both people share what they think the outcome of counseling should be. This often involves asking the client what they hope to achieve, with the counselor providing insight about the feasibility and steps needed to achieve that outcome. Although goals should be established early on in the counseling process, they can frequently change allowing different priorities to take place as time goes on.

Clients may come in with a set of goals already in mind. Other times, clients may come in uncertain of their preferred counseling outcomes. In both instances, the counselor helps discern positive outcomes. Oftentimes, positive counseling goals evolve as those that (a) both the client and the counselor agree on; (b) both the client and the counselor believe to be realistic; (c) remain within the client's ability to work toward; and (d) appear within the scope of competence of the counselor. Although it would be ideal for the client and the counselor to hold the same goals and priorities, they may frequently select different goals (Mackrill, 2011). These situations appear normal and can be constructive. For example, a situation might present whereby the client prioritizes a particular goal while the counselor thinks that the goal should be something different. In such instances, dialogue between the counselor and the client appears to be the best option. The counselor should listen, wholeheartedly and nonjudgmentally, to the client's rationale. The counselor should also share their thoughts about the alternative goals. This serves as an act of collaboration: listening to the client while sharing the counselor's thoughts. Working together, the client and counselor can develop healthy, attainable goals.

THE WORKING SECTION

With introductions and pleasantries completed, the client and the counselor find themselves in the working phase of the counseling session. In this stage, the client tries their best to articulate life experiences, thoughts, and feelings. During this time, the counselor pays attention to myriad facets of counselor–client disclosure. The counselor, actively listening to what the client says, pays close attention to expressed feelings, monitors client body language, and keeps track of the narrative that the client constructs.

The working section of the counseling session often seems taxing on both the counselor and the client. During this time, the client recalls and shares important, often emotional, details about their life. The counselor pays keen attention to the influx of information that the client shares. The counselor tracks and keeps the client oriented to the session; the client tries their best to discuss topics that would otherwise be kept private. The purpose of the working section, in addition to the natural catharsis that comes from sharing experiences with another person, involves the counselor's continuous gathering of information, incorporation of theory and appropriate interventions, engaging the client, and developing and implementing long-term strategies.

THEORY AND INTERVENTION

The importance of theory in the counseling process cannot be understated. Without a theory to guide the counselor, it becomes difficult—perhaps impossible—to create a road map for the conceptualization of the client's problems. As stated previously, theory offers tools that help conceptualize the client's problem. A myriad of theories remains available for CITs to become familiar with, and education and training on those theories do not end with graduate school.

A counselor should view the client, the client's concerns, and the nature of counseling from developmental, systemic, relational, and multicultural perspectives that inform theoretical lenses (Corey, 2017). For example, a counselor who views problems through the cognitive behavioral theory lens will most likely view client problems as being a function of faulty thinking (Corey, 2017). Counselors who use dialectical behavior therapy (DBT) will most likely consider client problems to stem from severe or chronic invalidation (Koerner, 2011). Theory serves as the foundation for how counselors will view client problems; how they will work with clients; and how they will create short- and long-term goals. Additionally, each theory comes with tools and interventions to use in session with the client.

Clients come from many different walks of life. As stated previously, it is crucial that counselors consider developmental, systemic, relational, and multicultural factors when incorporating theory and interventions. Developmental considerations would include utilizing age-appropriate (i.e., is the client old or young enough to benefit) and/or cognitively appropriate interventions. Developmental considerations can dovetail with systemic factors, such as the client's family, school, social network, and living arrangement. Counselors use interventions that seems compatible with, and even incorporate, systemic elements.

Counselors incorporate relational factors when developing wellness plans for clients. Asking questions about the client's positive and negative relationships helps the counselor tailor treatment plans. The counselor creates a plan that involves sources of support to bolster the strength of the counseling intervention. Multicultural perspectives should also be addressed when working with theory and interventions. Older counseling theories tend to be more Western-centric, focused on the norms set by the culture of the theorist. More contemporary theories address the norms on which they were created but still may be countercultural to some clients.

While in the working portion of the counseling session, the counselor can use various interventions. Interventions in counseling can be considered methods, tasks, or dialogue that help the client work through a problem, a thought, or a feeling (Halstead, 2015). Counselors make decisions about interventions; consider the timing of the intervention; assess the client and the client's readiness for the intervention; and determine the best modality to implement the intervention (Halstead, 2015). Counselors use some interventions to affect a client's cognitions (Wenzel, 2017). These types of interventions often come in the form of questions or statements that the counselor poses with the intended purpose for the client to think from a different perspective; this also enables the client to consider the statement from a new perspective. Cognitive interventions challenge thoughts and assumptions (Wenzel, 2017). Behavioral interventions target undesired or unhealthy behaviors and come in a wide range of options including assigning homework; making use of diaries or journaling; and deep breathing (Wenzel, 2017). Behavioral interventions also include methods to reduce clinical behaviors, such as hairpulling and skin picking, or purge behaviors. Creative, experiential interventions can be used to help clients work through various emotional blocks that may impede progress or interfere with quality of life (Corey, 2017). Experiential interventions involve the client actively participating in an in vivo (i.e., in the moment) action. An example would be the use of the two-chair/empty chair technique, or a role play where the client can interact within a hypothetical context. Another example would be the use of a sand tray, or other manipulatives, for the client to use in order to better express themselves or identify difficult thoughts or feelings.

In every case, interventions used need to be linked to theory, and the theory needs to be applied to each client (Corey, 2017; Halstead, 2015). Ideally, the counselor should be well versed in a given theory and, thus, quite familiar with the associated techniques and interventions. The theory suggests to the counselor when and how to deploy a particular intervention. Further, the theory would also help the counselor interpret the outcome of the intervention. It remains important to note, here, that an element of subjectivity within the counseling session remains present (Halstead, 2015). The manner in which a client reacts to an intervention may not apply to every other client who undergoes the same intervention. The counselor interprets the responses to intervention and incorporates their ideas back into the counseling session.

ENGAGING THE CLIENT

Client engagement (a relational perspective) becomes paramount to the counseling process (Karson & Fox, 2010; Rumsey & Milsom, 2019). Meaningful discussion between the client and the counselor, and thus meaningful change for the client, can only occur in the context of a strong therapeutic relationship. That therapeutic relationship develops as a result of client engagement. Counselors should consider client engagement as a necessary component to creating a therapeutic alliance. Research shows that one of the biggest predictors of client outcomes remains the relationship between the client and the counselor (Wampold, 2001). Therefore, counselors should take steps to engage the client in the counseling process.

Counselors engage with clients in several ways and consider many of these techniques basic attending skills. Basic attending skills, although easy to understand, appear difficult to master. They often involve the first set of skills that CITs learn and require the most amount of time and attention, basically for good reason in that attending skills help steer and steady the counseling session.

Basic Attending Skills

Ivey et al. (2019) designate paraphrases, summaries, reflections of meaning, and reflections of content as the most fundamental of the basic attending skills. Counselors paraphrase by taking what the client says and present that information back to them. For example, after a client describes a tumultuous divorce, the counselor might respond with "It sounds like the divorce was a difficult time for you." Importantly, clinicians do not intend for paraphrasing to be a recording of what the client said or exact repetitions of what the client said. Paraphrasing involves taking the content of what the client said and restating it back to the client while highlighting key points. This serves to make sure that the counselor tracks what the client says, as well as ensuring that the counselor understands what the client shares. Further, paraphrasing allows the client to expand further on the topic of discussion. They also provide an opportunity for clients to hear their talking points, which allows clients to reflect on what they share. This contributes to client engagement by helping the client feel confident that the counselor appears to be listening and understanding what the client says.

Summaries, similar to paraphrases, contain much more information (Ivey et al., 2019). Whereas counselors use paraphrases throughout the session, they use summaries typically at the beginning and end of sessions. Summaries can be considered a collection of paraphrases. They encapsulate much more breadth. This makes paraphrasing an ideal skill to use when a client shares quite a bit of information, and the counselor wants to make sure that they understand what the client says. Summaries appear to be wonderful tools to use to begin and end sessions by reviewing the content of the session. They also serve as great ways to open a session by reviewing information from the previous session. This helps to keep the client and counselor on track for achieving the established goals.

While paraphrases and summaries focus on the accuracy of the content, reflections focus on possible interpretations of what the client said. Reflections of feelings require counselors to "reflect" back what a client shares, along with what the counselor believes the client feels (Ivey et al., 2019). For example, when a client talks about difficulties at work due to negative interactions with a coworker, a possible reflection of feeling would be "You are feeling frustrated." Although the client never directly expressed an emotion, the counselor presents the feeling of frustration back to the client. The skill required for this technique appears to be an ability to accurately identify the feeling that the client shows or describes. Counselors can discern this information in a number of ways, including observing the client's body language, tone of voice, and affect.

Reflections of meaning denote interpretations of what the client says (Ivey et al., 2019). Whereas reflections of feelings focus on the experience and the emotions felt by the client, reflections of meaning focus on what the client truly means. Expanding on the example of the client who struggles with a coworker, imagine that the client states that he neither wants to confront the co-worker nor escalate the situation to a supervisor. A reflection of meaning, here, may be "You do not want to be seen as a difficult person" or "You do not like confrontation." Although the client never overtly stated this, the counselor presupposes the meaning behind what the client shared.

Counselors consider both types of reflections to be incredibly powerful counseling tools (Ivey et al., 2019). They both serve to further enhance client engagement and to strengthen the therapeutic relationship. Reflections continue to make clients feel heard, and they also serve as insight for the clients. Counselors should not rush to make reflections, and CITs should understand that reflective skills remain something that develop through experience.

Pacing

Many times, clients will come to counseling sessions with much on their mind, and a lot to say. However, counseling sessions can be inherently time-limited. The length of a counseling session varies, usually based on the type of setting or agency (e.g., a school, a community agency, and a hospital). Typically, a traditional counseling session lasts about 50 minutes. Clients may come to session, feeling overwhelmed with what they would like to share within the time constraint. The counselor should keep a healthy, productive pace within the session.

In the throes of emotion and narration, clients may spend a lot of time discussing superfluous events, and little time on experiences that warrant further discussion. The counselor must help regulate these discussions and make the most of the time in the session. At one end, some counselors may sit silently, listening to everything the client says but offering little to help guide the session. At the other end of the spectrum, counselors may interject often or may be overbearing with what the session should focus on. It appears easy to imagine how a counselor at either end of this spectrum can disrupt client engagement; session pacing can absolutely affect engagement.

Ideally, the counselor allows the client to lead discussion and lets the client bring up what they consider important. Yet, the counselor must also make sure that the counseling sessions consist of a sense of continuity, and that progress moves forward toward goals. This means that the counselor may need to verify if the client truly wishes to discuss topics that appear unaligned with the goals, or overall work with client. It also means that the counselor will need to slow down the client, asking more pointed questions to keep the client focused on the original concerns that brought the client to counseling in the first place.

Confrontation

When working with clients, it seems all too common for counselors to notice negative thought processes, behaviors, and attitudes. Sometimes, this comes in the form of a client not following through with an intervention suggested by the counselor. Other times, the client fails to see or denies that they themselves may be contributing to the very problem that they seek to solve in counseling. In these situations, counselors can make use of confrontation. This appears to be a skill that many CITs may feel trepidation about. Yet, when used effectively, confrontation can be one of the most powerful ways to engage clients, and to help them achieve their goals.

Many CITs join the profession in order to help people work through conflict. The word "confrontation" carries a negative connotation for the uninitiated. However, *confrontation* can be inherently different from *conflict*. Conflict occurs when two or more people cannot agree on something. To be clear, counselors do not view conflict as being fundamentally bad; it all depends on how the involved parties manage the conflict. Confrontation, in the counseling sense, refers to presenting a client with information or an idea that challenges what the client says or does (Ivey et al., 2019). For example, when working with a teenage client who states that she "badly wants to go to college," yet frequently skips school and does not complete assignments, the counselor might say "You are saying that you very much want to go to college and that education is very important to you, yet you do things that are directly opposed to that goal." Another client might express that they take their work in counseling seriously, and at the same time, they often cancel or no-show. The counselor here might confront the client by stating that "You're saying you take your work with me seriously, but you aren't doing all the things that we lay out in session."

Confrontation brings discrepancies to the client's attention (Ivey et al., 2019). Successful use of confrontation takes an understanding of the client's response, timing, tact, and ability to roll with resistance. Like everyone else, clients possess states and traits. Some clients will be incredibly open and receptive to being confronted; others may become defensive or defeated. Some clients would be able to handle confrontation, if not for *when* and *how* the counselor handled the confrontation. The way the counselor confronts (e.g., body language and tone) can greatly hinder (or enhance) the effectiveness of confrontation. The goal becomes to never be antagonistic. The counselor confronts the client to either (a) promote the betterment of the client (i.e., being part of the treatment) or (b) gain a better understanding of how and why the client sees the world.

Redirecting

Redirecting in a counseling session occurs when the counselor keeps the client from moving from topic to topic. Clients commonly feel compelled to share many details about various aspects of their lives. However, sometimes, those details can derail the counseling session; one experience can lead to another, which leads to another, thus taking the clients off track from what originally brought them to counseling. This can become a normal part of wanting to talk with a counselor. In these situations, counselors can *redirect* the client back on track.

Redirecting a client can feel uncomfortable for counselors. Moreover, redirecting certainly takes tact. However, if counselors do not keep clients on track, a risk emerges limiting the counseling session from staying on focus. In other words, the client might discuss numerous details, with only a small amount of attention given to truly pertinent details. No counselor wants to make a client feel as though what they share seem unimportant. Yet, counselors *must* redirect if the goals of the counseling session remain the focus.

Counselors can successfully redirect clients with simple statements and questions (Desole et al., 2006). A teenage client who struggles with her parents' impending divorce may state,

> *I have a friend whose parents divorced, and he is doing well. His parents got him a car, but they have the ability to afford it. His parents have a lot of money, and he doesn't need to have a job like I do. . .*

In this case, the client begins to spend more time describing the life of her friend and drifts away from the original concern, the divorce. A counselor in this situation might ask "And what would 'doing well' look like for you?" This brings the attention back to the client and her experience, without criticizing or dismissing what she voiced.

The importance of redirecting when thinking about working with children and adolescents seems apparent. It appears common for child clients' minds to wander causing distractions. The counselor takes a developmentally sound way of redirecting the child back to the topic at hand. Adolescents can also be distracted and also face a distinctly different set of pressures than children. Teenagers often seem overwhelmed and preoccupied with the happenings within their social circles and can be easily distracted with the activities of friends and romantic partners. Again, the counselor identifies when the adolescent client drifts too far from the presenting concern, and the counselor redirects in a developmentally appropriate way that honors the client.

Reframing

As clients share their experiences, counselors remain in a unique position to provide different perspectives on what the clients discuss. Clients may be somewhat myopic with their perspectives. This appears to be especially true for children and teenagers. As counselors hear clients' stories, they may notice negative thoughts and interpretations experienced by the client. This describes the empowerment of reframing. In a nonjudgmental fashion, and while being careful to not dismiss what the client appears to be thinking, a counselor might suggest other ways to process experiences (Desole et al., 2006; Kraft et al., 1985). For example, a teenage client might share with his counselor how his father constantly pressures the client to do well in school. The client states,

> *My dad is always on my case, telling me that I spend too much time with my friends and playing games. He is constantly quizzing me and asking about my schoolwork, and it feels like he does not care for any of my hobbies or interests.*

In response to this, the counselor may offer the following perspective: "Your father cares greatly about your academic success; he wants to see you succeed and reach your long-term goals." In this example of reframing, the counselor attempts to avoid dismissing the client's frustration, or challenging the veracity of what the client shared. Rather, the counselor provides an alternative way of viewing the experience.

As with other ways of engaging a client, reframing requires tact and awareness. Many clients may feel defensive if challenged too soon, or in a way that seems judgmental. Counselors must consider if reframing appears to even be appropriate for responding to what the client shared. However, when used effectively, reframing can help clients to view both current and future events from different points of view. In the context of client engagement, reframing also serves as another means to deepen the conversation, and even to help build rapport. In the context of the overall counseling process, reframing can serve as a tool that the client can use outside of the counseling session; it can be an exercise that the client can utilize in future situations.

Differentiating the skills described earlier is important. CITs often conceptualize using these skills the same way one would think about moving pieces in a game of chess; the counselor speaks, the client speaks, and now the counselor thinks of which skill to use, and then responds. However, in practice, the counseling exchange happens very seamlessly and conversationally. After practicing and gaining experience, counselors begin to carry out exchanges without analyzing what "the next move" should be. Take the following exchange between a counselor and an 8-year-old client:

Counselor:	*Tell me, Jonah. What is it like at home?*
Client:	*I have my mom and dad and sister.*
Counselor:	*And what is your relationship like with your parents?*
Client:	*It's good. They give me a lot of stuff. My dad plays video games with me, and mom does art stuff with me. My dad says that I can be a professional gamer when I grow up, and he will come to all my matches. I play a lot of Warzone but I haven't come in first place yet, but I'm getting better and I keep practicing.*
Counselor:	***(Redirecting)*** *Fun! Sounds like you've got a really great relationship with your parents.*
Client:	*Yeah, but sometimes they tell me what to do and I get mad.*
Counselor:	*Tell me about that.*
Client:	*Well, it's like they always tell me what to wear and they always want me to comb my hair. They're always telling me to read even though I already read a lot at school.*
Counselor:	***(Reflection)*** *You don't like that.*

Client:	*Not really. And they're always making me practice reading and writing even after I've been at school all day.*
Counselor:	*They give you a lot to do. They want you to do well with school.*
Client:	*I don't like it. They don't ever let me do what I want.*
Counselor:	*Do they support you being a gamer? And getting better at. . .Warzone. . .was it?*
Client:	*Well. . .yeah. They do. But. . .*
Counselor:	*(silence)*
Client:	*I just don't like it.*
Counselor:	***(Reflection)*** *It's hard being told what to do. You like making your own choices.*
Client:	*Yeah.*
Counselor:	*A lot of great leaders like to make their own choices.*
Client:	*Okay.*
Counselor:	*I bet making your own choices is important for being a pro-gamer. Don't you think?*
Client:	*Yeah. Like I need to be able to choose where to go and what to use and how to play.*
Counselor:	*I've heard there are videos online that help guide you to be a pro-gamer. Have you ever seen those?*
Client:	*Oh yeah! I watch them all the time and I started doing better.*
Counselor:	*They tell you how to do better? Training tips, maybe?*
Client:	*Yeah!*
Counselor:	***(Reframing)*** *Do you think, in a way, your parents are kind of like those videos? They are trying to guide you?*
Client:	*Maybe but it's different.*
Counselor:	*How so?*
Client:	*I don't know, it just is.*
Counselor:	***(Reflection)*** *Because you don't like it when they tell you what to do?*
Client:	*Yeah.*
Counselor:	***(Confrontation)*** *So it's really not so much about being told what to do, as it is not liking what you're being told to do. If your dad told you to go practice gaming, you probably would. Is that fair to say?*
Client:	*Yeah.*
Counselor:	*But if he told you to read, you wouldn't like that?*
Client:	*No.*
Counselor:	*Your goals, gaming, and your parents' goals, school, are different.*
Client:	*Yeah.*
Counselor:	*Does that make anyone wrong?*
Client:	*I guess not.*
Counselor:	***(Redirecting)*** *And that includes you! You are not wrong! You have a goal: gaming! Your parents' goal: school! No one is wrong here! We just need to find a way so that both goals are met. What do you think?*
Client:	*That makes sense. Like I can do some reading, and then game. Or game and then read.*
Counselor:	***(Goal setting)*** *There you go! That's good thinking! Do you think that you and I could come up with a schedule? Then we can show it to your parents and they can see that you are willing to do school or math or whatever, and you can see that there will still be time to practice. Sound good?*
Client:	*Yeah!*

Interventions and Strategies

The working portion of the counseling session involves a tremendous amount of effort from both the counselor and client. It involves a time where individuals experience a lot of emotion and processing. At times, a lot of behavior modification occurs. In all cases, the working section provides a time where the counselor can make use of counseling interventions and strategies.

The term "intervention" takes on many different meanings. In this context, the term intervention refers to an act or idea used by the counselor to positively affect the client in the counseling session. Counselors use countless interventions and even more ways to introduce and administer them. Counselors must select interventions and strategies that appear to be effective for the current client, and the specified problem or goal. Whereas interventions act as short-term techniques used or taught in session, counseling strategies refer to the longer-term plan to help the client.

When selecting an intervention, counselors must make many considerations. The appropriateness of the intervention becomes one of the first points that counselors should consider. As the old saying goes, "when all one has is a hammer, everything looks like a nail," meaning that just because a counselor seems aware of an intervention and may even be excellent at executing that intervention, this does not mean that the intervention would be the best tool at the present moment. Additionally, counselors should demonstrate confidence in the intervention that they select. Part of the treatment planning process becomes the investigation of potential interventions and long-term strategies that can help with the client's goals. Therefore, as counselors research potential options, they take advantage of the opportunity to review several different interventions, with some interventions being more supported than others.

Counselors must also consider the individual client and the presenting concern. Counselors tailor treatment plans to the unique needs of each client. While a particular intervention may work wonderfully on one (maybe even several) client, one must not conclude that the intervention will be effective for every client. The counselor must consider age and development, culture, and individual traits of the client. Regarding age, not every technique will be well suited for children, teens, or adults. What might be effective for an adult may be completely benign for a child. Techniques that work well for teenagers may be less effective for adults. Specifically, children may be more reliant on concrete thinking than adults, making discussions and techniques that rely on abstract thought processes difficult. For example, utilizing the two-chair/empty chair technique or asking how another person feels may be beneficial for an adult, but too complex for a child. However, many times the counselor can adjust an intervention to make it more age-appropriate. This can be as simple as adjusting the language needed to communicate the intervention. Other times, it can be more thought-provoking, with the counselor linking the intervention to the client. There will also be clients who may possess developmental differences; an adult client may be immature, or a younger client may be developmentally older than their chronological age. In these instances, the counselor, again, can find adjusting the intervention to be more effective (Kottman, 2016).

Culture plays a large role in the selection of interventions and strategies (Hays, 2016; Matsumoto, 2009; Sue & Sue, 2019). Different models exist to help extrapolate the cultural factors of a client (e.g., ADDRESSING, which will be discussed more in Chapter 15 [Hays, 2016]). Culture encapsulates such factors as ethnicity, socioeconomic status, and religion. These different cultural factors must be critically considered because a particular intervention, task, or strategy can appear antithetical to the client's cultural norms and values. Again, counselors find themselves needing to rely on the client to teach the counselor about themselves. This exemplifies the importance of establishing mutual respect, rapport, and an egalitarian relationship with the client; counselors rely on the client to inform them of cultural norms and values, and clients must feel empowered to educate the counselor (Sue & Sue, 2019).

Systemic factors that inhibit or promote the intervention will also need to be considered. Counselors will ask about the various systems that a client belongs to or is affected by. For example, a child or teenage client will be part of a school system. If a client encounters legal problems, they may be part of a legal system. Housing arrangements, support systems (e.g., community support and church groups), and managed care may all be factors that positively or negatively impact counseling goals. Thus, it is critical that counselors address these factors when implementing a strategy or intervention.

Similar to systemic factors, relationships can also influence counseling outcomes. Relational factors include the nature, positivity/negativity, and strength of the relationships that a client experiences with others. For example, a counselor asks if a client has a best friend or confidant; if the client experiences a positive relationship with family members; and if the client feels supported by friends or loved ones. Counselors do not only consider ways to work with these relational factors; they explain to the client that as the client changes (as a function of the strategy or intervention), other people may notice.

When implementing interventions and strategies, the client must feel comfortable with the task or idea being presented. When the intervention runs counterculture to the client, the client might appear less likely to participate. In fact, the client may think that the counselor appears ineffective, or even that counseling as a whole seems ineffective. Interventions and strategies must be culturally appropriate.

Finally, even if a counselor truly believes an intervention to be effective, and the intervention appears to be both age-appropriate and culturally appropriate, there can still be individual client differences that make the intervention more or less effective. Such differences can include personality, temperament, tolerance, and extraneous circumstances. Counseling can be an uneasy process for clients. Change, even when positive, can appear uncomfortable. For some clients, the discomfort of a given intervention may be more than they can handle. Other clients may be completely willing to participate but experience difficulty because of phase of life concerns (e.g., starting a new job). Some clients may not feel confident about the intervention, and thus a bias prevents the effect from occurring.

Selecting a counseling intervention appears to be a heavy undertaking (Halstead, 2015; Wampold, 2001). The difficulty lies in the abundance of counseling strategies and interventions (Halstead, 2015). Reflecting on the American Counseling Association Code of Ethics, counselors want to avoid harm to the client and wish to maximize benefit. That means wholeheartedly considering the client and the presenting concern in order to choose the appropriate intervention. Moreover, counselors want to choose the *most* impactful intervention.

Finally, effective interventions include measuring change. Counselors enhance their clinical work when they ask clients about the outcomes of counseling interventions. Asking questions about how the client feels or acts between sessions serves as a barometer of change.

The working section of the counseling session provides counselors with the opportunity to introduce and incorporate interventions and ask for feedback. These areas become part of the counseling process. When clients affirm that an intervention helps, counselors can ask why; and if needed, counselors can push for more change. If a client says that there appears to be no effect, the counselor can, then, ask for more information, and ask the client why the intervention appears unsuccessful. For strategies, counselors can track a client over time as well as solicit for information about progress to see if the overall plan for the client appears to present a positive effect.

THE CLOSING SECTION

As described earlier in the chapter, most counseling appointments last approximately 50 minutes in length. The first part of the appointment involves exchanging pleasantries and recapping the previous session. This part of the session involves the counselors and clients working to understand the clients' concerns and to develop a plan to reach client goals. Counselors refer to the final minutes of the counseling session as the *closing section,* where the counselor begins to prepare the client to leave the session and begins to plan for the next appointment.

SUMMARIZATION AND REVIEW

As the session comes to a close, the counselor may summarize the discussion that occurred. Recall that a summary connotes a basic attending skill, similar to paraphrasing, that the counselor uses to present back session content to the client. Summarizing at the end of the session becomes an excellent way to make sure that both the counselor and the client leave the session with similar understanding of what occurred. In addition to summarizing the content of the session, counselors can also review the session, and overall progress of counseling, with the client. Counselors can review the next steps that both individuals will take between sessions. This can serve to keep the client and the counselor unified in working toward the long-term goal. Summary and review serve as useful methods of closing the session, while preparing for the time between sessions.

Checking for Client Understanding

At the end of each session, it becomes imperative to ensure that the client understands what transpired (Desole et al., 2006). This can be said of the counselor as well. Checking for understanding becomes especially important when working with children and adolescents. Counselors should confirm that clients understand what happens in counseling, what happens in the session, and why the counselor approaches the situation in a particular manner. Regarding children and teens, counselors must keep in mind that these age groups may possess a faulty understanding of the situation (Sandberg & Spritz, 2009). This can be attributed, in some instances, to age and development. As described earlier, counselors must realize the role that human development plays in the counseling process. Therefore, counselors should work to confirm that child and teenaged clients accurately understand the work being done.

Establishing Continuity

For counseling to be effective, there must be a thread that follows through each counseling session (Young, 2017). Each session must work toward the ultimate goal for the client. Of course, there will be exceptions, such as an unexpected change or emergency in the client's life; but overall, counselors must work to ensure that each session builds on top of the last. Counselors can establish continuity of treatment by giving attention to goals (both short term and long term), future session dates, and preliminary plans for those future sessions.

During the closing portion of the counseling session, counselors can devote some time to discussing long-term goals with the client. Counseling can be described as a marathon; it takes time, and sometimes it takes a slower pace. In these instances, it becomes imperative to discuss with the client how what occurs in the current session contributes toward the future goal. In addition, clients may come into counseling with more immediate goals (i.e., short-term goals). The end of the session presents a great time to review those short-term goals.

A natural and necessary part of closing a session includes a discussion of the next (if not future) session. Most immediately, the counselor and client should plan when the next session will occur and what should be expected at that session. Counselors should also initiate conversations about changes to consider in those future sessions. For example, it seems common for clients and counselors to make travel plans during the holidays. Therefore, counselors should discuss when the next appointment will be and what clients can do during that time away if a situation should occur.

The close of the session also focuses on preliminary plans for the next session. The counselor might explain how they will prepare for the next session (e.g., find referrals and create worksheets). The counselor may also delegate a task to the client to be prepared for the next session (e.g., completing homework, imagining situations, and journaling behavior). This way the counselor and the client share the same understanding of what will happen before and at the next session.

Maintaining Continuity Between Sessions

Continuity between sessions ties each of the counseling sessions together. If a client attends counseling for five sessions, it would be best if each of those sessions worked toward the same goal, rather than having five appointments that each focus on separate concerns, though there may be exceptions; emergencies, life changes, and symptom relapse all become examples of when a session might deviate from working toward the long-term goal.

When sessions appear disjointed, focusing on something new each appointment, it becomes difficult to work toward the goals established at the beginning of the counseling process. Because of this, counselors strive to keep the client centered on those original goals. At the close of the counseling session, as part of the review, counselors might tie the session content back to the goals. In situations where the counseling session seems unfocused on the original or long-term goal, the counselor might acknowledge this and describe how the next session will revisit the original goal.

REFERRALS AND TERMINATION

When counselors believe that they can no longer provide a benefit to the client, they should provide a referral. However, the counselor should not simply create a list of just any professionals whom they find on the internet. Counselors make effective referrals by appropriately vetting other professionals that may help clients. When providing referrals, the counselor should explain the reason for referring the client to another professional, and why each of those professionals would be a good fit for the client.

Termination refers to the process of ending the counseling relationship with a client (Headley et al., 2015). Several reasons lead to termination. The most common ones appear to be (a) the client no longer needs counseling (i.e., the counselor addressed the client's concerns) and (b) the client's concerns appear to be beyond the scope of the counselor's competence. Careful consideration goes into the decision to terminate or refer. Termination is tantamount to ending a relationship, and clients experience a multitude of emotions. The counselor plans on when and how to begin the termination process so that clients feel prepared to stop counseling. Regarding referrals, counselors carefully consider *why* they are referring the client elsewhere. Referral should occur only in those situations where the counselor might be working out of the scope of training with a particular *issue*, not because the counselor does not want to work with a particular *client*. In these situations, counselors should seek consultation and professional growth opportunities and supervision to expand their capability.

The end of a counseling relationship can greatly impact the client (Goodyear, 1981; Piselli et al., 2011). Frequently, clients grieve the end of the relationship, or feel a certain level of anxiety or fear when leaving their counselor. In fact, it can be just as emotionally difficult for the counselor (Goodyear, 1981). The process of termination involves telling the client that concluding the counseling process may be appropriate, or even necessary. The end of the counseling relationship involves discussing the work completed and the goals achieved (Table 7.2). Finally, there should be time and space given to the client, so that they can express and process their feelings and thoughts about the end of the counseling process.

TABLE 7.2 SECTIONS, PURPOSE, AND GOALS OF THE COUNSELING PROCESS

Section	Overall Purpose	Specific Goals
Opening	Establish counseling relationship. Build rapport. Identify outcomes.	Provide informed consent. Identify client concerns. Establish concrete goals for counseling. Establish baseline for client concerns.
Working	Work with client, through client issues. Modify treatment plan as needed.	Identify appropriate, client-specific interventions. Track changes in client concerns (e.g., improvement, lessening of severity).
Closing	Reduce need for counseling. Help client rely on self without counselor. Plan for future concerns.	Monitor and report changes in client's behavior. Plan for termination. Discuss plans for life after counseling (e.g., how to handle future problems, when to consider returning).

CHAPTER SUMMARY

The counseling session can be a dynamic, collaborative process equally involving the counselor and the client. Counselors can utilize fundamental skills and ideas to outline the counseling process. Counselors, trained on the importance of development, systems, relationships, and culture, emphasize wellness and prevention in their work with clients, across multiple settings.

During the counseling process, the counselor implements strategies and interventions after considering various aspects about the client. Developmental factors include age and cognitive abilities of the client. Additionally, the client and the counselor address multicultural factors, such as sex, ethnicity, and religion. Counselors will also explore systemic influences in the client's life, including school, work, and legal systems. Finally, counselors incorporate relational attributes such as romantic, familial, and social relationships into treatment planning.

Counselors can work in a variety of settings, including schools and clinical mental health centers. In these settings, counselors work with clients with a myriad of issues. Based on their training and education, counselors approach clients through the lens of a wellness model; counselors look at clients holistically, considering age, development, culture, context, and individual traits or characteristics. In addition to work in different settings, counselors can also utilize technology to conduct online counseling.

When opening a counseling session, the counselor leads with a nonjudgmental stance and aims to establish rapport. The counselor gives space and attention to what the client describes. Counselors set goals and establish roles for this egalitarian, professional relationship.

In the working portion of the counseling session, the client shares more details about their life; and the counselor helps direct the flow and navigation of the session. The counselor draws upon the basic attending skills to help steer the session, and to further enhance rapport with the client. During this working phase of the session, the counselor may also make use of theory and interventions.

In the closing part of the session, the counselor aims to establish continuity of care, and helps to keep the client working toward their original goals. The counselor describes next steps and delegates tasks to the client that would aid the therapeutic process during the closing section. In some instances, the counselor may utilize referrals and termination.

Counselors should continue to distinguish themselves from other mental health professionals. Every counseling relationship is unique and counselors should not take a one-size-fits-all approach. New counselors may feel overwhelmed and lost when they begin to see clients. However, the basic attending skills can greatly enhance how counselors communicate with clients. Once the counselor establishes rapport, the counselor and client can take incredible strides toward working on the client's goals.

POINTS TO REMEMBER

- Counselors work from a wellness model, considering each client's systems, development, culture, and unique traits and relations with others.
- The counseling relationship should be collaborative, with deference given to the client's expertise on their own life.
- Rapport serves as the foundation upon which the counseling relationship can be established.

- Basic attending skills can be used early and often with clients.
- The beginning stage (the opening) of counseling lays the foundation for trust and rapport.
- The middle stage (or working section) of counseling introduces interventions from the counselor and requires much effort from the client.
- The ending stage (or closing stage) of counseling calms the client and prepares them for the next session.
- Treatment planning should involve the client and incorporate theory.
- Counselors must terminate appropriately to avoid client abandonment.
- Effective referrals involve an intentional selection of other professionals for the client to work with.

OTHER HELPFUL INFORMATION FOR CONSIDERATION

- American Counseling Association: www.counseling.org
- American School Counseling Association: www.schoolcounselor.org
- A Brief Guide to Cognitive Behavioral Therapy: depts.washington.edu/dbpeds/therapists_guide_to_brief_cbtmanual.pdf
- Session Goals and Guidelines handout: hhs.texas.gov/sites/default/files/documents/doing-business-with-hhs/provider-portal/behavioral-health-provider/cognitive-behavioral-therapy-resources/session-goals-guidelines.pdf

QUESTIONS FOR FURTHER DISCUSSION

- Reflect on past conversations where you felt truly heard by the other person. What did they do to help you feel heard?
- Regarding the skill of confrontation, how uncomfortable would you be confronting a client (if at all)? What would make you feel more comfortable? If you feel comfortable, where does that confidence come from?
- What drew you to the counseling profession? Why counseling/school counseling, and not one of the other mental health professions?
- How would you request privacy from a client's family?

KEY REFERENCES

Only key references appear in the print edition. The full reference list appears in the digital product on Springer Publishing Connect: connect.springerpub.com/content/book/978-0-8261-4764-6/part/part02/chapter/ch07

Brammer, L. M. (1973). *The helping relationship: Process and skills.* Prentice Hall.
Corey, G. (2017). *Theory and practice of counseling and psychotherapy* (10th ed., Student ed.). Brooks/Cole/Cengage Learning.

Halstead, R. W. (2015). Designing the counseling intervention: Framing the client's living story. In R. W. Halstead (Ed.), *Assessment of Client Core Issues* (pp. 53–67). American Counseling Association. https://doi.org/10.1002/9781119222798.ch4

Ivey, A. E., Daniels, T., Zalaquett, C. P., & Ivey, M. B. (2017). Neuroscience of attention: Empathy and counseling skills. In T. A. Field, L. K. Jones, & L. A. Russell-Chapin (Eds.), *Neurocounseling: Brain-based clinical approaches* (pp. 81–100). American Counseling Association.

Ivey, A. E., Packard, N. G., Ivey, M. B., Bailey, D. F., Santiago-Rivera, A. L., Lyons, K., & Microtraining Associates. (2019). *Basic attending skills*. Cognella Academic Publishing.

Karson, M., & Fox, J. (2010). Common skills that underlie the common factors of successful psychotherapy. *American Journal of Psychotherapy, 64*(3), 269–281. https://doi.org/10.1176/appi.psychotherapy.2010.64.3.269

Mackrill, T. D. (2011). Differentiating life goals and therapeutic goals: Expanding our understanding of the working alliance. *British Journal of Guidance and Counselling, 39*, 25–39.

Piselli, A., Halgin, R., & Macewan, G. (2011). What went wrong? Therapists' reflections on their role in premature termination. *Psychotherapy Research, 21*(4), 400–415. https://doi.org/10.1080/10503307.2011.573819

Wampold, B. E. (2001). *The great psychotherapy debate: Models, methods, and findings* (2nd ed.). Routledge.

Young, M. E. (2017). *Learning the art of helping: Building blocks and techniques*. Merrill.

PART III

Bridging Gaps: Special Populations (Children, Adolescents, and Parents)

CHAPTER 8

Contemporary Issues and Counseling Tropisms: Leaning Toward Promise With Children and Adolescents

Deborah Healy and Kristin O'Donnell

LEARNING OBJECTIVES

After completing this chapter, the reader should be able to:

- Express familiarity with social challenges to healthy child development.
- Recognize the crucial role of professional school and clinical mental health counselors in the cultivation of positive school and community contexts.
- Hypothesize counseling from a strengths-based, curious, and creative stance.

CACREP STANDARDS FOR THIS CHAPTER

- CACREP 2016: 2.f.3.e.f.h.i.; 5.c.d.e.f.j.k.m.; School Counseling: 5.G.2.a.b.g.; 3.d.f.h.; Clinical Mental Health Counseling: 5.C.3.b.e.
- CACREP 2009, Section II: 2.G.1.b.; 2.a.b.c.e.f.; 3.f.h.; 5.a.b.; School Counseling: III.A.3.6.d; C.3; D.; E.2.3.4; K.1.2; M.1.2.3.5; Clinical Mental Health Counseling: III.C.1.8.9; E.1.2.

INTRODUCTION

Viewing a plant leaning toward the nourishment of sunlight causes many to wonder. Seemingly, no one taught the plant to do that. Scientists call that tropism. Plants and people hold a natural proclivity to reach for cultivating environments that support healthy growth and development. Professional school counselors, clinical mental health counselors, and educators must ask, "How nourishing is the soil of our families, school communities, neighborhoods, classrooms, and larger cultural contexts?" "How will we gather and mobilize collective support to bring about positive change in the lives of our students?" Professional school counselors and clinical mental health counselors play a vital role in preventing, addressing, and mitigating the effects of many contemporary social concerns, including the problems of family discord, violence, substance abuse, suicide, youth depression, immigration stress, bullying, and more.

The counseling profession makes available numerous opportunities to foster healthy contexts that invite "leaning toward promise." What might change if school counselors and educators stopped speaking of students as "at risk" and began to think of them as "at promise" (Craig, 2015; Walker, 2015)? This should foster a first step toward a more optimistic and strengths-based approach to working with students—a contextual tropism. "At risk" may be the systemic *environments* that do not support healthy youth development. The greater number and scope of positive supports we provide to students, the greater the likelihood they will flourish academically, interpersonally, and socially. More information about the "at-risk"/"at-promise" population will be provided in Chapter 10.

When professionals believe that the problem resides within the student, they then think that the student must be changed. When professionals adopt a strengths-based approach indicating that "the problem is the problem" (White & Epston, 1990, p. 40), *then the person is not the problem.* The person possesses strengths that can be leveraged both toward and against the problem, since not all problems need to be extinguished; some can be transformed. This stance helps to reduce stigma and widens the scope of change. The counselor and client tackle the problem, not the person. The targets of change become the patterns between and among people and within systems. The emphasis shifts from individual blame to strategic solution building for positive contextualized, sustainable change (deShazer et al., 2007). White and Epston (1990) termed this concept *externalization* and viewed the problem as residing outside of the person and, therefore, much more available for change. This also promotes the development of a success identity for students rather than a failure identity and allows students to invite teachers and counselors a glimpse of their "quality world" or meaningful personal space (Glasser, 1997). Glasser indicates that students hold the right to be in control of their learning. Educators would be wise to respect and support students and avoid coercion. Students will exercise their curiosity to learn when educators uphold their rights to succeed and fail and when the relationships and quality of instruction meet their needs.

Through the years, professional school counselors have continuously intervened to combat the labeling of students. Commonly heard school labels include the bully, the "special-ed" student, the troublemaker, the class clown, the slow learner, the smart kid, and more. Labels produce impact. Students distinguish themselves through the many roles and identities they occupy. Since labels appear to be one dimensional, they "totalize" students—as though this represents holistically this young person. These sticky labels appear as singular, thin descriptions (Morgan, 2000) and pose obstacles to the full expression of student's learning, growth, self-concept, and development.

Developmentally, systemically, relationally, and multiculturally speaking, virtually all codes of ethics in mental health (American Counseling Association, 2014; American Psychological Association [APA], 2016) call upon mental health providers to uphold the highest levels of respect for clients and avoid any language, label, or action that may be perceived as demeaning. For example, nonbiased or person-first language became an initiative of the APA (2015) and stipulated that no label should precede the name of the person. This model would speak of children with autism, not autistic children, or students in special education programming, not special-ed students.

The American School Counseling Association (2020) advances a similar wide-scope view in the Preamble to the Code of Ethics:

> *School counselors are advocates, leaders, collaborators, and consultants who create systemic change. . . . School counselors demonstrate their belief that all students have the ability to learn by advocating for an education system that provides optimal learning environments for all students.* (p. 1)

Activity 8.1

Using a glass jar, place a stick figure of the student in the jar. On the outside of the jar, place sticky notes indicating all of the factors that impact the development of this youth (e.g., environmental, familial, cultural, health related, socioeconomics, nutrition, gender, religion, era in history, generational, weather factors, education, sexual orientation).

Debrief. Discuss the impact of the many factors that influence youth development and how mental health professionals may embrace these influences in a way that acknowledges and benefits student clients. Discuss how these multifaceted factors defy labeling of the student.

CONTEXT

Bronfenbrenner (1979) underscores the importance of viewing students contextually in the Ecological Systems Theory Model. This model reminds us that children develop in concentric, nested, and interactive systems, not in isolation. The systems described include the following: The *microsystem*, the innermost circle—family, household, and school; the *mesosystem* contains the tangled relationships between and among the microsystems; the *exosystem* influences actions and occurrences in the microsystem; the *macrosystem* holds the cultural, social, and rhythmic realm; the *chronosystem* refers to aspects of time and era; and the *technosystem*, which no one saw to be more salient than in the coronavirus disease 2019 (COVID-19) world, refers to how technology became a virtual lifeline. Brief systemic approaches to counseling allow for the conceptualization of children "in motion" in familial–cultural systems and therefore invite larger units of study beyond viewing the student singularly. Furthermore, Paat (2013) applies Bronfenbrenner's systems to work with children in immigration situations, adding legal, cultural, and sociopolitical considerations. This becomes especially relevant to children in resettlement communities and unaccompanied minors.

Students live in complex systems that continue to be dynamic, multilayered, intersectional, and interactional. As noted from the "student in a jar" activity, the factors that influence change appear more likely to surround our therapy clients than to be solely situated within them. Professional school and mental health counselors would be wise to consider and understand systems and advocate for change at systemic, interpersonal, and intrapersonal levels. How can this be accomplished? Working with families and teachers and groups, advancing advocacy skills, and noting aspects of social justice concerns inherent in procedures and policies will be an important aspect of supporting positive change.

THREATS TO HEALTHY YOUTH DEVELOPMENT

Data from a variety of sources underscore the imperative to mitigate the effects of threats to our nearly 77 million school-age students in the United States. Reviews of findings from the U.S. Census Bureau (2018), Gambon et al. (2020), and the Centers for Disease Control and Prevention (CDC; 2018) all point to the crucial need for educators to be aware of and plan for student success in the backdrop of social concerns that threaten student development and well-being. According to Curtin and Heron (2019) of the National Center for Health Statistics (2016), suicide ranks as the second leading cause of death for persons aged 10 to 14, 15 to 19, and 20 to 24. Signs and symptoms of suicidality include expressing hopelessness, having made a previous attempt at suicide or having a close relative or friend who died by suicide, giving away prized possessions, unable to speak of or imagine a future, writing a goodbye letter or note, and being preoccupied with death, dying, and highly depressive content. Other data from the CDC (2020) indicate challenges to healthy youth development in the United States (Table 8.1).

The profession recognizes an increase in diagnoses over the years. The diagnosis of depression and anxiety increased over time among children aged 6 to 17 years. The CDC (2020) noted an increase from 5.4% in 2003 to 8% in 2007 and to 8.4% in 2011 to 2012. School-based personnel should be especially mindful of these statistics since mental, behavioral, and developmental disorders that begin in early childhood and early intervention appear to be associated with better outcomes. Counselors report one in six U.S. children aged 2 to 8 years (17.4%) to be diagnosed with a mental, behavioral, or developmental disorder (CDC, 2020). The rate of diagnosed mental health concerns differs among various age cohorts. Depression and anxiety occur more commonly with increased age, and behavior problems occur more commonly in younger children (6–11). Noting these trends continues to be important for professional school and clinical mental health counselors and others to gain familiarity with the characteristics of these conditions and identify student needs.

These data indicate that mental health counselors diagnose children and adolescents more often with depression and anxiety and therefore may need additional treatment from outside school resources to address early interventions that mitigate the severity of these disorders. Data (CDC, 2020) indicate that youngsters with depression appear more likely to receive timely treatment. Nearly 8 in 10 children (78.1%) aged 3 to 17 years with depression received treatment, while only 6 in 10 children (59.3%) aged 3 to 17 years with anxiety received treatment. Counselors report that fewer children with behavior disorders receive treatment. Only about half of youth (53.5%) aged 3 to 17 with behavior disorders received treatment. Children may be less likely to receive treatment outside of school, which makes schools a prime place for mental health services to occur.

The presence of mental health disorders in children and adolescents evidences an increase over time, necessitating a call for action. Evidence suggests significant increases in mental health concerns among young people in Western nations between the early 20th century and the early 1990s (Twenge, 2011). More recently, research points to elevated numbers of anxiety and panic attacks (Goodwin, 2003; Scollon & Diener, 2006; Swindle et al., 2000; Twenge, 2000). While there have been reductions in the overall numbers of

TABLE 8.1 ATTENTION DEFICIT HYPERACTIVITY DISORDER

ADHD, behavior problems, anxiety, and depression represent the most commonly diagnosed mental disorders in children aged 3 to 17

Condition	Percent
Attention deficit hyperactivity disorder	9.4% (approximately 6.1 million)
Behavior problem	7.4% (approximately 4.5 million)
Comorbid Conditions	
Depression and anxiety	73.8% (3 in 4)
Depression and behavior problem	47.2% (1 in 2)
Anxiety and behavior problem	37.9% (1 in 3)
Anxiety and depression	32.3% (1 in 3)
Behavior problems and anxiety	36.6% (1 in 3)
Behavior problems and depression	20.3% (1 in 5)

ADHD, attention deficit hyperactivity disorder.

Source: National Alliance on Mental Illness. (2019). *Mental health by the numbers*. https://www.nami.org/learn-more/mental-health-by-the-numbers

individuals who report mental health conditions since the peak in the 1990s, a very large percentage of the population continues to report having a mental health diagnosis that impacts their functioning and can lead to other concerning behaviors (Twenge, 2011).

One in 5 U.S. adults experience a mental health condition each year and one in 25 U.S. adults experience serious mental illness each year (National Alliance on Mental Illness [NAMI], 2017). As mentioned previously, mental health conditions in youth also appear more common than one might think. According to studies conducted by the Substance Abuse and Mental Health Services Administration (SAMHSA, 2018), the CDC (2020), Bronson and Berzofsky (2017), and the NAMI (2019), one in six U.S. youth aged 6 to 17 experience a mental health disorder each year, equating to 16.5% or 7.7 million youth. The need for youth to seek psychological services exists; however, few youth with a mental health concern receive services (NAMI, 2017). This statistic varies by diagnosis. Seventy-eight percent of individuals diagnosed with depression receive therapeutic services. However, anxiety falls within the next highest area, with about 53% of diagnosed individuals receiving services. In most cases, this leaves about half of youth diagnosed with a mental health condition without services to assist with their mental health needs. The lack of service provision can lead to larger and more systemic issues. An increase in suicide and dropout rates continues to occur, and 70% of youth in the juvenile justice system receive a diagnosis of a mental illness (NAMI, 2017). Adolescence, the time in which many of these mental health conditions become diagnosed, evidences trials of its own, which include such daily tasks as navigating school and family life, physical changes of maturation, pressures of friendships, and concern of the future. Chillag (2019) considers Mental Health First Aid to be a highly research-based, protocol-driven model that assists parents, teachers, community members, and nonmental health individuals to sharpen their observation skills and take effective action to identify youth who may be struggling with risk factors and might be considering suicide.

ADOLESCENT DEVELOPMENT AND BEHAVIOR

Adolescence (roughly ages 12–18) portends many changes mentally, physically, and emotionally. So many changes occur at any given time that might leave youths feeling overwhelmed by the multitude of thoughts and feelings they experience. These types of changes in thinking and behaving seem common and developmentally appropriate. However, while typical adolescents experience mood swings and changes to their behavior, the mental health concerns discussed in this chapter seem more significant than developmental changes to mood or behavioral shifts. Concerns ensue when these thoughts and feelings impair an adolescent's ability to function normally in their day-to-day activities.

Fear and nervousness manifest at school, especially as educators require youth to engage during the typical school day. Imagine students being assigned a research paper that will culminate in an oral classroom presentation. These students worked for weeks on the report and practiced reciting it all night long prior to the big day. When the students enter the school on the report's due date, they develop "butterflies" in their stomachs and sweaty palms. As the students wait in their seats, they find it difficult to listen to the other students reading their reports. Instead, the students sit and think about what it will be like when they get up in front of the class with all eyes looking at them. The time finally comes to present, and the teacher calls the students' names, in turn. The students stand up, feel a rush of nervousness, and ponder running from the room; but instead, the students take a big gulp and begin to read their reports with shaky voices. Before long, the students finish the report reading. Some can relax and give a big sigh of relief. Others remain anxious and unsettled.

Giving a report in front of a class, asking a group to join their activity, or entering a crowded, loud cafeteria can cause feelings of dread, nervousness, and worry. Sometimes, this uneasiness works as a motivator—a term called *eustress* (Selye, 1965). This feeling helps to propel a person into action and serves as the energy needed to accomplish a difficult task or keep one safe when danger arises (Tocino-Smith, 2020). This type of anxiousness seems common and experienced by many. However, when this stress and fear shifts to intense distress that impairs a student's ability to engage in the tasks asked of them in the school, a more significant distress may be present. Behavior rehearsals and scaffolding (Waite, 2019) can prepare the student for success.

CONTEMPORARY MENTAL HEALTH CONSIDERATIONS IN ADOLESCENCE

ANXIETY

Approximately 7% of children aged 3 to 17 experience anxiety disorders (NAMI, 2017). Most individuals who develop an anxiety disorder receive a diagnosis prior to age 21. The *Diagnostic and Statistical Manual of Mental Disorders*, Fifth Edition (*DSM-5*; American Psychiatric Association, 2013) classifies Generalized Anxiety Disorder, Social Anxiety Disorder, Panic Disorder, and Phobias under Anxiety Disorders. Characteristics of these disorders include chronic exaggerated worry about everyday life, intense fear in social interactions, feelings of panic and sudden terror that can strike repeatedly and without warning, and avoidance of certain objects, activities, or situations that make a person uncomfortable or fearful. The *DSM-5* classifies Anxiety Disorders as a group of related conditions with common symptoms. According to the *DSM-5*, these symptoms can be both emotional and physical. Emotional symptoms include feelings of apprehension or dread, feeling tense or jumpy, restless or irritable, anticipating the worst, and being watchful for signs of danger. Physical symptoms include pounding or racing heart and shortness of breath, sweating, tremors and twitches, headaches, fatigue and insomnia, upset stomach, and frequent urination or diarrhea.

The emotional and physical symptoms of anxiety can create challenges to optimal student performance in the school environment. In the preceding example, the student feeling anxious prevails over these feelings, performs the task, and moves on to the next activity. However, a difference transpires between typical feelings of fear and worry and those that require more specific and targeted intervention approaches. Clinically, significant levels of anxiety do not typically propel students into action but instead can cause inaction, lethargy, or "freezing." A student experiencing clinical levels of anxiety might not be able to begin their report or may complete the report but not show up to school on the due date. Students diagnosed with anxiety may or may not show signs of distress in school. The distinction between common forms of anxiousness and clinical forms of anxiousness lies in the symptomatic interference with daily activities. The former provides some fuel for action, and the latter often ceases action as the individual appears overwhelmed by the multiple steps needed in the assignment, along with managing the symptoms of their mental health condition.

DEPRESSION

Feelings of sadness and withdrawal may also be common during the period of adolescence. Typical development brings times of sadness and isolation as youth move from childhood pursuits to adolescent interests, and they experience both social and emotional changes linked to this change (National Council for Behavioral Health, 2016). Everyone experiences sadness and difficult times. Parents and school personnel may witness youth who do not interact with adults as much as they used to and instead rely on their peers for support through tough times. Youths may also spend more time alone or experience significant mood changes as they figure out their standing in this changing world. Such hurdles can be uncomfortable for individuals as they move through these events; however, they do not appear to be the same as depression. Youth, while experiencing changes in their relationships, continue to engage in social interactions (National Council for Behavioral Health, 2016). Though they may be sad for a time or experience mood swings, these passing moments do not impede their ability to function in their daily tasks (National Council for Behavioral Health, 2016).

Approximately 1.9 million children in the United States experience depressive disorder (Wesley, 2019). Common symptoms include changes in sleep and appetite, lack of concentration, loss of energy, lack of interest in activities, hopelessness or guilty thoughts, changes in movement (less activity or agitation), physical aches, and suicidal thoughts (NAMI, 2017). In order for an individual to be diagnosed with depressive disorder, a person must experience a depressive episode lasting longer than 2 weeks (American Psychiatric Association, 2013). Depression presents significant impacts on academics and social interactions for youth as well as impacting their eating and sleeping patterns along with social, emotional, and cognitive development (Wesley, 2019). Students who experience depression may encounter difficulty sleeping at night or getting up in the morning, which, in turn, will directly impact their attendance and exposure to curriculum. The symptoms of depression can also cause students to face difficulty interacting with others, which will increase their feelings of social isolation and cause them to withdraw from others more. In severe cases, suicide may be a concern. In 2018, suicide became the second leading cause of death, after accidental death, for people aged 10 to 34 (NAMI, 2017). Additional concerns for students with depression involve school persistence. High school students with severe depression become two times as likely to drop out of school as their peers (NAMI, 2017).

While anxiety and depression appear to be the most commonly diagnosed mental health conditions in youth, other threats to healthy mental health development exist. Mental health considerations for youth entail supporting them through events that may be related to external events, internal events, or both. Internal factors refer to a person's traits, feelings, or overall ability to recover. These factors may be genetic or tied to an individual's emotional health (NAMI, 2020). External factors depict environmental events that may impact a youth's development, such as home and family circumstances, exposure to media or social media, or the availability of a support network. These factors may be due to the environment, which include cultural pressures from family or popular culture pressure found in society (NAMI, 2020) and psychosocial factors (Russell-Mayhew et al., 2012). Professional school counselors hold a unique position to intervene. They can observe behaviors of students in their natural environments as they interact with their peers. Counselors may talk one on one with students, and they can talk with parents to gather an ecological picture of the youth's environment. This helps to determine effective methods and modes of intervention for youth and their families.

ADOLESCENT SUBSTANCE USE

According to the National Center for Drug Abuse Statistics (NCDAS, 2019), 86% of teenagers know someone who smokes, drinks, or uses drugs during the school day. Additionally, 47% of teenagers report that by the time they graduated from high school they had used an illegal drug. These statistics reveal the ever-growing concern that substance use presents in our schools and communities. A majority of teenagers get exposed to substance use, and 30% report seeing illicit drug use while on school property (NCDAS, 2019). Based on NCDAS's findings, 78% of teens reported that neither their doctor nor their dentist (the medical personnel who see adolescents the most) ever talked with them about dangerous or addictive properties of prescription drugs. This indicates that students, exposed at a young age, do not receive education on the many dangerous aspects of both illicit and prescription drug use.

Professional school counselors and other school personnel hold a unique position to engage youths in prevention, detection, and referral to intervention with adolescents. Schools and the counseling profession also see school mental health professionals to be best trained in working with adolescents and addressing them from a developmental perspective. Teens need individuals who will discuss the dangers and consequences associated with substance use in a manner also reflective of the many pressures that students face. It remains important that schools and communities work collaboratively with parents as well. According to research, 55.8% of teens point to their parents' disapproval or their fear of parental punishment as the main deterrent to using alcohol or drugs (NCDAS, 2019). These statistics can serve as driving forces to implementing programs aimed at helping adolescents to understand not only the pitfalls and dangers of substance use but also how to manage the peer pressures inherent in these circumstances.

Statistics also highlight alcohol and substance use as a contributing factor among the top three leading causes of death in youth aged 15 to 24. This includes accidents, homicides, and suicides (NCDAS, 2019). Alcohol consumption in this age range can most often be seen in binge drinking episodes, where an adolescent will consume a great deal of alcohol in a short period of time. Statistically, 11% of American teenagers consume alcohol through binge drinking annually.

NCDAS (2019) designates marijuana as the most commonly used drug among youth, with 36% of high schoolers reporting frequent use. Continuous marijuana use can increase the possibility of addiction. Individuals who use marijuana daily appear to be 25% to 50% more likely to become addicted (NCDAS, 2019). Habitual use can also cause an increase of comorbid conditions such as depression, poor educational outcomes, and memory difficulties. Professional school and clinical mental health counselors can be helpful in identifying students at risk and intervene early for the best overall outcomes.

Very few adolescents seek treatment for substance use. In 2018, only 0.3% of adolescents who needed substance use treatment actually received treatment from specialty facilities (NCDAS, 2019). This small number of individuals who received help further highlights the significant role schools and communities can play in helping those who need support to obtain support. Counselors can help students, parents, and school staff and the community by educating all regarding the dangers and warning signs of substance use. Once professionals or parents identify students as needing support, school counselors can refer them to services in the community that will best support them in their endeavors for treatment. Some schools use the national SBIRT model (Screening, Brief Intervention and Referral to Treatment) and other programs such as Mental Health First Aid for Youth (www.mentalhealthfirstaid.org/population-focused-modules/youth/) or programs provided through SAMHSA (www.samhsa.gov/find-help/national-helpline), which serve as a guide for schools, youth, and parents for noticing characteristics so they may seek support. Schools working collaboratively with parents demonstrate the best chance for success in decreasing the lasting effects of substance use in adolescents.

BODY IMAGE

Body image (how individuals view their own physical appearance) can appear as a complex concept and display many different aspects of self-perception. Developmental, systemic, relational, and multicultural influences impact self-perceptions. How individuals view their own appearance can be influenced by cultural and familial factors, for example. Body image includes satisfaction with appearance, as well as disturbance or dysmorphia influenced by biological, psychological, and social factors (Cash & Pruzinsky, 2002). An individual may be upset with their appearance and engage in activities such as exercising or eating a healthy diet, which will help them to feel better about themselves. These activities enhance a person's life in that they represent practices that enrich their overall well-being. However, when a person's belief about what they perceive their body to be does not match the reality of how they actually view their body, a disconnect occurs. This may lead to engaging in behaviors around weight loss that hurt or harm their physical and emotional well-being.

When body image leads to harmful behaviors, counselors typically term these as eating disorders. Eating disorders affect people of any age or gender but more often occur in women and typically begin in adolescence (NAMI, 2020). Eating disorders occur in 3% of adolescents (U.S. Department of Health and Human Services, 2018). An eating disorder can be characterized as a psychiatric illness that encompasses extreme fear of gaining weight and strong desire to be thin (Keca, 2004). This desire to be thin encompasses all that an individual does and often impairs the ability to engage in social situations, especially those that involve food. Counselors classify eating disorders into three different categories that are similar in that they involve severe food and weight issues but vary based on symptoms.

Counselors associate anorexia nervosa with refusal to maintain a normal body weight, characterized by 85% of expected body weight as defined by national norms (Keca, 2004). This condition may be characterized by extreme weight loss due to restricting food intake or binge and purge eating. Anorexia often represents an ongoing activity where the client consistently withholds or purges food to succeed in weight loss.

In contrast, bulimia nervosa represents a condition that reoccurs but does not happen consistently. Bulimia nervosa may be characterized by eating large amounts of food in a short period of time and then purging the food through vomiting, abusing laxatives, or excessive exercising (NAMI, 2020). Counselors diagnose youth twice as often with bulimia nervosa as anorexia, despite the fact that individuals with bulimia nervosa often appear to be of average body weight and cannot easily be detected by appearance alone (Gordon, 2000). Individuals with bulimia nervosa seek treatment more often than those with anorexia nervosa, leading to higher numbers of identification and interventions.

Counselors characterize binge-eating disorder by a loss of control over eating, and often an individual will eat large amounts of food in a short period of time (NAMI, 2020). This eating takes place in the absence of hunger and, at times, in the presence of already feeling overly full. After binge eating, a person with a binge-eating disorder will not attempt to purge the food. Individuals with binge-eating disorder appear commonly overweight; however, some maintain an average weight (Keca, 2004).

Eating disorders can produce physical effects in individuals. Due to the lack of food intake, individuals may experience loss of energy, lower or irregular heart rate, loss of menstruation, stomach issues, issues with digestion, and trouble sleeping (NAMI, 2020). Nutritional deprivation can present the initial effect of weight loss that leads to an individual appearing thin. However, the prolonged effect of this deprivation can lead to the body slowing down as it works hard to conserve its energy. While a person's physical well-being appears affected, a significant toll may also be taken on an individual's emotional well-being.

Individuals with eating disorders often feel a loss of control linked to feelings of lower self-esteem due to body image (NAMI, 2020). Guilt and shame also emerge as predominant emotions, which lead to individuals slowly withdrawing from others. This social isolation can be seen in interactions with peers and family and may continue to contribute to feelings of low self-worth.

Treatments for eating disorders often include a combination of medical treatment and therapy (Keca, 2004). While eating disorders often appear to be hard to diagnose, once determined, more than half of the individuals who seek assistance show significant improvement (Gordon, 2000). Due to the difficulty in diagnosing, it remains important that people in the lives of youth monitor the physical and emotional factors that may be signs of an eating disorder. Noticing the signs may lead to saving a life.

ABUSE

The CDC (2020) describes child abuse as a "serious public health problem" and further documents that one in seven children experienced abuse in the past year (para. 1). Annually, nearly 2,000 children die as a result of abuse. Schools hold a unique position to serve as a safety net for both prevention and intervention. Teachers, counselors, and other school professionals can be attuned to the indicators of child and adolescent well-being.

The schools call on professional school and mental health counselors to work with systems of care on behalf of children (e.g., social workers, police, Child Protective Service caseworkers). This also includes educating teachers on sharpening their observation and reporting skills. More information on abuse will be covered in Chapter 11.

SELF-INJURY

According to the U.S. Department of Health and Human Services, Centers for Disease Control and Prevention, National Center for Health Statistics (2017), clients make nearly 500,000 ED hospital visits annually in the United States for self-injury. Boyles (2012) indicates nearly 8% of third-grade students engage in some form of self-injurious behavior. Kress and Drouhard (2006) outline the legal and ethical concerns that counselors need to consider when working with clients who self-injure. While professional school and clinical mental health counselors strive to maintain confidentiality with students, they must balance this with a parent's right to know. This often appears to be a difficult circumstance when working with minors. Nevertheless, assessment continues to be important in these situations to gage the likelihood of serious harm. Often through clinical interview, the practitioner can determine the frequency and severity and make sound ethical and legal choices in the best interest of the student. The distinction between suicidal and nonsuicidal self-injury (NSSI) remains an important one. DeAngelis (2015) defines self-injury as a variety of behaviors that may include cutting, burning, scrapping, and skin picking and distinguishes NSSI from those behaviors meant to cause loss of life. According to Whitlock (2011), about 15% of college students engaged in self-injurious behavior at least once while compared to about 17% of teens (Muehlenkamp et al., 2012).

BULLYING

Bullying provides a significant challenge in schools and spans across all grade levels, from elementary schools to high schools. According to the National Center for Education Statistics and Bureau of Justice Statistics (2017), about 20% of students aged 12 to 18 report that they experienced bullying. This demonstrates a decrease from 29% to 20% from 2005 to 2017. However, the prevalence rates continue to be between one and four and one and three students who report that they have been bullied at some point during their school career. According to the CDC's Youth Risk Behavior Surveillance System Report (CDC, 2017a), most bullying occurs in middle school (Figure 8.1).

In 2014, the federal government released a uniform definition of bullying to provide guidance to schools and other entities in determining which characteristics to look for in terms of intervention and consequences. Gladden et al. (2014) determined unwanted aggressive behavior, power imbalances (perceived or observed), and the repetition of these behaviors to be the core elements of bullying. Bullying can be either direct or indirect. Direct bullying occurs in the presence of the youth and may include fighting, verbal threats to a student, stating an untruth to damage their reputation, or destruction of the youth's possessions. Indirect bullying occurs outside of the youth's presence and may come in the form of spreading rumors to damage the youth's reputation, getting another person to engage in physical aggression against them, or not allowing someone to be a part of a group by excluding them from an activity. Both boys and girls experience bullying directly

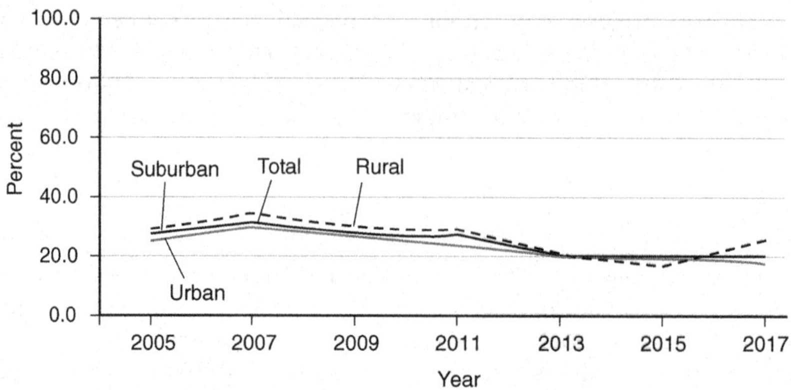

FIGURE 8.1 Youth risk behavior surveillance system report.

Source: U.S. Department of Justice, Bureau of Justice Statistics, School Crime Supplement (SCS) to the National Crime Victimization Survey, 2005 through 2017.

and indirectly; however, boys appear to be more often bullied through physical aggression and girls seem more likely to engage in relational aggression, where they spread rumors and engage in social exclusion or isolation (Robison, 2010).

Bullying can occur in direct person-to-person interaction or in a virtual setting. Based on data found in the 2017 School Crime Supplement (SCS) to the National Crime Victimization Survey, 42% to 43% of students report that bullying occurred in the school setting inside a classroom or hallway/stairwell; 26.8% report being bullied in a cafeteria; and 12.1% in a bathroom. Nearly 22% of students report being bullied outside the school grounds and 8% state they experienced bullying on a bus. Around 15% of students reported that they experienced bullying online or by text (National Center for Educational Statistics, 2017). These data indicate the majority of students who report being bullied experience these incidents in the school setting.

Cyberbullying, which involves the use of electronic forms of communication via phone, text, email, or websites to harass or harm individuals, appears common most often in high school settings (Feinberg & Robey, 2010). According to the SCS to the National Crime Victimization Survey, ethnic differences occur, in that 17.3% of White students and 16.0% of students who identify as two or more races reported being cyberbullied in the past year. This compares to 10.9% of Black students and 10.0% of Asian students who report being cyberbullied. Additionally, female students in grades 9, 10, and 11 experienced bullying much more often (20%–22%) than students in sixth grade (7%); see National Center for Educational Statistics (2017).

Bullying presents long-lasting effects on students involved, whether representing the role of a bystander, who witnesses the bullying events, or an active participant in the bullying event. Barriers to learning and other negative outcomes such as decreased academic performance, increased risk of substance abuse, delinquency, suicide, truancy, mental health problems, and physical injury all relate to involvement with bullying (Robison, 2010). Bullying represents broad effects in schools, impacting students at all different socioeconomic levels, in all communities, across gender and ethnic lines. For this reason, it remains imperative that school personnel implement programs to address prevention and intervention.

While counselors note bullying to occur in all grade levels and across genders, they recognize differences in the types of bullying that students experience based on age and gender. No one bullying prevention program fully eradicates bullying in schools. Schoolwide prevention programs appear to be effective at educating students and adults about the definitions of bullying and signs of distress and actions to take. Best practices for schoolwide prevention programs include comprehensive policies and procedures that foster a safe and supportive learning environment focusing on acceptance and inclusion (Lazarus & Pfohl, 2010).

Olweus (1993) examined school climate and its impact on bullying. His findings determined that changing the school climate to one that appears more positive, inclusive, and accepting significantly reduced the prevalence and impact of bullying. This substantive body of research led to the development of four key steps to implementing effective schoolwide bullying prevention programs (see Table 8.2).

Programs such as *Bully Proof Your School*, *Bully Busters*, and *Steps to Respect* teach students, witnesses, and targets on how to intervene in bullying situations. These represent examples of full comprehensive programs that effectively focus on knowledge, attitudes, and skill development through the use of role play and modeling (Lazarus & Pfohl, 2010). While school officials often use these programs to implement schoolwide practices, other best-practice suggestions for creating a positive school climate exist. These practices include surveying students to determine their feelings about bullying in their school; developing specific, clear, and concrete antibullying policies; and encouraging students to sign a proclamation that they will not bully and that they will take action by reporting when they witness bullying. Protective factors can be best nurtured through relationship building in the school between and among adults and students (Lazarus & Pfohl, 2010; Pelligrini & Long, 2004). The results of efforts may not be immediately apparent. Patience may be needed throughout the implementation and revision processes in order to see lasting change. Professional school counselors and other members of school mental health teams (e.g., school psychologists, school social workers) serve in an ideal position to work as change agents in endeavors to increase the positive aspects of school climate. School mental health personnel hold a duty to help students who represent the

TABLE 8.2 FOUR STEPS TO CHANGING SCHOOL CLIMATE TO REDUCE THE IMPACT OF BULLYING

Step	Action to Be Taken
1	Create both school and home environments characterized by warmth, positive regard, and involvement with adults.
2	Establish firm limits against unacceptable behavior.
3	Apply nonphysical, nonhostile negative sanctions if a student breaks a rule.
4	Expect that all adults in the school hold a responsibility for maintaining a safe and supportive school climate.

Source: Olweus, D. (1993). *Bullying at school: What we know and what we can do.* Blackwell.

bully, the bullied, and those who witness bullying by providing meaningful, influential interventions and support individualization to the school and student needs. This can help to increase positive behaviors, alleviate negative behaviors, and reduce student suspension and expulsion.

BUILDING EMPATHY

A key strategy to the prevention of bullying takes place when counselors amplify its opponent process; in other words, emphasize empathy, kindness, character education, and social-emotional learning. Educators need to teach and model desired behavior, rather than focusing chiefly on eradicating undesirable behavior. Focusing on the presence of something rather than on its absence leads to positive, observable, and actionable goal setting and change. Teaching empathy continues to be an imperative:

> *Without empathy, justice-making and peace-keeping are impossible. So, cultivating empathetic practices among ourselves and our students must be among our highest priorities.* (Shushok, 2015, p. 2)

School leaders can take five steps to teach empathy in schools: modeling, teaching, practicing, setting clear expectations, and making school culture and climate a priority (Jones et al., 2018). Many teachers and counselors promote student empathy skills through schoolwide caring campaigns, character education, service-learning opportunities, advisory programs, positive behavior initiatives, and class meetings (Leachman & Victor, 2003). Newstreet et al. (2019) address cultivating empathy with a multicultural emphasis deconstructing Islamophobia using children's literature. Sivaraman (2017) offers specifics on building empathy in children with autism. In Texas, professional school counselors provide weekly classroom guidance via direct instruction in four strategic areas: (a) intrapersonal effectiveness; (b) interpersonal effectiveness; (c) postsecondary education and career readiness; and (d) personal health and safety aimed at perspective taking, empathy building, personal and ethical decision-making, interpersonal and cross-cultural effectiveness, and more (Texas Education Agency, 2018, p. 84).

Again, the programs listed earlier under bullying teach students, witnesses, and targets how to intervene in bullying situations and demonstrate examples of full comprehensive programs that effectively focus on knowledge, attitudes, and skill development through the use of role play and modeling (Lazarus & Pfohl, 2010).

SCHOOL SUSPENSIONS AND EXPULSIONS

School officials do not consider misbehavior in school as a new phenomenon. Students of all ages engage in conduct that results in classroom or out-of-classroom consequences. For the most part, teachers typically will maintain their own classroom behavior management system that will, in some cases, culminate in a student being sent to the principal's office. Once school personnel refer a student to the principal, they follow the schoolwide rules for behavior management. Schools typically seek to offer consequences to students that will allow them to stay in school while rectifying the situation. School suspensions and expulsions occur when students engage in behaviors that significantly violate the code of conduct. In some cases when an egregious offense occurs or when misbehavior persists, the school suspends students; in some extreme cases, when students bring a weapon to school, they can be expelled.

Systemically and relationally speaking, evidence in the literature shows that out-of-school suspensions or expulsions appear to negatively affect student outcomes and the overall learning environment (APA, 2008; Healy & O'Donnell, 2018; Minnesota of Department of Education, 2012). Suspensions also affect how supported students feel in their educational environment. When schools suspend or expel students, students become less able to learn prosocial behaviors that will help to alleviate the difficulties they experience. Often, the school suspends them because of persistent misbehavior. It would seem that in order to help students, they should stay in school to learn appropriate behaviors with supportive personnel to teach and guide them along the way. Instead, when the school suspends them, or in extreme cases, expels them, students become removed from the environment that would offer this support and guidance. A correlation exists between student suspensions, the overall dropout rate, and a link to incarceration later in life in that a high percentage of those incarcerated also dropped out of school (New York Civil Liberties Union, 2008).

Schools use systemwide supports to help individuals with behavioral difficulties through remediation and support instead of punitive actions only. Despite the need for more social-emotional support in school settings, 1.6 million students attend schools that employ police officers and no professional school counselors (Blad & Harwin, 2017). Lack of professional school counselors can lead to differences in the ways that the school handles discipline and remediation of behavior.

In schools where school officials employ safety officers over employing school counselors, this represents a marked movement toward punitive strategies as opposed to prevention and intervention. When students become exposed early to the legal system, this can lead to continued interactions and involvement within the system. Additionally, students tend to view school as places of punitive actions instead of places where they can thrive and learn. There also happens to be an ethnic and socioeconomic aspect to this issue. School districts require schools located in lower socioeconomic areas with less funding supports to make this hard staffing decision more often than schools located in more affluent areas, where adequate funding to employ both a professional school counselor and safety officers exists.

School counselors and other school mental health professionals serve as the only individuals within a school setting who hold training on how to properly infuse mental wellness into the learning environment by supporting optimum conditions of learning through social-emotional and learning supports (Cowan et al., 2013). In order for students to thrive academically, they first need to be able to thrive emotionally. This emotional wellness paves the way for learning to occur. In addition to behavioral supports, school counselors also provide guidance in other aspects of growth and development.

SEXUAL IDENTITY

Murchison (2016) developed a guide, *Supporting and Caring for Transgender Children.* Social gender transition may be an initial step in which children can be permitted to hold power over their gender expression through naming, dressing, and moving in the world in a manner consistent with their understanding of their authentic and preferred gender. The literature defines helpful terms such as "gender expansive," "intersex," "nonbinary," and more. Specifically, respecting children's understanding of self in terms of gender can be lifesaving. Gender and sexual identity differ from sexual orientation. Identity does not denote an attraction to others but rather about how one understands oneself. Transgender individuals could be gay, lesbian, bisexual, heterosexual, or questioning. Identity becomes central; and children experiencing gender incongruence deserve to be heard and understood in order to mitigate the effects of dissonance, shame, and dysphoria. More information on sexual identity will be covered in Chapter 10.

SEXUAL ORIENTATION

The APA help guide entitled *Just the Facts about Sexual Orientation and Youth: A Primer for Principals, Educators, and School Personnel* (Just the Facts Coalition, 2008) cautions against conversion therapies and other methods shown to be injurious. The consensus of half a million practitioners confirms the rejection of conversion therapy as an ethical practice. The authors assert that sexual orientation can be conceptualized along a continuum, though often described as binary—either heterosexual or homosexual. This oversimplifies sexual identity. The authors also point out that gay and lesbian students experience more discrimination, violence and family rejection, and isolation. All students deserve a safe school and learning environment where they can feel respected and welcomed (Abreu et al., 2018). The CDC (2017b, 2018) documented the following:

"According to data of surveyed LGB students from the 2015 National Youth Risk Behavior Surveillance (YRBS),

- 10% experienced being threatened or injured with a weapon on school property,
- 34% experienced bullying on school property,
- 28% experienced bullying electronically,
- 23% of LGB students who dated or went out with someone during the 12 months before the survey experienced sexual dating violence in the prior year,
- 18% of LGB students experienced physical dating violence, and
- 18% of LGB students experience being forced to participate in sexual intercourse at some point in their lives."

Specifically, 98.1% of LGBT students heard the word "gay" used in a derogatory manner, 85.2% reported verbal harassment, and 34.7% reported being physically harassed in the past year. The Trevor Project cites research from the CDC (2015), indicating that LGBT youth appear nearly five times more likely to attempt suicide than youth who identify as heterosexual.

The formation of Gay–Straight Alliances (GSAs) represents one way that many school communities acknowledge that schools can be inclusive and welcoming to all. The National Association of Gay-Straight Alliance Networks (Buehler et al., 2011) offers an advisor handbook that clearly outlines how to get started. Since 1973, advocacy and support to families continue to be the mainstays of the not-for-profit Parents and Friends of Lesbians and Gays (PFLAG) organization. Additionally, bullying cannot be tolerated. Respect for all efforts remains crucial. The signing of the Declaration of Respect in the Northside Independent School District (2019) in San Antonio, Texas, represents one such effort, where over the past decade, more than 500,000 students and teachers added their signatures to declare their respect for all on Unity Day each October. These include outreach efforts, rainbow coalitions, character education, and an expectation of respect for all!

COVID-19

In the spring of 2020, COVID-19 upended the rhythms of daily life globally. This virus revealed and magnified underlying health disparities, which compounded the difficulties in accessing resources and care, illuminating all of the other stressors children and families already faced. Nearly 56 million school-age students plunged into virtual education with only a few days to prepare. According to Younger (2020), Division 43 of the APA, children and adolescents benefit from stabilizing routines during times of sustained uncertainty and disruption. The profession calls on adults to provide grounding in the face of sudden and jarring change. Counselors worked with families to help some secure the internet, a computer, a quiet place, and guided an adult at home on how to assist. Counselors show sensitivity when assessing dangers of domestic violence, which by some reports spiked during "stay at home" orders (Taub, 2020). Teachers and parents pivoted, multitasked, and accepted different roles and responsibilities while grappling with economic and health threats unparalleled in over a century.

Separated and divorced parents who share custody during any crisis such as the pandemic must construct routines that allow their children to feel calm and safe. Younger (2020) suggests that parents need to work together whether coparenting, parallel parenting, or living together. A unified approach helps to stabilize family life and offer some predictability in the midst of chaos and uncertainty. Bartlett et al. (2020) indicate that children can be "keen observers" of their social world and seem more susceptible to the reactions of the adults who set the tone for their emotional effects of the pandemic. Therefore, the profession encourages parents and counselors to pay special attention to their own well-being since they represent potential models of coping and resilience (Seligman, 2007). Children and teens appear better able to cope and make sense of their experiences when the adults lead the way. Bartlett et al. (2020) recommend the *new* "3 Rs: reassurance, routines, and regulation."

In the spring of 2020, nearly four million high school seniors faced postponing graduation celebrations or participating in virtual meetings to acknowledge their accomplishments. The emotional impact of this upheaval merits substantial attention as society slowly returns to life after stay at home orders though in new and different ways. As covered in Chapter 1, Maslow (1943) emphasized the fundamental imperative to meet human needs prioritized in a pyramid with physiology and safety as the primary platforms upon which self-actualization can be predicated. Restoration of safety (psychologically, medically, and economically) represents a priority and likely more of a process, than an event. Counselors stand prepared to assist.

Mental health professionals quickly pivoted to becoming telecounseling providers, despite a lack of prior training or supervision in telehealth. During 2020, the profession relaxed many legal requirements of telehealth in order to make counseling and other health services far more widely available. These changes in access to care may lead to more permanent modifications in how mental health delivers services in the future.

THE IMPACT OF MENTAL HEALTH ON EDUCATIONAL FUNCTIONING

While effects of mental health disorders can severely impact a student's ability to keep up with their academic and social pursuits in school, it can still be overcome. School staff can assist students in helping to ensure their success academically and emotionally by first being on the lookout for the symptoms mentioned earlier. The ability to identify when a student needs help can be the first step to mental wellness for the student. With treatment, wellness appears not only possible but likely.

Knowing these trends in children's mental health and the effects emphasizes the importance of easy access to prevention and intervention services. Professional school counselors, embedded in the school building, can be wonderful first responders for mental health services. In the school counseling office, students receive "on-the-spot" walk-in services (Slive & Bobele, 2011) and might be seen many times or only once. Knowing that students and families move away, it remains crucial to be strategic and make the most of every session.

Working in multidisciplinary teams within the school may be another outlet for school counselors. In the majority of states, professional school counselors served as former teachers well versed in assessment, behavioral interventions, classroom management strategies and in working on teams with teachers, school nurses, after-school program staff, ancillary service providers, administration, parent groups, and community stakeholders. Professional school counselors hold a master's degree in mental health and know the importance of a collective and collaborative approach to building a healthy school community. Professional school counselors also hold experience in needs assessments, interpretation of career and interest inventories, academic testing, and student remediation plans through Response to Intervention (to be discussed fully in Chapter 9) and other programs. School counseling and school psychology work collaboratively, predicated upon united and multidisciplinary efforts. Providing appropriate mental health services to students within the context of the school can be a challenging task and one that requires a pooling of resources. Mental health teams that include professional school counselors, school psychologists, and school social workers present an effective method for supporting student success. Professional school counselors and school psychologists receive training to identify how behavior can affect learning and success in school. Each field showcases unique training in assessing for need and determining intervention strategies. School social workers receive unique training in finding services outside of the school that will help to build stronger students and families. While the training received differs, they maintain a common goal in providing social, emotional, and behavioral support to students with the intent of assisting the student in being successful in school.

THE COMMON FACTORS RESEARCH

Lambert (2005) researched the variables that account for positive counseling outcomes. Resoundingly, it appears that the working alliance, a sense of hope and expectancy, and the extratherapeutic client factors account for 85% of the counseling or therapy outcomes. Only 15% appears to be attributable to the theoretical approach. The relationship, the sense of optimism, and the strengths and resources of the client account for 85% of the outcomes. Therefore, it remains crucial that professional school and clinical mental health counselors pay attention to the rapport, the relationship, the hopeful and affirming possibilities, and the strengths the client already possesses. This involves determining what seems to be going well, in addition to determining how counselors can magnify this while serving the clients.

THE RELATIONSHIP–ISOLATION DILEMMA

Historically, the increase in electronic means of communication permits the sharing of ideas on a global scale. The internet and social media present ways in which people share their views and stay connected with others by sharing pictures and stories of their day. People can stay in contact with those who live far away through these relatively free and easy electronic means. However, what can be done about the fact that this means of interaction seems, in some ways, to replace face-to-face communication? In the midst of the COVID-19 pandemic, the paradigm shifted. Technology actually became a lifeline for connection, schooling, and securing basic food and durable goods. One wonders if the rhetoric around the role of technology will evolve from the popular belief that electronic modes of communication exist to help keep people connected but may be contributing to more social isolation and less social interface that warrants addressing. Research beginning in the 1990s and continuing into the 2000s examined the impact that social isolation and disconnection from each other subsists on the increase in mental health conditions (Eckersley & Dear, 2002; Myers, 2000; Seligman, 1990; Twenge, 2006, 2011).

THE FINDINGS OF THE SEARCH INSTITUTE

The Search Institute, a nonprofit research agency founded in 1958, became solely dedicated to documenting the factors (or positive assets) that lead to the reduction of risk and the promotion of health and well-being of children, teens, families, and communities. Their research spans 25 years with six million students responding to their surveys. The Search Institute (2020) outlines its history in a timeline entitled *Our Story,* documenting decades of commitment to healthy youth development. Students who obtain a greater number of "assets" acquire greater protective factors against the use of drugs, involvement in violence, and early sexual contact. The Search Institute describes these assets in eight domains: *External Assets* represent Support (e.g., mentorship from family and teachers), Empowerment (opportunities for youth to be of service to others), Boundaries and Expectations (rules and structure), Constructive Use of Time (leisure activities, sports, music); *Internal Assets,* which speak to Commitment to Learning (taking pride in school achievement), Positive Values (having a sense of purpose larger than self), Social Competencies (developing interpersonal effectiveness and positive relationships), and Positive Identity (instilling self-esteem and goals), acquire greater protective factors against the use of drugs, involvement in violence, and early sexual contact. At the same time, these protective assets also appear to be associated with great leadership skill demonstration. These external and internal developmental assets cannot be purchased in a packaged curriculum. However, Ragsdale and Saylor (2014) offer ideas on how to work with youth from a strengths-based perspective based on the 40 assets. These 40 developmental assets provide collective power and work synergistically to foster a nurturing environment for children and teens. School professionals, parents, and community members all play an important role in the development and maintenance of this asset-rich context. Students consistently supported in this way appear to be much more likely to set and accomplish goals. Students who self-define as capable appear more likely to demonstrate their abilities in their social worlds to an "appreciative audience" (Winsglade & Monk, 2007) who will cheer them on. Again, this underscores the importance of understanding student behavior systemically, rather than in isolation. The profession calls upon mental health counselors, professional school counselors, and psychologists to lead the efforts toward healthy youth development. These data from the Search Institute underscore the importance of prevention and intervention efforts and community outreach. Only 3% of students who perceive themselves as possessing 30 to 40 developmental assets (which include connections to a positive social environment) report involvement in violent behavior as compared to 53% of students who rate themselves as holding 0 to 10 assets (Search Institute, 2018; Table 8.3).

TABLE 8.3 DEVELOPMENTAL ASSETS AND HIGH-RISK BEHAVIORS

Behaviors That Involve Risk to Youth	0–10 Assets	30–40 Assets
Engagement in sexual contact—experiencing sexual intercourse three or more times in their lifetime at the time of the survey	31%	3%
Use of alcohol—using alcohol three or more times in the past month or becoming intoxicated one or more times in the previous 14 days	39%	2%
Alcohol and driving—driving after drinking or being a passenger with an intoxicated driver three or more times in the past year	27%	2%

Source: Data from Search Institute. (2018). Developmental assets among LGBT youth. https://www.search-institute.org/wp-content/uploads/2018/01/DataSheet-Assets-x-LGBT-2018-update.pdf—chart paraphrased by author.

CASE STUDY 8.1: STORY OF MICHAEL

Michael is a 13-year old African American male student who maintains high grades in middle school. He is described as socially awkward and has few friends. His teachers report that Michael seeks attention by talking loudly and often "out of turn." Michael's teacher escorts him into the Counseling Office while expressing anger and frustration and openly criticizing Michael in front of others.

Case Study Activity

In groups of four, discuss the following and develop your plan.

1. Specifically, how will you work with the teacher who openly criticizes Michael and uses the Counseling Office for disciplinary action?
2. What is the "Wonderfulness Interview"?
3. Who are the possible clients in this scenario?
4. How will you build rapport with your client/s?
5. How will you learn more about Michael's strengths?
6. What resources will you explore to help Michael develop more friendships and use his strengths at school?
7. Who else will you involve in your plan?
8. What actions *besides counseling* might address the school social climate?

GROWTH-FOSTERING APPROACHES

"The basic premise of positive psychology is that the happiness and fulfillment of children and youth entail more than the identification and treatment of their problems" (Park & Peterson, 2008, p. 4). What if there existed an official taxonomy that recognized and declared what seems to be going well with a student? Might students be "diagnosed" with curiosity, bravery, kindness, or other such strengths? Narrative therapy approaches indicate that how counselors name and know and circulate their understanding seems likely to set a trajectory for what comes next. How shall counselors set the stage to know students as filled with self-agency, capability, and competence? The work of professional school counseling does not represent a matter of subtraction and alleviation and cannot only serve to "zero out" problems. Taken a step further, professional school counselors and clinical mental health counselors also hold the special charge of helping students to realize their potential, maximize their educational opportunities, and move from surviving to thriving. Research emerges serving as a dedication to understanding thriving in young people (Lerner et al., 2011).

JOINING AND BUILDING RAPPORT

Activity 8.2: The Paper Plate

Use paper plates that can be written on easily (not wax coated).

1. Provide the student with a plate and ask them "What's on your plate these days?" Have them write everything that comes to mind.
2. On the underside of the plate, ask them to write what helps hold their plate up. What helps them to thrive? What gets them up in the morning? What makes "their heart sing?"

Typically, students write multiple stressors or problems on the face of the plate and social support and extratherapeutic factors on the underside. This serves as an easy, time-efficient, and externalized way to gain a glimpse of their daily landscape. Ask them what "of all of that" they would like to talk about now and how we can be most helpful to them today. *What might be the first step to let you know that things appear to be getting better? What do you call this thing that you labeled "anxiety"?* Externalizing anxiety safeguards students from being defined by their label. The anxiety represents a condition they experience and does not define them. Clients identify with more than the conditions they grapple. The profession defines *"externalizing"* as teaching the clients to view problems as existing outside themselves (Roth & Epson, 1996). Anxiety also represents something that they experience and also does not define them. Additionally, counselors encourage clients to see that mental health conditions do not necessarily remain permanent. Even in weather patterns, change occurs. It does not rain forever, nor does the sun shine permanently. Variability becomes part of the human experience. Client identity must not be overtaken by diagnostic labels. Counselors may want to ask clients, *"What name do you call this difficulty?" How might you send it away, break up with it, unfriend it, hang up on it, delete it, unsubscribe to it, chase it off, block it,* and so forth? Students can brainstorm the many contemporary ways of detaching from something unwanted. The client maintains power and control when the client can unfriend the problem! Freeman et al. (1997) and Smith and Nylund (1997) suggest some creative ways to address children's problems that involve metaphors and story work.

Activity 8.3: Empowered Drawing

Using strengths-finder cards or a strengths-finder inventory such as the Values in Action (2020), the VIA strengths finder, for students aged 10 to 17, provides a time-efficient example:

1. Identify signature strengths—the ones they rely on as their "go to" strengths.
2. List the strengths of their family, cultures, supportive beliefs, neighborhoods, school community, and more.
3. Describe how they use their strengths to "stand up" to the difficulties they face.
4. Make a drawing, collage, or a visual display of how they will overcome the problem using their strengths.

STRENGTHS-BASED DRAWING

Figure 8.2 depicts a drawing from a middle school student who experienced chronic bullying and drew the realization that he would live at 100% even though he knew that in order to get there, he needed to "count on himself, his family, and his community."

The same student, who later described himself as "a powerful fish" and who learned that he would sink or swim and decided to swim, also drew the picture in Figure 8.3. Clients can be invited into empowered drawing to depict their pathways toward success!

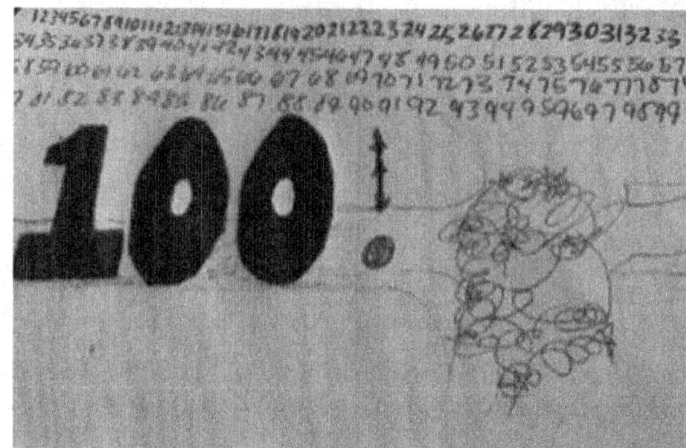

FIGURE 8.2 Middle school student's drawing.

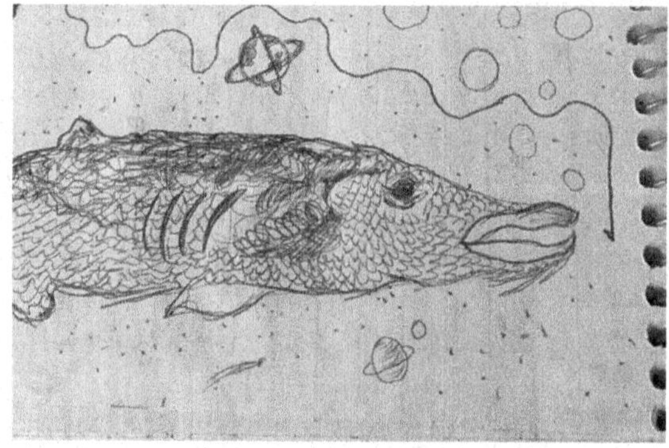

FIGURE 8.3 Middle school student's drawing after intervention.

CHAPTER SUMMARY

Mental health professionals who work with students must be well versed in the protective factors that maximize youth academic, social, and personal success. We can and must cultivate healthy communities and teach youngsters to advocate for themselves as we advocate for them. Significant research points to strategic ways we can strengthen schools, families, and communities. All too often, violence, substance abuse, bullying, sexual assault, suicidal ideation, and more threaten student well-being. The profession calls upon professional school and mental health counselors to be ethical, skilled, culturally attuned, and ready to engage in prevention and intervention as they work with students and families. The American School Counseling Association, the CDC, the Search Institute, and the American Academy of Pediatrics represent just a few organizations that carry out a goal to set their trajectories on reducing risk and amplifying student success.

POINTS TO REMEMBER

- Addressing students as "at promise" rather than as "at risk" communicates high expectations. Research indicates that holding high expectations leads to more positive outcomes for students.
- Externalization is a narrative therapy concept that views problems as existing outside of people, therefore, reducing stigma and blame.
- Person-first, nonhandicapping language is an initiative of the APA aimed at upholding respect and avoiding the labeling of children and adults.
- Statistics of interest in working with youth:

In 2018, suicide became the second leading cause of death, after accidental death, for people aged 10 to 34 (NAMI, 2017).
The diagnoses of depression and anxiety have increased over time among children aged 6 to 17 years. An increase from 5.4% in 2003 to 8% in 2007 and to 8.4% in 2011–2012 is noted (CDC, 2020).
One in six U.S. children aged 2 to 8 years (17.4%) are reported to have a diagnosed mental, behavioral, or developmental disorder (CDC, 2020).
Nearly eight in ten children (78.1%) aged 3 to 17 years with depression received treatment, while six in ten children (59.3%) aged 3 to 17 years with anxiety received treatment.
Only about half of youth (53.5%) aged 3 to 17 with behavior disorders received treatment.
One in five U.S. adults experience a mental health condition each year and one in 25 U.S. adults experience serious mental illness each year (NAMI, 2017).
An increase in suicide and dropout rates continues to occur, and 70% of youth in the juvenile justice system receive a diagnosis of a mental illness (NAMI, 2017).

Approximately 7% of children aged 3 to 17 experience anxiety disorders (NAMI, 2017). Most individuals who develop an anxiety disorder receive a diagnosis prior to age 21.   Approximately 1.9 million children in the United States experience depressive disorder (Wesley, 2019).
Despite the need for more social-emotional support in school settings, 1.6 million students attend schools that have police officers but no school counselors (Blad & Harwin, 2017).

- Protective factors are those experiences and resources that help to safeguard students against the effects of risk factors and build resilience. Protective factors are best nurtured through relationship building in the school between and among adults and students (Lazarus & Pfohl, 2010).
- The APA Help Guide entitled *Just the Facts about Sexual Orientation and Youth. A Primer for Principals, Educators, and School Personnel* cautions against conversion therapies and other methods shown to be injurious. Nearly half a million practitioners have come together to document their disagreement with conversation therapies.
- The formation of GSAs is one way that many school communities acknowledge that schools are inclusive and welcoming to all. The National Association of Gay–Straight Alliance Networks (2011) has an Advisor Handbook that clearly outlines how to get started.
- Professional school counselors, embedded in the school building, can be wonderful first responders for mental health services. Counselors need to be aware of single-session and one-at-a-time counseling session skills (Slive & Bobele, 2011).

OTHER HELPFUL INFORMATION FOR CONSIDERATION

WEB INFORMATION

- American Academy of Pediatrics: https://www.aap.org/en-us/Pages/Default.aspx
- American Association for Marriage and Family Therapy: https://aamft.org
- American Counseling Association: https://www.counseling.org
- American Psychological Association Help Center: https://www.apa.org/helpcenter
- American School Counseling Association: https://www.schoolcounselor.org
- CDC Resources in Languages Other than English: https://wwwn.cdc.gov/pubs/other-languages?Sort=Lang%3A%3Aasc
- Centers for Disease Control and Prevention: https://www.cdc.gov
- Mental Health First Aid: https://www.mentalhealthfirstaid.org/about
- National Association of Gay–Straight Alliance Networks: https://gsanetwork.org/national
- National Association of GSA Networks. GSA Advisor Handbook: https://gsanetwork.org/wp-content/uploads/2018/09/GSA_Advisor_Handbook-web.pdf

- National Association of School Psychologists: https://www.nasponline.org
- National Center for Education Statistics: https://nces.ed.gov
- PFLAG: https://pflag.org
- Positive Psychology Center: https://ppc.sas.upenn.edu
- Search Institute's 40 Developmental Assets: https://www.search-institute.org/our-research/development-assets/developmental-assets-framework
- StopBullying.Gov: https://www.stopbullying.gov

QUESTIONS FOR FURTHER DISCUSSION

- What is the importance of using person-first language when talking about children and adolescents in the school setting?
- How can Bronfenbrenner's Ecological Systems Theory Model inform the work of counselors and other mental health professionals when considering the challenges students encounter?
- Functional implications are the observable results of a condition that may impact typical development. What are some indications that a student is experiencing atypical development that may warrant assistance?
- What is the significance of the 40 Developmental Assets model as it pertains to healthy youth development?
- What steps can school personnel take to make a more inclusive and welcoming environment for all students?
- Consider Emily, a sixth grader who has made good grades most of her school career and has always had a small group of friends. Recently her teachers have noticed that her grades are dropping and she no longer seems to be with the same group of friends. As a school counselor, discuss the characteristics that you are noticing and determine what areas should be considered to help Emily.
- What are Olweus's four steps to changing school climate to reduce the impact of bullying? What is the role that a school counselor might take in implementing these steps?
- How can schoolwide mental health teams create and shape a safe and secure place for a student to learn?
- How might Mental Health First Aid benefit both school and larger communities?

KEY REFERENCES

Only key references appear in the print edition. The full reference list appears in the digital product on Springer Publishing Connect: connect.springerpub.com/content/book/978-0-8261-4764-6/part/part03/chapter/ch08

American Counseling Association. (2014). 2014 ACA code of ethics. https://www.counseling.org/knowledge-center/ethics

Bartlett, J. D., Griffin, J., & Thomson, D. (2020). *Resources for supporting children's emotional well-being during the COVID-19 pandemic.* https://www.childtrends.org/publications/resources-for-supporting-childrens-emotional-well-being-during-the-covid-19-pandemic

Centers for Disease Control and Prevention. (2017a). Youth risk behavior surveillance system. https://nces.ed.gov/programs/crimeindicators/ind_10.asp

Chillag, A. (2019). Why you should learn mental health first aid. CNN. https://www.cnn.com/2019/06/20/health/iyw-mental-health-first-aid-classes-trnd/index.html

Freeman, J. C., Epston, D., & Lobovits, D. (1997). *Playful approaches to serious problems: Narrative therapy with children and their families*. W. W. Norton & Company.

Just the Facts Coalition. (2008). *Just the facts about sexual orientation and youth: A primer for principals, educators, and school personnel*. American Psychological Association. https://www.apa.org/pi/lgbt/resources/just-the-facts.pdf

Morgan, A. (2000). *What is narrative therapy? An easy-to-read introduction*. Dulwich Centre Publications.

National Center for Education Statistics and Bureau of Justice Statistics. (2017). *School crime supplement*. https://nces.ed.gov/programs/crime/surveys.asp

Olweus, D. (1993). *Bullying at school: What we know and what we can do*. Blackwell.

Search Institute. (2018). *Developmental assets among U.S. youth: 2018 update*. https://www.search-institute.org/wp-content/uploads/2018/01/DataSheet-Assets-x-Gender-2018-update.pdf

CHAPTER 9

Addressing the Needs of Children and Adolescents With Disabilities and Those Classified as Gifted

Dianne P. Hengst, Brigitte Rauschuber, Kimberly Stewart, and Brenda Jones

LEARNING OBJECTIVES

After completing this chapter, the reader should be able to:

- Identify the disability categories under the Individuals with Disabilities Education Act and the common characteristics of giftedness.
- Recognize legislative mandates that apply to the education of children and adolescents with disabilities and giftedness in grades pre-K through 12.
- Describe postsecondary transition issues for adolescents with disabilities entering postsecondary institutions.
- Express the connection between identity and disability.
- Explain the role of the professional school counselor and clinical mental health counselors when working with students with disabilities and those classified as gifted.

CACREP STANDARDS FOR THIS CHAPTER

- CACREP 2016: 2.F.1.b.e.; 2.a.c.d.f.h.; 3.c.e.f.h.i.; 4.b.c.d.e.f.g.h.i.j.; 5.f.j.k.; School Counseling: 5G.2.a.b.c.d.g.; Clinical Mental Health: 5.C.2.d.g.; 3.b.e.
- CACREP 2009: II.g.1.b.i.; 2.a.b.e.f.; 3.3.f.; 4.g.; School Counseling: III.A.2.3,6.; E.1.,2.,3.,4.; M.1.2., 3.,4.5.; O.4.; Clinical Mental Health Counseling: III.C.8.,9; E.1.,2.,4.,5.,6.

INTRODUCTION

For professional school counselors and clinical mental health counselors to serve students with disabilities and adequately advocate within the comprehensive school and community contexts, they must first understand the legislation that exists. Congress set these legislations in place to protect the rights of students with disabilities and assure them access, inclusion, and a free and appropriate public education.

The Disability Rights Movement, starting in the early 1970s, joined other civil rights movements by promoting a culture of inclusion, diversity, and the capacity to appreciate and value individual differences. While the concept of diversity encompasses acceptance, inclusion, and respect, ultimately, society benefits with the inclusion of individuals with disabilities as part of our diversity discussion. Today, people with disabilities rank among one of the largest protected class of minorities (U.S. Census Bureau, 2018).

Many challenges exist when examining disability as part of the diversity discussion. Despite advances precipitated by the Disability Rights Movement, the portrayal of individuals with disabilities in some literature and popular media still depicts stereotypes, some of which evoke pity, inspire admiration constructed out of guilt, or portrayal of a character centered on visible disabilities (Vaughn, 2003). Some theorists describe disability identity development as an all or nothing concept in which the medical model assigns a diagnosis as an aspect of an individual rather than a focus on the disability (Johnstone, 2004; Werner, 1994). The Disability Rights Movement promotes a paradigm shift from the medical model, where the understandings of professionals move from viewing disability as a problem that resides with the individual, to an interactive model, where disability occurs through the interaction between the individual and society and barriers. This paradigm shift presents a neutral viewpoint of disability meaning neither negative nor positive, but simply as the interaction of a person with their environment that fails to accommodate a condition (Hutcheon & Wolbring, 2012). Other identity development studies recognize disability as an aspect of human experience that crosses all boundaries of race, class, and gender. Thus, the definition of a person with a disability remains complex and changing and can result from a social/cultural construct, stemming not from individual disability differences but from a cultural expectation of normality (Putnam, 2005).

Historically, the Disability Rights Movement parallels the civil rights movements, which provided clarification for the ideal "all men are created equal." The disability civil rights movement protests unequal treatment and limited access and demanded recognition of human equality and value. In order to protect and advance disability equality, the educational community must progress to meet the needs of students with disabilities in the classroom. This challenges educational institutions to develop new ways of teaching that endorse an inclusive classroom culture and which ensures that all students receive equal opportunities to explore their interests, discover new academic and extracurricular pursuits, and learn from each other (Colker & Grossman, 2014; Rose & Meyer, 2002; Vaughn, 2003).

The Council for Exceptional Children (2005) mandated *inclusion as* the process of involving and valuing all people in an environment regardless of their differences. *Inclusion* requires a proactive strategy that reflects a conscious decision to respect individuals by affording them the opportunity to become a valued part of an organization. With regard to postsecondary education, being inclusive can actually help campuses develop a competitive edge by cultivating a diverse student body. Today, more than ever, students, faculty, and staff must demonstrate an ability to adapt to different situations and skill sets in a quickly evolving workforce. By promoting an inclusive educational community, pre-K through 12 and postsecondary education welcomes and values individuals and their differences including differences in race, socioeconomic status, gender expression and identity, sexual orientation, ethnicity, national origin, first language, religion, gender, age, and, of course, disability (Madaus et al., 2009; Rothstein, 1991).

LEGISLATIVE MANDATES

INDIVIDUALS WITH DISABILITIES EDUCATION ACT

Congress enacted the *Education for All Handicapped Children Act* (Public Law 94-142) in 1975, currently known as the *Individuals with Disabilities Education Act* (IDEA; Colker & Grossman, 2014), to support states and localities in protecting the rights of, meet the individual needs of, and improve the results for infants, toddlers, children, and youth with disabilities and their families. Amended in 1997 and reauthorized in 2004, IDEA ensures services to children with disabilities throughout the nation. IDEA governs how states and public agencies provide early intervention, special education, and related services to millions of eligible infants, toddlers, children, and youth with disabilities. Infants and toddlers with disabilities (birth to age two) and their families receive early intervention services under IDEA, Part C. Children and youth (ages 3 through 22) receive special education and related services under IDEA, Part B.

ACCOMPLISHMENTS UNDER INDIVIDUALS WITH DISABILITIES EDUCATION ACT

The majority of children with disabilities attend school in their neighborhood in regular classrooms with their peers with no disabilities. As a result, high school graduation rates and employment rates among youth with disabilities increased dramatically (Colker & Grossman, 2014). For example, graduation rates increased by 14% from 1984 to 1997. Today, postschool employment rates for youth served under IDEA are twice those of older adults with similar disabilities who did benefit from the IDEA mandate (Colker & Grossman, 2014). Postsecondary enrollments among individuals with disabilities receiving IDEA services also increased sharply, and the percentage of freshmen reporting disabilities tripled since 1978 (American Council on Education, 2008).

The expanding demographics of students create greater diversity in pre-K through postsecondary-level classrooms (Colker & Grossman, 2014; Davis, 1993). Today's typical classroom might include students with a first language other than English, students reading at different levels, students with attention and motivational problems, students from varied cultural backgrounds, students with different learning styles, and students classified as gifted (Council for Exceptional Children, 2005; Rose & Meyer, 2002). Because the definition of diversity in education includes students considered to be historically underrepresented, students with disabilities become part of that diverse student population. Prior to the inception of federal mandates in 1992, Rothstein (1991) indicated that between 1980 and 1990, the number of students with disabilities attending postsecondary institutions tripled. Today, the U.S. Department of Education estimates that over 11% of freshmen in postsecondary institutions enter with some type of disability (Colker & Grossman, 2014).

Current laws that guide disability rights in the classroom began as late as the 1960s despite historical timelines and significant milestones in disability legislation beginning as early as the 1800s. Pre-K through 16 now appears to be more accessible for historically underrepresented groups such as students with disabilities with the inception of legislative mandates and educational accommodations in the classroom (Colker & Grossman, 2014).

One additional legislative mandate, Child Find, supports this free and appropriate public education. Federal mandates define Child Find as "a legal requirement that schools find all children who have disabilities and who may be entitled to special education services" (Lee, 2019, para. 1). IDEA guarantees children aged 3 through 22 with disabilities a free and appropriate public education in the least restrictive environment (LRE) designed to meet their unique needs (Hancock, 2019). Under IDEA, LRE intends that students with disabilities spend as much time as possible in the classrooms with their peers who do not receive special education services (Morin, 2019). In the LRE, students with disabilities should make appropriate progress with educational services and support. A student qualifies for free and appropriate education under IDEA once the school conducts an evaluation to determine if the student presents with a disability, and if that disability inhibits progress in the general curriculum (Morin, 2019).

The evaluation starts with *Response to Intervention* (RTI). The RTI, a process provided by general education teachers, special education teachers, and specialists, addresses both the learning and behavior of the student (Fenell et al., n.d.). The RTI process consists of three tiers (1–3), and each tier should take 6 to 9 weeks to complete. Each tier varies in interventions with *tier 1* having the least intensive interventions and *tier 3* having the most intensive interventions (Fenell et al., n.d.). A variety of assessment tools and learning strategies must be used to gather relevant information in each tier. This evaluation period includes the student's teacher(s) implementing different scientifically based learning strategies and accommodations in the classroom(s). If needed, the teacher may modify the curriculum in a way to see if this makes a difference in the student's success in the classroom (Morin, 2019). Parents or guardians should be contacted throughout the RTI process, and teachers/specialists will collect data throughout the tiers evaluating the effectiveness of the interventions used. Table 9.1 summarizes the differences between each of the tiers in the RTI process.

TABLE 9.1 SUMMARY OF FACTORS THAT SHOW THE DIFFERENCES BETWEEN TIERS 1, 2, AND 3

Factor	Tier 1	Tier 2	Tier 3
Description	Implementation of scientifically based strategies	Support now supplemental of specific needs of the student	Most needed intensive interventions and individualized and strategically structured instruction
Who Implements	Core curriculum teacher	Core curriculum teacher and specialist	Specialists or special education teacher
Time Set Aside for Instruction	No extra time	Extra 30 minutes two to three times per week	Extra 45 minutes three to five times per week
Grouping	Whole class	Five to eight students	One to three students
Where	Core curriculum class	Core curriculum class or outside the class	Outside the core curriculum class

Note: Information for factors that show the difference between tiers 1–3 from Shapiro, E. (n.d.). Tiered instruction and intervention in a response-to-intervention model. http://www.rtinetwork.org/essential/tieredinstruction/tiered-instruction-and-intervention-rti-model

After the RTI process takes place and should educators determine that none of the interventions help the academic success of the student, they conduct a formal evaluation (Morin, 2019). School personnel, including administrators, specialists, the professional school counselor, and the general and special education teacher initiate this formal evaluation and determine if the student needs special education services. Parents or guardians must give consent before a formal evaluation occurs, and the parents or guardians exercise their right to refuse special education services. A formal evaluation may include speech and language testing, behavior inventories, observations, history of the student (provided by the parent), and related medical information (Lee, 2019). Sometimes, an outside evaluation must be done by specialists to diagnose the student with a disability.

Once special education services become necessary for student success and the parents or guardians give permission for the student to receive special education services, an *admission, review, and dismissal* (ARD) process takes place using a developmental, systemic, relational, and multicultural approach. The ARD represents a specific meeting where "teachers and other support staff bring their expertise on education, and parents bring their expertise on their child—their needs, abilities, and desires, and their expectations" (Hohl, 2016, para. 2). The parents and support staff write and develop an *Individualized Education Plan* (IEP) in the ARD. The IEP serves as written documentation that outlines the student's functioning, strengths, needs, and measurable goals for the school year. The IEP also outlines the programs and services offered to the student (Hancock, 2019). To qualify for special education services and an IEP, the student must hold one of IDEA's 13 disability categories: Autism, Deafness, Blindness, Hearing Impairment, Emotional Disturbance, Intellectually Disabled, Multiple Disabilities, Orthopedic Impairment, Other Health Impaired, Specific Learning Disability (SLD), Speech or Language Impairment, Traumatic Brain Injury, and Visual Impairment (Lee, 2019).

Autism, a developmental disorder, consists of challenges with social skills, communication skills (both verbal and nonverbal), and repetitive behaviors (Lee, 2019). *Deafness* may be defined as a hearing impairment so severe that the person cannot understand linguistic information, even with the assistance of hearing aids (Center for Parent Information & Resources, 2017). *Visual Impairment,* including *Blindness,* refers to someone who can see partially or not at all; and the vision cannot be corrected by eyewear (Lee, 2019). The *Hearing Impairment* disability can be described as permanent hearing loss or one that can change over time. This affects a child's educational performance (Lee, 2019).

Counselors associate *Emotional Disturbance* with mental health or severe behavioral issues that adversely affect a child's educational performance. Some examples of emotional disturbances include anxiety disorders, bipolar disorder, conduct disorder, eating disorders, obsessive-compulsive disorders (OCD), and psychotic disorders (Special Education Guide, 2016). Lee (2019) describes *intellectual disability* as below-average intellectual ability including poor communication, self-care, and social skills. A child with more than one condition covered by IDEA reflects *Multiple Disabilities* (Lee, 2019). *Orthopedic Impairment* describes a child who lacks function or ability in their body (Lee, 2019). *Other Health Impaired,* an overarching term, covers conditions that limit a child's "strength, energy, or alertness" (Lee, 2019). A *Specific Learning Disability,* another overarching term, "covers a specific group of learning challenges. These conditions affect a child's ability to read, write, listen, speak, or do math" (Lee, 2019, para. 7). Dyslexia, dysgraphia, dyscalculia, auditory processing disorder, and nonverbal learning disabilities serve as examples of SLDs. *Speech or Language Impairment* refers to a child who experiences trouble pronouncing words or making sounds with their voice (stuttering), and language problems that make it hard for kids to understand words or express themselves (Lee,

2019). *Traumatic brain injuries* encompass brain injuries caused by accidents or some kind of physical force to the child (Lee, 2019).

Professional school counselors, through individual counseling, play an important role in working with students with learning disabilities. Their interventions must be intentional and time efficient in order to effect positive change within the student. "The time constraints of the academic calendar and daily school schedule, the number of students for which school counselors are typically responsible, and the variety of roles a school counselor must assume on a typical day are indicative of brief counseling episodes" (Davis & Osborn, 2000, p. 19). Therefore, the focus of the professional school counselor remains on the educational need behind the disability of the student rather than on the disability itself. Professional school counselors use bibliotherapy, solution-focused brief therapy (SFBT), and cognitive behavioral therapy (CBT) as interventions when counseling students with learning disabilities.

Bibliotherapy refers to the use of stories, both fiction and nonfiction books, poetry, plays, short stories, and self-help materials, to help students gain a deeper understanding of the concerns that brought them to counseling in the first place (Lindberg, 2020). The professional school counselor must consider the student's developmental level when choosing which source of literature to use in the counseling session. Backed by literature that allows for coverage of a wide range of issues and problems and can readily adapt when working with students, bibliotherapy can easily be used with any of IDEA's 13 disabilities. The literature being used should directly relate to the student's difficulty so that the student can identify with the protagonist of the story (Lindberg, 2020). After the story, the professional school counselor and the student should talk about the way the protagonist handled their problems and the "applicability of the solution or solutions in the book to the client's situation" (Lindberg, 2020, para. 6). Bibliotherapy helps students understand the issues they experience, amplifies the effects of other treatments, normalizes experiences with mental health concerns, and offers hope to positive change (Telloian, 2016).

As discussed in Chapter 5, SFBT focuses on the present moment and future circumstances. SFBT, a short-term, goal-focused approach, allows professional school counselors to help students change by focusing on solutions, rather than problems (de Shazer & Berg, 1997, as cited in Lee, 2013; Psychology Today, 2020). SFBT, used to treat students of all ages, may work well with students in any of IDEA's 13 disabilities. Clinicians do not consider SFBT to be a cure for psychiatric disorders; rather, SFBT can help improve the quality of life for the students with these disorders (de Shazer & Berg, 1997, as cited in Lee, 2013; Psychology Today, 2020). SFBT focuses on the student's resilience and the number of different ways that they cope with the challenges in their life. The professional school counselor can also use a technique called the "miracle question" with SFBT to help students envision a future in which the problem does not exist. The professional school counselor can modify the miracle question based on the student's developmental level. For example, the professional school counselor or the clinical mental health counselor can ask, "If you had an app on your phone that when clicked the app would erase everything, as if the problem did not exist, what would be different?" The counselor can, then, help the student identify small steps or changes that they can take to make change happen. *Scaling questions* provides another more time-sensitive approach that counselors can use with SFBT. This technique can be used when students experience trouble verbalizing their experiences in a less challenging and quite versatile manner (de Shazer & Berg, 1997, as cited in Lee, 2013; Psychology Today, 2020). For example, when a student comes into the office with a problem, the counselor can draw a scale of 0 to 10 on a piece of paper or even with a dry erase marker on a desk. The counselor can then ask, "On a scale of 0 to 10, 10 meaning you have confidence that this problem can be solved and 0 meaning that you have no confidence at all, where would you put yourself?" The student can then make a mark showing where they rank on the scale. After the student establishes their number on the scale, the counselor can ask questions that elicit the student to start thinking about solutions to their problem. For example, "What would it take for you to increase, by just one point on the scale, that this problem can be solved?" The counselor can either ask the student to write or draw what this change looks like and then revisit the scale.

Because of its structured and systematic nature, CBT, covered in Chapter 5, can be adapted to use with many of IDEA's 13 disabilities (Gillihan, n.d.). Through CBT, counselors can help students recognize the way they think about themselves and how their experiences influence how they feel (Reif, 2019). Depending on the developmental level of the student, some popular techniques to use with CBT include reframing negative thoughts, progressive muscle relaxation, and relaxed breathing. Reframing negative thoughts with a student with anxiety can be powerful because it requires the student to take a step back and look at their thinking objectively. This technique requires the student to write down their situation or problems, write down their thoughts pertaining to the situation, write down what feelings and emotions they feel, create alternative thoughts, and write down what feelings and emotions they feel post reframing (Ackerman, 2020). For students with cognitive limitations, it becomes important for the counselor to make CBT equal parts talk therapy and hands-on activities (Ackerman, 2020). For example, a counselor can ask the student to stand; and as they stand, the counselor instructs the student to voice their negative thoughts. For each of the student's negative thoughts, the counselor can hand a book to the student to hold as they stand. The more negative thoughts they verbalize, the more books they will hold; therefore, the heavier the books will become (Jacobs & Schimmel, 2013). The counselor and student can then make the connection that although one book seems tough to manage, a whole stack of books may be quite uncomfortable and heavy, just like negative thoughts or worries that the student never addressed. Cognitive behavioral play therapy (CBPT), an adaptation of CBT, can be used with younger students or with students who function at a lower developmental stage (Ackerman, 2020). For example, modeling can be a technique used in CBPT. During modeling, the counselor can use puppets to teach more adaptive responses for social skills. The student can then rehearse the new skills learned with the puppets while the counselor gives feedback (Ackerman, 2020). Social stories for students with autism provide another example of CBPT that can be used. Social stories may be adaptable to the student's specific social problems so that the student can successfully participate in peer activities (Auger, 2013).

OTHER LEGISLATIVE MANDATES

SECTION 504 AND THE REHABILITATION ACT OF 1973

The Rehabilitation Act of 1973 became the first federal legislation to address the notion of equal access for individuals with disabilities through the removal of architectural, employment, and transportation barriers. Title VI of the Civil Rights Act of 1964 provides the framework for key information within the legislation. The Rehabilitation Act created rights of persons with disabilities through affirmative action programs by authorizing formula grant programs of vocational rehabilitation, supported employment, independent living, and client assistance. It also authorized a variety of training and service discretionary grants administered by the Rehabilitation Services Administration. In addition, the legislation attempted to address some of the societal barriers faced by individuals with disabilities, including isolation by placement in institutions, limited access to buildings, and discrimination in education and employment. Section 504 of the Rehabilitation Act specifically states,

> *No qualified individual with a disability shall, by reason of such disability, be excluded from participation in or be denied the benefits of the services, programs or activities of a public entity, or be subjected to discrimination by any such entity.* (Rehabilitation Act of 1973, Pub.L. 93-112, 87 Stat. 355, enacted September 26, 1973)

Congress designated Section 504 as a civil rights law that became part of the Rehabilitation Act of 1973 (U.S. Department of Education, 2020). A student who receives services for Section 504 does not benefit from the same mandates as a child who receives services under IDEA, including funding. Section 504 provides access to programs and encompasses students diagnosed with a disability that affects them in school but does not require the student to receive special education services. Section 504 defines disability in terms of "physical or mental impairment" that "substantially limits a major life activity" like walking, dressing, feeding oneself, working, or seeing and supports the provision of needed accommodations (Hancock, 2019). Like obtaining an IEP, parents can request the school to evaluate their child for these services. The school can consider diagnoses from doctors, test results, comments from teachers, parents, and others to determine the appropriateness of a 504 plan (Mauro, 2018).

An example of a student who receives 504 accommodations rather than an IEP could be a child with an average ability to learn academically who presents with a mobility impairment or medical conditions such as epilepsy and attention deficit hyperactivity disorder (ADHD). Another example could be a child under a doctor's care for psychological conditions such as anxiety and depression (Hancock, 2019). Notably, all students who qualify for an IEP also qualify for a 504 plan. However, not all students with a 504 plan qualify for an IEP (Jones, 2019). Table 9.2 highlights the differences between an IEP and a 504 plan.

SECTION 508 OF THE REHABILITATION ACT

On August 7, 1998, President Clinton signed into law the Rehabilitation Act Amendments of 1998, which covers access to federally funded programs and services. The law strengthens Section 508 of the Rehabilitation Act and requires access to electronic and information technology provided by the federal government. The law applies to all federal agencies when they develop, procure, maintain, or use electronic and information technology. Because of this legislation, federal agencies and those who receive federal funding must ensure accessible technology to the extent that it does not pose an "undue burden." Section 508 speaks to various means for disseminating information, including computers, software, and electronic office equipment. The U.S. Access Board assumes responsibility for developing information and communications technology (ICT) accessibility standards to incorporate into regulations that govern federal procurement practices. On January 18, 2017, the Access Board issued a final rule that updated accessibility requirements covered by Section 508, and refreshed guidelines for telecommunications equipment subject to Section 255 of the Communications Act. The final rule went into effect on January 18, 2018. The rule updated and reorganized Section 508, Standards, and Section 255, Guidelines, in response to market trends and innovations in technology. The refresh also harmonized

TABLE 9.2 INDIVIDUALIZED EDUCATION PLAN FOR ECH AND PRE-K THROUGH 12 COMPARED TO 504 PLAN

IEP for ECH and Pre-K Through 12	504 Plan
Based on federal special education law	Based on civil rights law
Applies to assessed students who qualify for special education services (IDEA)	Applies to students with a disability that inhibits a major life function, but do not qualify for special education services
Students use special education services, accommodations, and modifications	Students use accommodations
Applies to students through grade 12. Does not transfer to postsecondary institutions	No age limit and will transfer to postsecondary institutions

ECH, early childhood handicapped; IDEA, Individuals with Disabilities Education Act; IEP, Individualized Education Plan.

Source: Celletti, E. (2018). *IEP vs. 504 Plan:* What's the difference? https://www.niche.com/blog/iep-vs-504-plan-whats-the-difference.

these requirements with other guidelines and standards both in the United States and abroad, including standards issued by the European Commission, and with the World Wide Web Consortium (W3C) Web Content Accessibility Guidelines (WCAG 2.0), a globally recognized voluntary consensus standard for web content and ICT (Section 508 of the Rehabilitation Act, 29 U.S.C. § 794d).

AMERICANS WITH DISABILITIES ACT AND THE AMENDMENTS ACT

Congress enacted the Americans with Disabilities Act (ADA), a civil rights law that prohibits discrimination against individuals with disabilities in all areas of public life, including jobs, schools, transportation, and all public and private places open to the general public (Americans with Disabilities Act of 1990, Pub. L. No. 101-336, § 2, 104 Stat. 328). Congress created this law to ensure that people with disabilities receive the same rights and opportunities as everyone else. Congress enacted the ADA to establish a clear and comprehensive prohibition of discrimination based on disability. Although Section 504 of the Rehabilitation Act of 1973 previously addressed the rights of individuals with disabilities, the ADA extends this coverage to a wider array of areas. Specifically, the ADA outlines five areas ("Titles") in which persons with disabilities hold legal rights: employment, public services, public accommodations, telecommunications, and other miscellaneous provisions (Colker & Grossman, 2014).

In 2008, President Bush signed the unanimously passed Amendments to the ADA, called the Americans with Disabilities Act Amendments Act (ADAAA). Changes to the ADA included a broadening of the scope of the definition of disability, the elimination of the mitigating measures, a new definition of the term "substantially limits," and an inclusion of episodic conditions. With the passage of the ADAAA, postsecondary institutions experienced a significant increase in the number of graduating seniors with disabilities seeking accommodations at the postsecondary level (Colker & Grossman, 2014).

ROLE OF PROFESSIONAL COUNSELORS

Through developmental, systemic, relational, and multicultural roles, professional school counselors and clinical mental health counselors need to advocate for students with disabilities. Through advocacy, counselors can genuinely help all children achieve their highest potential. Advocacy can occur on an individual or systemic level. Counselors advocate mostly on an individual level. For example, if made aware that one individual shows little to no respect for another individual diagnosed with a disability, the counselor can take steps to amend the situation. The professional school counselor and clinical mental health counselors could take steps to present classroom guidance lessons or psychoeducational programs on respecting individual differences. Counselors could also offer small-group counseling that deals with conflict resolution strategies (Barrow & Mamlin, 2016). Using this same example, professional school counselors may realize that teachers could experience difficulties working with students with disabilities. Through systemic advocacy, professional school counselors can provide teachers and parents in-service training to enhance their understanding of the needs of students with learning disabilities (Barrow & Mamlin, 2016).

Through professional school counselor's service delivery system components, students with learning disabilities must be included. The delivery system components include guidance lessons, individual planning, responsive services, and system support (American School Counselor Association, 2019; Texas Education Agency, 2018). Professional school counselors provide genuine inclusion by modifying lesson plans for guidance lessons so that they apply to students with learning disabilities. Professional school counselors and clinical mental health counselors utilize students' IEPs and 504 plans and then individually formulate plans and make short-term goals and goal-focused strategies. Students' IEP and 504 plans could also be used in assisting with transitioning through individual planning with a professional school counselor. Counselors may also respond to the specific needs of students with disabilities through both individual and group counseling.

Parental involvement transpires into a positive and direct impact on academic achievement (Castro et al., 2015). Professional school counselors must garner parent/guardian support to create opportunities for students with learning disabilities. Professional school counselors can create positive school environments for students with learning disabilities by cultivating collaborative parental involvement, helping teachers communicate and work with parents, and serving as liaisons between home and the school. A key focus for the professional school counselor is creating a shared power dynamic with the parent/guardian. Also, the professional school counselor needs to remain unbiased and maintain a positive attitude emphasizing what is in the best interest of the student (Castro et al., 2015).

The role of the professional school counselor appears broad and encompasses many areas. However, limitations of the professional school counselor's role may be evidenced when working with students with disabilities. The professional school counselor's role does not involve administrative roles, including

- being the sole decision maker on the placement of the students with disabilities,
- deciding on the execution of IDEA,

- writing, putting together, or ensuring adherence to the IEP plan,
- performing educational or psychological assessments, and
- providing long-term therapy (American School Counselor Association, 2016).

As mentioned in Chapter 8, counselors must also, in their systemic, relational, and multicultural role, become familiar with the preferred language and disability etiquette for students with learning disabilities. Logsdon (2019) states, "Person first language is often considered the most respectful way to talk about disabilities and differences. It focuses on the individual and not the issue he or she has" (para. 1). For example, someone might say "She is dyslexic" to describe someone diagnosed with dyslexia. Using person-first language, this would change to "she has dyslexia." Another example would be saying "person who uses a wheelchair" instead of "wheelchair-bound person" and saying "student who receives special education services" instead of "special education student." By using person-first language, counselors understand that they define someone as a whole person, not their disability. Logsdon (2019) describes person-first language as using the person's name or pronoun first, following it with an appropriate verb, and then stating the name of the disability.

Professional school counselors and clinical mental health counselors can help the student with learning disabilities navigate their identity formation by first understanding the Disability Identity Development Model (Lovell & White, 2019). Gibson identifies three stages of identity development for people with learning disabilities (Lovell & White, 2019). The first stage, *passive awareness,* signifies that the individual fails to connect to or gain awareness of their disability. The second stage, *realization,* brings awareness to the disability, which could result in possible anger and devaluing of one's self. The last stage, *acceptance,* points to where the individual with the disability begins to accept their disability identity (Lovell & White, 2019). By understanding this identity model, professional school counselors and clinical mental health counselors can understand where an individual student may be on their journey of developing a sense of one's self and identity. Professional school counselors can help normalize the development process for students and facilitate movement through the different stages via individual counseling.

TRANSITION AND SERVICES IN HIGHER EDUCATION

Life at postsecondary institutions poses different challenges for students with disabilities. An accurate knowledge about their civil rights becomes an important factor in their successful transition from high school to postsecondary education. These institutions view all students as responsible adults and expect that students will assume responsibilities for meeting admission standards and essential elements of academic program requirements. This added responsibility, coupled with a change in environment, makes transitioning from high school to postsecondary education challenging. Whereas the high school environment appears very structured with a set schedule, the schedule of postsecondary institutions can vary dramatically. For the first time, the school may allow many students considerable time between classes and frequently need assistance in managing their time wisely. Students must enforce their own attendance policies and prepare to realize personal consequences if they choose not to attend class. Managing life as a student with a disability requires attending to many details. Counselors and educators encourage students to be proactive and to plan ahead. Requesting academic accommodations becomes an important aspect to the success of students with disabilities because it takes time to arrange services.

SELF-ADVOCACY

Students leaving high school must become adept at realistically assessing and understanding their strengths, weaknesses, needs, and preferences. As self-advocates, they must become experts at communicating this information to other adults including instructors and service providers. Ultimately, the postsecondary institution will hold the student responsible for seeking out disability services and supports as well as follow institutional policies and procedures. Good communication skills and knowledge about oneself become crucial to success in postsecondary institutions.

ADMISSION TESTS AND ADMISSION TO POSTSECONDARY INSTITUTIONS

Although some institutions of higher education produce their own entrance exams, the majority use commercially available tests. Admission tests may not be selected or administered in a way that tests a disability; rather, they assess the achievement or aptitude of an individual. Federal law requires standardized test organizations to change testing conditions through accommodations that allow a student with disability to participate, given those changes do not fundamentally alter the examination or create an undue financial or administrative burden. Postsecondary institutions do not identify students with disabilities and generally they cannot make preadmission inquiries about an applicant's disability status. If an applicant meets the essential requirements for admission, an institution may not deny admission based on a disability, nor may they categorically exclude any applicants with a particular disability to a program. However, postsecondary institutions may require an applicant to meet any essential technical and academic standards for admission to or participation in the institution or a program. A student holds no obligation to inform an institution of postsecondary education of their disability; however, if the student wants an institution to provide an academic adjustment or assign the student to accessible housing or other facilities, or if a student wants other disability-related services, the student must identify and explain the nature of their disability (U.S. Department of Education, 2011).

SELF-DISCLOSURE AND DOCUMENTATION

Unlike early childhood programs and pre-K–12, federal laws do not require postsecondary educational institutions to conduct or pay for an evaluation to document a student's disability and/or need for an academic adjustment. Postsecondary educational institutions may set their own requirement for documentation as long as they appear reasonable. Frequently, documentation standards vary from institution to institution. Thus, students with disabilities must research documentation standards at those institutions they plan to attend. Generally, a student's documentation must explain how their disability substantially limits a major life activity and supports the need for an academic adjustment since a diagnosis of impairment alone does not establish a disability under the law. Although an IEP or Section 504 plan may help identify services used by the student in the past, postsecondary institutions do not view them as sufficient documentation to support the existence of a current disability and need for an academic adjustment. Assessment information and other material used to develop an IEP or Section 504 plan may be helpful to document a current disability or the need for an academic adjustment or auxiliary aids and

TABLE 9.3 SERVICE COMPARISON BETWEEN INSTITUTION LEVELS

High School	Post-Secondary Institutions
Services must be delivered to the student	Students must seek out services
Services based on an agreed upon menu of choices	Services based on situational and/or individual needs/requests
Counselors act as advocate	Student acts as self-advocate
Annual review of services and Individualized Education Plan completed	No annual review or Individualized Education Plan completed
Regular parent interactions	No regular parent contact

services. High school personnel can help a student with a disability identify and address the specific documentation requirements of the postsecondary institution that the student will be attending (Table 9.3). This may include assisting the student to identify existing documentation in their education records that would satisfy the institution's criteria, such as evaluation reports and the summary of the student's academic achievement and functional performance. If the student's disability and need for an academic adjustment appear obvious, less documentation may be necessary. If the documentation a student submitted for the institution's consideration does not meet the institution's requirements, someone at that institution should notify the student in a timely manner of what additional documentation the student needs to provide (U. S. Department of Education, 2011).

THE ROLE OF DISABILITY SERVICES IN POSTSECONDARY EDUCATION

Students with disabilities bring different experiences to the classroom, which may vary from the traditional ages of postsecondary students. Postsecondary institutions must collaborate with students with disabilities and "think outside the box" to eliminate barriers to education and counter misconceptions and stereotypes that contribute to those barriers. Generally, postsecondary institutions provide no one standard option to students with a disability. Disability service providers in postsecondary institution encounter many unique issues when it comes to helping students with disabilities adjust to this environment. Disability service programs must work in close collaboration with other services throughout the campuses (e.g., counseling and mental health programs) and seek out opportunities to provide outreach for various high school groups off campus.

ACCOMMODATIONS

Although students may request academic adjustments at any time, students needing services should notify the institution as early as possible to ensure that the institution can review their request in a timely manner and provide an appropriate academic adjustment. Postsecondary institutions, in general, expect students with disabilities to be responsible for their own academic programs and progress in the same ways that students without disabilities do. No legislation requires postsecondary institutions to provide an academic adjustment that would alter or waive essential academic requirements. No law requires them to provide an academic adjustment that would fundamentally alter the nature of a service, program, or activity or result in undue financial or administrative burdens considering the institution's overall resources. The law does require postsecondary institutions to give primary consideration to the auxiliary aid or service requested by the student, but can opt to provide more effective alternative aids or services. They can also opt to provide an effective alternative if the requested auxiliary aid or service would fundamentally alter the nature of a service, program, or activity or result in undue financial or administrative burdens.

The postsecondary institution holds the student responsible for knowing and following procedures for requesting reasonable academic adjustments. If the academic adjustments provided do not meet the student's needs, the student must notify the institution as soon as possible. The student and the institution should work together to resolve the problem. Upon request, a designated disability official/office may prepare notifications for students and their instructors. The letters provide verification of the student's disability and list the approved accommodations. Students who want to use accommodations must engage in an interactive discussion with those appropriate officials and discuss arrangements for accommodations. Students who employ positive skills as a self-advocate find that this system results in a good working relationship with their instructors. Some tips on how to employ self-advocacy skills include the following. First, students must understand how their disability may affect their ability to meet the course and program objectives. Disability accommodations and services modify barriers caused by a disability to provide equal access to education. The student's ability to discuss anticipated barriers and effective modifications will provide the best opportunity for success in the course. Further, discussion with instructors about effective study strategies may also be productive. When meeting with professors to request accommodations, students should be prepared to review exams and identify areas for improvement and further study. Students who experience difficulty in a course often find instructors helpful in suggesting ways to study and improve on assignments. Instructors may also appreciate suggestions from students that may improve understanding of the course material (U.S. Department of Education, 2019).

COUNSELING CHILDREN AND ADOLESCENTS WITH DISABILITIES: SUMMARY

The professional school counselor holds many responsibilities and plays an active role in planning a comprehensive guidance and counseling program for all students. Professional school counselors transform a school counseling program so that it facilitates competency development for students with disabilities through advocacy, leadership, and collaboration. Postsecondary education, disability service officials, and personnel in higher education talk about equal access for students with disabilities in the context of inclusion and diversity. Today, the definition of diversity extends far beyond the legally protected categories that we grew accustomed to acknowledging. Postsecondary education can be described as communities of learning enriched by a wide variety of experiences and perspectives of its students, faculty, and staff. Educational institutions must be accessible to students from a broad range of cultural, ethnic, ability, and economic backgrounds. Today, students who graduate from institutions of higher education must demonstrate an ability to adapt to different situations and overcome difficult circumstances. Now, more than ever, postsecondary institutions must work together and value human differences in order to provide the kind of quality education students expect when they attend an institution of higher learning and be inclusive of all populations including students with disabilities.

ADDRESSING COUNSELING NEEDS OF GIFTED CHILDREN AND ADOLESCENTS

THE SIGNIFICANCE OF GIFTEDNESS

The professional literature identifies giftedness as one of the most misunderstood concepts in education (Kessler, 2018). Educators frequently categorize gifted students as high achievers. Other words and phrases often associated with giftedness include "creative," "smart," "out of the box thinking," and, sometimes, "social awkwardness." Educators use an ever-present and usually unspoken idea, "elitist," as another description. The very word "gifted" tends to be perceived as "better than" when it actually serves as an educational diagnosis. Too often, educators assume that their brightest students will "be okay" without specific interventions and focus their time and energies on students who function below the gifted levels. Professionals never argue that students functioning at and below grade level need instruction appropriate to their abilities. However, addressing the needs of these students must not come at the expense of others, specifically, gifted learners. When schools identify students as "*gifted,*" it connotes an educational need that interventions for advanced instruction become necessary. Too often, educators use gifted students as peer tutors and teaching assistants, causing limitations in their intellectual growth, presenting cause for concern to many. These bright minds with the ability to solve global issues, cure diseases, and truly improve the world in which we live cannot do this alone. Educators and counselors will need to guide *all* students and equip them with the tools needed to maximize their innate potentials. We cheat ourselves out of the gifts these special students offer the world when we do not address their academic and social needs. Xiang et al. (2011) conducted a study at the Thomas B. Fordham Institute and examined performance trends of top students. Researchers found that about two in five students who excelled in early grades failed to continue that upward trajectory as they progressed through the school system. Not only does the profession consider this a loss to the individuals experiencing such decline, "every casualty among this group is a loss in human potential capital" (Xiang et al., 2011, p. 4). Educational programs must not only continue to improve the performance of low-achieving students, but also support and advance the performance of high-achieving students. Researchers indicate that the future prosperity of our nation depends on it (Xiang et al., 2011).

GIFTEDNESS DEFINED

While an absolute definition for giftedness does not exist, the National Association for Gifted Children (NAGC; 2019) defines the term in the following way:

> *Students with gifts and talents perform . . . at higher levels as compared to others of the same age, experience, or environment in one or more domains. They require modification to their educational experience(s) to learn and realize their potential.* (p. 1)

These students come from all racial, ethnic, and cultural populations across all economic strata. Other definitions used to describe gifted youth include *asynchronous development*. Essentially, this means that an individual appears *out of sync* with oneself, typically showing advanced cognition while other aspects of development (such as social or fine motor skills) appear on level, or even delayed (NAGC, 2019). Figure 9.1 further explains *asynchronous development*.

LEGISLATION RELATING TO GIFTED EDUCATION

The National Commission on Excellence in Education (1983) presented *A Nation at Risk*, a report published during the Reagan presidency, which detailed the scores of American students indicating an inability to successfully compete with their international

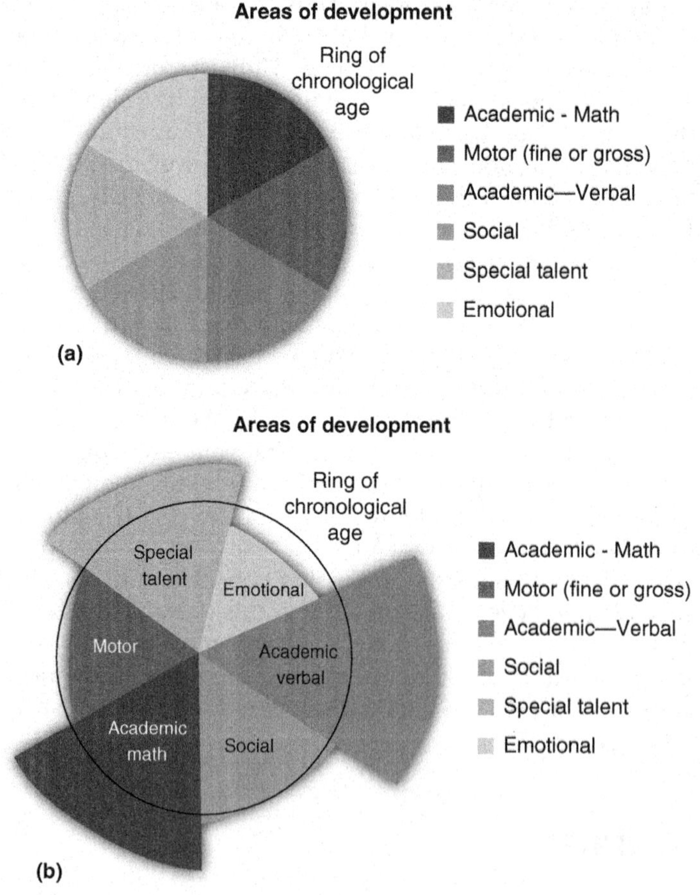

FIGURE 9.1 Typical versus asynchronous development.

Source: Reproduced with permission from Newitt, S. (2014). Asynchronous development. Gilbert Supporters of the Gifted. http://gilbertgifted.blogspot.com/2014/04/asynchronous-development.html?spref=pi&m=1

counterparts. This report provided evidence that unmet educational needs appeared to produce substandard results including boredom, apathy, and mediocrity in the most capable students. As a result, the federal government established policies for gifted education and increased academic standards. While legislation in gifted education increased since that landmark event, the commission did not provide standards for districts to follow when identifying and serving gifted students—only federal mandates require that they do. Therefore, the ways in which schools identify students for participation in gifted programs vary from district to district. Typically, school personnel administer achievement and ability tests. In consideration of the previously listed definition of giftedness, which addresses *the superior performance of students in comparison to others of the same age, experience, and environment* (NAGC, 2019), qualifying scores vary from district to district, and sometimes, from school to school.

In 2015, Congress passed *Every Student Succeeds Act (ESSA),* which included mandates for school districts to address gifted and advanced learners developmentally, systemically, relationally, and multiculturally. Prior to this, Congress required states to report achievement data disaggregated by subgroups for students performing at the proficient level and below. ESSA ensures inclusion of advanced student achievement levels in this report. Therefore, schools become more incentivized to consider the social, emotional, and academic needs of gifted learners and to adjust instruction allowing these students to reach their maximum potential. Further, due to the disaggregation of subpopulation data, districts must work to ensure their identification methods remain inclusive of all students, regardless of race, ethnicity, and economic status.

GIFTED PROGRAM IDENTIFICATION

As mentioned earlier, no one universal standard exists to qualify students for gifted programs. Mensa, a well-known, established high intelligence quotient (IQ) society, certifies membership based on IQ; however, most districts rely on standardized group assessments to identify students for gifted programs. Some common instruments used include the Cognitive Abilities Test (CogAT) (Lohman & Lakin, 2011), Iowa Achievement Test (Welch & Dunbar, 2017), the Stanford Achievement Test (Harcourt Assessment, Inc., 2020), Naglieri Nonverbal Ability Test (Naglieri, 2008), and the Woodcock–Johnson Tests of Cognitive Abilities (Woodcock & Johnson, 2014). Sometimes, schools administer creativity tests, such as the Torrance Test of Creative Thinking (Torrance, 2018), to screen students. These tests yield national percentile ranking scores, which compare the performance of each student to all students of their same age who took that same test. Previously, we learned that "gifted and talented" refers to a child or youth who performs at or shows the potential for performing at a remarkably high level of accomplishment *when compared to others of the same age, experience, or environment* (NAGC, 2019). The consideration of *environment* suggests that national norms may not be the most appropriate way to identify underserved populations (Peters et al., 2019). Consequently, school districts may use local norms as one strategy to combat low identification among minorities and economically disadvantaged students. Local norms help to achieve equity and access in gifted education.

IQ AND GIFTEDNESS

Searches for hard data in what qualifies an individual as *gifted* yield limited reliable results; however, current research indicates that an IQ of 130 or higher constitutes a person

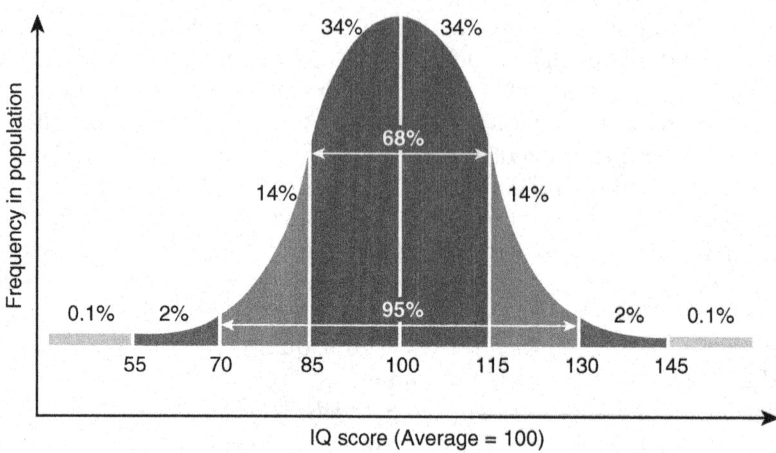

FIGURE 9.2 Frequency distribution of IQ scores.

as *gifted* (Mensa, 2019). Roughly 2% of the population score at the 98th percentile on a valid, standardized IQ test, which serves as the qualifying score for Mensa (2019). Figure 9.2 shows the normal intelligence distribution among the total population.

Figure 9.2 shows that 68% of people demonstrate an average IQ, ranging between 85 and 115. Mensa requires membership exclusive to the top 2% (130+); however, most gifted programs in today's schools encompass students commonly called *mildly gifted* with IQs ranging from 116 to 129. While the terminology remains somewhat inconsistent, schools identify individuals with an IQ of 145 to 159 as *highly gifted*, while considering those over 160 *exceptionally gifted*, and 175+ as *profoundly gifted*. Diagnosticians classify students with an IQ of 145+ as genius. They estimate that .04% of the population demonstrate an IQ over 145 (Mensa, 2019). Educators and counselors working with individuals who possess high intelligence should be trained to recognize characteristics that often lead to struggles and to help these students to overcome the obstacles often associated with giftedness (some of which include anxiety, perfectionism, and even underachievement).

CHARACTERISTICS OF GIFTEDNESS

SIX PROFILES OF GIFTEDNESS

After years of interviews, observations, and literature reviews, Betts and Neihart (2010) outlined six profiles of gifted/talented (GT) youth that seek to bring awareness to educators and counselors that giftedness should not be viewed as a "one-size-fits-all" approach; in fact, giftedness looks extremely different among individuals depending on their interactions with family, educational institutions, relationships, and personal development. The model proposed by Betts and Neihart seeks to help educational professionals identify different types of gifted students, as well as to provide a framework for better understanding these students by studying their feelings, behavior, and needs.

Type I: The Successful Learner

Betts and Neihart (2010) estimated that as many as 90% of the identified gifted students appear to be *type Is*. These students figured out how to play the game of school. They listen to parents and teachers, and they follow directions. These conformers make good grades, score high on standardized tests, and seek approval from others, thereby rarely exhibiting behavior problems. This can become problematic. *Successfuls* often learn to use the system by exerting minimal effort. Rather than pursuing their own interests and passions, these individuals go through the motions and achieve; but they do so at the expense of creativity and autonomy. While they generally become competent adults, *type Is* do not possess the skills and attitudes of lifelong learners. It becomes imperative that educators and counselors challenge these students by implementing appropriate curriculum, teaching assertiveness skills, and promoting autonomy. Increased rigor and opportunities for self-selected learning will help these students become the independent problem solvers needed in today's world.

Type II: The Creative Learner

Suffice it to say these students do *not* play the game of the school! Betts and Neihart (2010) describe these students as impulsive and defensive. They sometimes even challenge teachers in front of the class. They tend to possess a high degree of creativity and become frustrated with the system for not recognizing their gifts and talents. While some stand up for their convictions, others struggle with social interactions, elevating their negative self-concepts. Betts and Neihart suggest that these hard-to-identify students may be in danger of dropping out of school if the school fails to implement interventions by junior high. Tolerance is key when working with creatives. Affirming their strengths and embracing nonconformity will help these students to maximize their gifts. It remains critical that the educators and counselors who work with these students do not allow their difficult behaviors to mask the gifts that lie beneath their rough exteriors.

Type III: The Underground Learner

These insecure, anxious students hide their talents, often in efforts to belong to a nongifted peer group. *Type IIIs* appear most commonly among middle school females, although high school males can also retreat underground as they long to belong to a specific group, usually athletics. Generally, these students start out as highly motivated achievers in pursuit of academic and/or creative endeavors, but they undergo a transition whereby they lose interest in their previous passions. Parents and teachers often react to these changes in ways that only increase the student's struggles and denial. Pushing resistant adolescents to continue their educational programming may only alienate them further from the people who can help them attain their needs and long-term goals. Rather, adults who work with these students should honor this transition; and while these capable individuals should not abandon all advanced coursework, efforts should be made to find alternatives while they work to figure themselves out and what they want out of life. Aiding these students through these difficult times will send the message that one accepts them holistically and not just as a high-achieving student.

Type IV: The At-Risk Learner

Feeling rejected by the system, these students might appear angry and will retreat emotionally, appearing disengaged from academic and extracurricular activities that schools offer. Their gifts and interests often appear to be rooted in areas not typically associated with traditional curriculum options (such as art or music); and therefore, they see school as irrelevant and, at times, even hostile. At-risks appear most frequently among high school students, although elementary students could also withdraw mentally from school for the same reasons. Nontraditional, alternative educational options are preferable for *type IVs* (Betts & Neihart, 2010). It becomes critical that these students receive individual counseling to work on building self-esteem. Ideally, at-risk students find an adult with whom they form a close working relationship and build trust so that they can learn to manage their anger, enabling them to realize and develop their gifts and talents. Without such interventions, *type IVs* remain at risk of criminal behaviors. Criminologist Joseph Schwartz from the University of Nebraska found a slightly elevated rate of criminal behavior among individuals identified as highly, or even profoundly, gifted (Oleson, 2016).

Type V: The Twice/Multi-Exceptional Learner

Betts and Neihart (2010) find *type V* students typically difficult to identify for gifted programs; therefore, the vast majority do not receive the services that would help them to maximize their potential. This may be due to learning disabilities and/or behavior disorders that tend to offset giftedness. These students exhibit behaviors that do not align with what many believe gifted students to be, including frustration with assignments, not completing work on time, and coping with feeling of inadequacy, among other issues. Further, their gifted characteristics can sometimes mask the deficit, resulting in no services or interventions at all. Also called *twice-exceptional*, these "2E" learners can be highly creative and strong problem solvers but may also struggle with the pace and rigor of coursework, causing inconsistent academic performance and frustration. It remains imperative that educators work to differentiate learning experiences for these students. Betts and Neihart recommend eliminating rote or repetitive tasks, allowing alternative products to demonstrate learning, and building in scaffolding to minimize weaknesses while focusing on strengths as ways to help double-labeled students succeed in school.

Type VI: The Autonomous Learner

Betts and Neihart (2010) classify *type VIs* as self-directed and confident. They work effectively in the school system, navigating ways to make the system work for them. They learn how to create change in their own lives, expressing needs and feelings freely and appropriately. Autonomous learners possess strong self-concepts and often become the kinds of individuals needed in today's schools and world. Well respected by the adults in their lives, these students most always receive the support they need to be successful while nurturing a strong sense of personal power.

USE OF PROFILES

Betts and Neihart (2010) consider the intent of these profiles of the gifted and talented framework for educators and counselors to understand the many facets of giftedness. Adults in the lives of these special individuals should share this insight with the students themselves to help them gain an understanding and appreciation of themselves and help them develop the gifts they could share with the world.

CASE STUDY 9.1: TWICE EXCEPTIONAL

Kevin is a 6-year-old first grader. His teacher, Ms. Smith, cannot figure out what is going on with him. The majority of her students are progressing as readers, but Kevin does not seem to understand the connection between letters and sounds. Ms. Smith consults with Kevin's kindergarten teacher and learns that Kevin had been considered for retention, but due to the fact that he had mastered math facts far beyond that of an average kindergartener, he was placed into first grade. Ms. Smith notices that Kevin is always talking about science experiments he conducts at home. Ms. Smith also notices that Kevin understands mathematical concepts that most first graders cannot. Ms. Smith is perplexed why a student who seems to be advanced in some areas is unable to read.

Activity 9.1

Consider the characteristics that Ms. Smith has observed in Kevin. Discuss with your group the following:

1. What are potential reasons as to why Kevin has not learned to read?
2. What support services would be of benefit to Kevin? Explain.

DABROWSKI'S OVEREXCITABILITIES

Dabrowski (Bailey, 2010; Dabrowski & Piechowski, 1972) identified five types of "overexcitabilities" that he believed connect strongly to giftedness. Dabrowski believed these intensities to be important for some to reach "higher levels" in life. He called this his *Theory of Positive Disintegration.* They can help students experience a much richer life. These overexcitabilities, especially the last three, cause a person to experience day-to-day life more intensely and to feel the extremes of the joys and sorrows of life profoundly. They can help students experience a much richer life. They can experience much higher highs but also, conversely, much lower lows (thus Dabrowski's reference to overexcitability as "the tragic gift"). These characteristics can make it difficult for students to work within the confines of a classroom or small-group counseling.

Dabrowski (as cited in Bailey, 2010) characterizes *intellectual overexcitability* as the "stereotypical" behavior often associated with giftedness. Students who display an intellectual overexcitability crave knowledge, sometimes about one subject (which can be challenging when working in areas not studied). These students ask questions constantly, sometimes unanswerable questions, such as *What if God isn't real? Why is the sky blue? Why do bad things happen to good people*? They may also make connections not considered by the teachers. Further, these students appear likely to move through content at a faster pace than their peers. Counselors or teachers working with students who display an intellectual overexcitability should consider allowing them time to look for some of the answers to their questions or concerns as one way to alleviate stress for all involved. Independent study projects appear to be helpful to students who constantly crave to know more.

Dabrowski (as cited in Bailey, 2010) often associated giftedness with creativity, which fuels *imaginational overexcitability.* Students who appear deeply drawn to fictional worlds (stories, movies, even art) may display what Dabrowski calls an imaginational overexcitability. These individuals often daydream and doodle and get lost in their own minds. They need open-ended, creative opportunities, such as writing their own stories or producing unique art, in order to fulfill their overactive imaginations. Guiding students to distinguish between fantasy and reality with patience and understanding will go far in helping students who tend to blur those lines.

Educators frequently observe another excitability that Dabrowski identifies as *psychomotor overexcitability*; however, they do not often recognize psychomotor overexcitability as a characteristic of giftedness. Students who possess psychomotor overexcitability exhibit an abundance of energy. These traits can manifest as excessive talking, fidgety behavior, and overactive physical movement. Schools often misdiagnose psychomotor excitability as ADHD. However, these students really do need more movement than others. Providing opportunities for hands-on learning, extra recess, running errands (even nonessential ones), alternative seating options, and alternative counseling styles (e.g., experiential and interactive counseling interventions) can all become helpful strategies when working with a student who exhibits psychomotor overexcitability (Figure 9.3).

Another overexcitability not typically associated with giftedness relates to the senses. *Sensual overexcitability* appears to be somewhat common, but Dabrowski's (as cited in Bailey, 2010) research found it occurs more frequently among gifted individuals. Essentially, these students strongly react to light, sounds, textures, and tastes. The reaction could be positive, as in a continued desire to experience the stimulus, or negative, driving the student away from the stimulus. A wide range of stimuli affect students with sensual overexcitability, including tags on clothing, seams on socks, fluorescent lighting, strong odors, and loud noises. Adults can validate student reactions in these situations. For example, encourage parents to try different socks or cut the tags out of the clothing. Schools could offer alternative lighting and be sensitive to students genuinely bothered

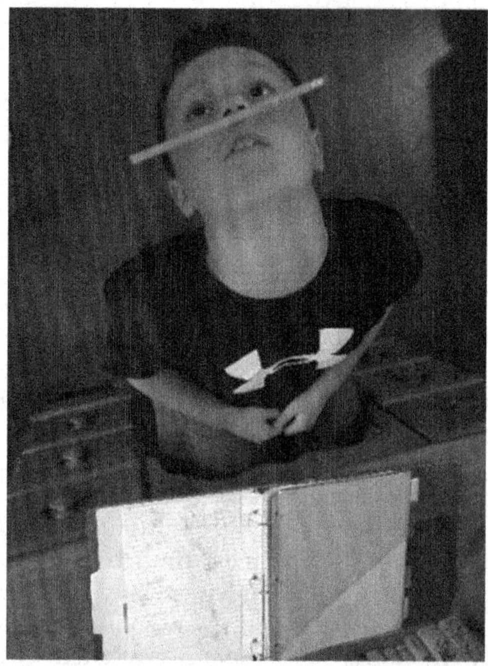

FIGURE 9.3 A child exhibiting psychomotor overexcitability.

by loud sounds. Students will likely continue to show strong reactions to certain stimuli; however, knowing that the educators and counselors working with them care enough to address the given impetus will go a long way in ensuring their comfort, allowing them to better focus on instruction.

Finally, Dabrowski (as cited in Bailey, 2010) discovered that some individuals feel tragedies, injustices, and reminders of mortality deeper and greater than others, a sign of *emotional overexcitability*. Adults may display a tendency to discount the feelings of these students, as they appear to be overly dramatic and in search of extra attention. However, these students often appear to be our most compassionate and empathetic students. While some children will want to take action to help others, they often feel powerless to make the difference they so badly want to make. Educators and counselors can help these students by offering a nonjudgmental stance and validating their feelings. Sharing stories of children who participated in amazing feats to improve the lives of others can also alleviate the feeling of helplessness and empower students to believe that they can and do make a positive difference.

While it may be difficult to live and work with individuals who exhibit any of these overexcitabilities, general strategies identified by professionals can help children and adults deal more effectively with these characteristics and even capitalize on their strengths. First, counselors and other educators can encourage youth to talk about these characteristics. They can ask individuals if they recognize these intensities as personal traits. They may emphasize that others perceive their behaviors to be acceptable and validate the way they feel about them. Acceptance frees people from feelings of isolation, and it becomes critical that professionals impart inclusiveness to all students. A focus on the positive aspects highlights another strategy for working with overexcited students. Sometimes, benefits can be difficult to recognize, since children and adolescents present with all of these extreme tendencies. Overactive imaginations give way to amazing creativity, and the quest for knowledge leads to new innovations and discoveries (i.e., a strong moral compass can lead to solutions for injustices). Even *psychomotor overexcitability*, arguably the most challenging of the five when dealing with classroom management, can be favorable when students channel excess energy into productive means. These individuals display enthusiasm and energy, which can be motivational for others. Finally, people who exhibit overexcitabilities need to be able to share their intensities in order to thrive. Educators and counselors must embrace these behaviors and treat students with understanding and patience, which will result in greater self-acceptance and appreciation from and for others (Bailey, 2010).

SOCIAL AND EMOTIONAL IMPLICATIONS

Counselors and educators who work with gifted students should be knowledgeable about several unique affective conditions commonly found among gifted individuals, including multipotentiality (Ibanez, 2015), perfectionism (Pyrt, 2004), underachievement (Smutney, 2004), and introversion (Cain, 2012). While multipotentiality appears as the only one listed specific to the field of GT, the other three illustrate a high frequency of occurrence among the gifted population. It remains important that professionals be equipped to work with students as they struggle through issues associated with each of these social/emotional issues.

Ibanez (2015) highlights multipotentiality in the literature as the term used to describe individuals who show interest in a wide variety of disciplines and possess the ability to be highly successful in every one of them. This aspect does not surprise most educators who work with gifted individuals, which accounts for the reason professionals often reassure highly talented students that they can do and be anything they want. Few people view being good in several areas to be problematic. It can, after all, appear like feeling sorry for the rich. Can there really be drawbacks for students who demonstrate varied interests and the capacity to pursue any one of them with a high degree of success? The answer might be surprising. These students may feel a great amount of pressure and stress. They may experience decision fatigue at a young age, conflicted as to how to use limited time. They fill their schedules with self-imposed, stressful academic, social, and extracurricular activities. Colangelo (2002) emphasized the importance of forming groups and holding peer discussions with others who possess multipotentiality to normalize their experiences, feelings, and concerns. Further, he suggests that these diverse individuals use leisure activities as a way of continually developing their abilities and interests apart from their career and believes it to be helpful to remind youth that more than one career can be possible in a lifetime.

PERFECTIONISM

Pink (2012) writes about the current trend to hire individuals with multifaceted abilities as opposed to those with fixed skills, a single skill set designed to perform a specific job, as historically being sought after by employers. Today, in our ever-changing, fast-paced world, there appears to be more of a demand for elastic skills that stretch across boundaries. This presents good news for students who fit the multipotential profile.

The quest for excellence can be an admirable trait to which many aspire. We encourage children to "reach for the stars" and strive to get what they want out of life. However, unhealthy perfectionism occurs when individuals strive toward unrealistic goals, causing them to feel defeated and unworthy. Perfectionism occurs for all types of people but correlates most closely with those who never seem satisfied and the gifted population (Pyrt, 2004). For many, it appears to be an inherent trait, present from birth, recognizable in a person's insistence to always be the best and their continual disappointment that they never seem to be good enough. However, for others, it becomes a learned behavior from the excessive expectations of others around them—parents, teachers, and peers. While professionals expect students to be their best, every effort they make may not be perfect. A gifted student may score 90% on an assessment instrument, and some parents tend to focus on the incorrect 10% rather than on the mastered 90%. In addition, gifted students frequently express the pressure they feel from peers who make comments like "I thought you were smart" or "I can't believe you missed that and you're in GT." Even teachers sometimes make comments indicating that GT students should know better and do better. Extreme cases of perfectionism can result in health problems, including depression, eating disorders, addiction, and more. These key concepts used by educators and counselors can prove helpful for children and adolescents to internalize as they learn to cope with perfectionism: (a) Educators and counselors should encourage students to separate their self-worth from their grades or products; (b) they should encourage youth to focus on improvement rather than the "end game"; (c) they may lead students to concentrate on small, incremental improvements on their way to excellence; (d) they may share the lives of eminent people because very few of them achieved without struggle; (e) they can inform students that it takes hard work and persistence in the face of obstacles; and (f) they can highlight that failure can be constructive on the road to accomplishing goals.

UNDERACHIEVEMENT

A myriad of reasons explains why a student might underachieve (Smutney, 2004). Professionals see underachievement as a major concern or risk for gifted individuals. Underachievement manifests when students refrain from submitting what they perceive to be imperfect. As a result, grades fall and the performances of these individuals are not commensurate with their abilities. The literature suggests that a nonnurturing environment may inhibit gifted students from optimal achievement. Students can appear to not be motivated to perform their best. In some instances, disabilities or learning deficits mask their gifts. Individuals who underachieve often struggle with low self-esteem, appearing to develop an aversion to risk, which may cause social isolation (Smutney, 2004). It remains important for counselors to discover the root cause for each individual underachiever in order to know how to proceed with interventions. Collaboration between parents and teachers often yields insights into why a student does not work to full potential, as well as revelations into the child's gifts. By keeping an emphasis on their strengths and involving individuals in the pursuit of their interests and talents, counselors can help students build confidence and equip them with the tools they need to manage their difficulties. Finally, advocacy can be considered one of the most critical keys to someone overcoming underachievement. Having a caring adult who guides and supports them through self-doubt and fears of inadequacy appears to very often function as the component an underperforming child needs to get back on the track to success.

INTROVERSION

Introversion, a social and emotional consideration, comes up as a component in discussion about optimizing gifted students. Introverts focus on their internal thoughts and feelings as opposed to external stimuli (Burruss & Kaenzig, 1999). They need time alone to recharge because people tend to drain their energy as opposed to extroverts who generally feel energized by being around others. Statistics characterize one third to one half of the U.S. population as introverts (Hassell, 2013); however, researchers report introverts to be the majority among the gifted population. This becomes an important finding as we continue to trend toward collaboration and group work in schools (Burruss & Kaenzig, 1999). While the ability to work well with others appears to be a skill that seems beneficial for all, educational professionals and counselors need to keep in mind that some gifted students require more processing time and reflection than others. Cain (2012) stresses that schools should teach children to work with others; however, she emphasizes that professionals must also provide the time and training for them to deliberately practice on their own since introverts appear to need quiet environments in order to do their best work. Cain makes a provocative point that many often see talkers as leaders, which she warns could be cause for concern. She writes:

> *If we assume that quiet and loud people have roughly the same number of good (and bad) ideas, then we should worry if the louder and more forceful people always carry the day. That would mean that an awful lot of bad ideas prevail while good ones get squashed.* (p. 51)

Counselors and educators should implement balanced instructional strategies that address the needs of all types of learners. Additionally, extending wait time following questions and offering students choice in how they will deliver their products and responses will help to nurture the gifts that our quieter, more reflective students can offer.

Educators and counselors working with gifted students might consider using Gardener's theory of multiple intelligences when planning appropriate counseling and instructional experiences. These students should be afforded open-ended opportunities that allow for greater depth of study on how they solve complex problems and how they demonstrate learning. Because of the focus on active learning based on student interest and learning styles, Basak and Birgili (2013) specifically list Gardener's theory of multiple intelligences as a highly preferable approach in gifted and talented children's education. Allowing students to engage in real-world problems and experiences increases the chances that they will be more likely to stay motivated to learn.

COUNSELING GIFTED STUDENTS: SUMMARY

In this section, we learn about the importance of allowing gifted students options that capitalize on their interests and intelligence. Creativity serves as another key factor that should be incorporated into counseling when working with gifted individuals. Designing opportunities in which students can express their original ideas by producing and sharing something new can promote creative thinking. Flexible thinkers see mistakes as opportunities. The ability to break apart from mental fixations and reorganize experiences and concepts requires flexibility of thought.

CHAPTER SUMMARY

Ralph Waldo Emerson (as cited in Osborn, 1945) once said, "Unless you try to do something beyond what you have already mastered, you will never grow." Too often, students who come to school with the potential to learn the most actually learn the least. Educators and counselors focus concentrated efforts on kids who openly struggle, both academically and socially/emotionally, and must not assume that gifted individuals possess some superhuman resiliency that propels them forward and away from so many of the intensities and social/emotional issues discussed in this chapter. Indeed, some of the smartest and most creative people get lost in their quest for idealism and excellence. Without guidance from teachers, counselors, and parents, whom we charge with enhancing the lives of children and adolescents, these individuals may never find their way. Gifted students, like all others, reflect uniqueness and do not demonstrate giftedness in the same areas. In fact, sometimes, their gifts present in ways that schools do not always value. During his childhood, comedian Robin Williams suffered from loneliness. In a biographical story, he recalled being tormented by bullies; and in order to cope, he created characters and conversations in his head. Williams evolved as a creative genius and masked his pain with humor. His gifts would probably not yield high scores on standardized achievement or ability tests. Yet he went on to receive many awards and accolades throughout his successful career. We now know, though, he continued to struggle with existential depression, which stemmed from his early years as a lonely child who entertained himself with his imagination. Our schools and communities need counselors to serve the needs of advanced and gifted students. The prosperity of our nations depends on this. Gifted students can be an asset or a detriment to themselves or our society if not properly cared for.

POINTS TO REMEMBER

- Disability identity development remains complex and continues to change.
- The Disability Rights Movement parallels other civil rights movements.
- Disability accommodations in education promote inclusion and diversity in the classroom.
- The school delivers services to students based on annual reviews, IEPs, and parental interactions.
- Key legislations such as the IDEA and Section 504 promote inclusion of children and adolescents with disabilities in the classroom.
- The ADA, a civil rights law, prohibits discrimination against individuals with disabilities.
- Professional school counselors and clinical mental health counselors advocate for students with disabilities and students classified as gifted.
- Adolescents with disabilities must develop self-advocacy skills and understand their disability in order to successfully transition to postsecondary educational settings.
- Disability services in postsecondary educational institutions work collaboratively with students with disabilities and the postsecondary community.
- Gifted students must receive instruction appropriate to their abilities in order to maximize their full potential.
- Counselors and teachers must address the unique social and emotional needs of gifted learners to ensure their optimal development.

OTHER HELPFUL INFORMATION FOR CONSIDERATION

- U.S. Department of Justice—ADA Assistance: https://www.ada.gov
- U.S. Department of Education, Office of Civil Rights: https://www2.ed.gov/about/offices/list/ocr/disabilityoverview.html
- Texas Education Agency (TEA) Texas Transition: https://www.texastransition.org
- Going to College: http://going-to-college.org
- The Davidson Institute recognizes, nurtures, and supports profoundly intelligent young people and provides opportunities for them to develop their talents to make a positive difference. The website contains information and resources that guide parents and educators as they seek to support highly gifted students. https://www.davidsongifted.org
- Mensa, a society of high IQ individuals, provides a forum for intellectual exchange among its members. The Mensa website offers criteria for membership, as well as opportunities for members to engage in intellectual and social events. https://www.mensa.org
- Hoagies' Gifted Education Page consists of articles, books, resources, and links to help parents and teachers support gifted children. https://www.hoagiesgifted.org

QUESTIONS FOR FURTHER DISCUSSION

- How can counselors assist children and adolescents in transitioning from high school to postsecondary institutions or employment?
- What exemplars highlight the significance of diversity and inclusion?
- What strengths and limitations do professional school counselors and clinical mental health counselors encounter when working with children and adolescents with disabilities and those designated as gifted?
- How do legislative mandates for children and adolescents in pre-K through 12 differ from one another?
- What constitutes the difference between legislation for children in pre-K through 12 and those for postsecondary institutions?

KEY REFERENCES

Only key references appear in the print edition. The full reference list appears in the digital product found on Springer Publishing Connect: connect.springerpub.com/content/book/978-0-8261-4764-6/part/part03/chapter/ch09

American School Counselor Association. (2019). *ASCA national model: A framework for school counseling programs*. American School Counselor Association.

Bailey, C. (2010). Overexcitabilities and sensitivities: Implications of Dabrowski's theory of positive disintegration for counseling the gifted. https://www.positivedisintegration.com/Bailey2010.pdf

Betts, G., & Niehart, M. (2010). Revised profiles of the gifted & talented. https://sciencetalenter.dk/sites/default/files/revised_profiles_of_the_gifted_and_talented_-_neihart_and_betts.pdf

Colker, R., & Grossman, P. D. (2014). *The law of disability discrimination for higher education professionals*. Matthew Bender & Company, Inc.

Dabrowski, K., & Piechowski, M. M. (1972). *Multilevelness of instinctive and emotional functions: Volume 2 – types and levels of development*. Unpublished manuscript, University of Alberta.

Lee, A. M. I. (2019). The 13 disability categories under IDEA. https://www.understood.org/en/school-learning/special-services/special-education-basics/conditions-covered-under-idea

Madaus, J., Miller, W., & Vance, M. L. (2009). Veterans with disabilities in postsecondary education. *Journal of Postsecondary Education and Disability*, *22*(1), 10–17.

National Association for Gifted Children. (2019). A position statement. https://www.nagc.org/sites/default/files/Position%20Statement/Definition%20of%20Giftedness%20%282019%29.pdf

Putnam, M. (2005). Conceptualizing disability: Developing a framework for political disability identity. *Journal of Disability Policy Studies*, *16*(3), 188–198. https://doi.org/10.1177/10442073050160030601

Pyrt, M. (2004). Helping gifted students cope with perfectionism. Parenting for High Potentials. http://www.davidsongifted.org/search-database/entry/a10459

Rehabilitation Act of 1973, Pub.L. 93-112, 87 Stat. 355, enacted September 26, 1973.

Shapiro, E. (n.d.). Tiered instruction and intervention in a response-to-intervention model. http://www.rtinetwork.org/essential/tieredinstruction/tiered-instruction-and-intervention-rti-model

CHAPTER 10

Addressing the Needs of Children and Adolescents of Special Populations

Naderia T. Hartley, Ruby R. Bible, and Brenda Jones

LEARNING OBJECTIVES

After completing this chapter, the reader should be able to:

- Recognize how personal bias may impact the counseling process.
- Apply culturally competent, theory-based techniques in counseling children and adolescents of special populations.
- Identify how socioeconomic status, poverty, race, gender, and sexual orientation impact children and adolescents.
- Demonstrate practical strength-based approaches to counsel youth of special populations.

CACREP STANDARDS FOR THIS CHAPTER

- CACREP 2016: 2.3.e.f.i.; 5.d.f.; School Counseling: 5.G.2.a.; 3.b.d.f.h.j.k.l.; Clinical Mental Health Counseling: 5.C.2.a.g.j.
- CACREP 2009: II.G.1.b., i.; 2.a.b.f.; 3.e.f.; 5.b.; School Counseling: III. A.3., 6; C.2.3; E.2.3.4; Clinical Mental Health Counseling: III.A.3.C.8.; E.3.

INTRODUCTION

This chapter emphasizes counseling strategies and techniques that address the needs of children and adolescents of special populations. Until recently, counseling services often underserved or did not serve the needs of marginalized youth. Counseling children and adolescents from special populations requires a different set of skills, with cultural competence as a central focus. These special populations include children and adolescents identified as at risk (or at promise), as marginalized statuses, as military youth, and as English language learners (ELLs) or those with limited English proficiency (LEP).

According to Arredondo and Arciniega (2001), strength-based counseling addresses the needs of all youth and provides positive impacts and outcomes. Counselors who use a strength-based perspective to deliver counseling services focus on promoting and advocating for all youth, as well as focus on positive development (Dollarhide & Saginak, 2012). Multicultural awareness continues to be essential for a strength-based approach. Multicultural counselors should remain aware of their biases and how they may impact the counseling relationship with children and adolescents. Luby (2012) defines multicultural counseling as a relationship between youth and counselors who experience different cultural backgrounds, gender, worldviews, sexual orientation, and social class. Multicultural counselors continuously self-reflect and remain aware of their biases, knowledge, and skills (Sue et al., 1992). They also remain aware of hidden factors that impact the well-being of children. Legal status, sexual orientation, homelessness, and language barriers serve as examples of hidden factors that may not be obvious when first working with youth. McAuliffe (2013) uses an analogy of an iceberg to describe culture not observed by outsiders. The larger part of the iceberg (under the water) consists of the cultural identity of the youth. That identity corresponds to more intense emotional experiences that may require extensive counseling services and support from the school counselor (McAuliffe, 2013). It continues to be important to note that youth from these special populations can be members of more than one special population; for example, a child can be homeless and an ELL, which creates compounding hardships and a need for support.

The counseling profession challenges mental health counselors and professional school counselors with the task of intervening sensitively and responsibly with children and adolescents from these populations. Clinicians must enter the counseling relationship with the notation of praxis, where cultural understanding, acceptance, and critical awareness meet advocacy and intervention. The learning objectives in this chapter will aid counselors-in-training in understanding the unique mental health needs of special populations, expanding the therapeutic relationship, and increasing the effectiveness of interventions when counseling children and adolescents from special populations.

CHILDREN AND ADOLESCENTS AT RISK: SOCIAL AND CULTURAL DESCRIPTION

As discussed in Chapter 8, the literature defines children and adolescents at risk as youth who appear likely to fail at school (U.S. Department of Education, National Center for Education Statistics, 1992). These youth come from varying economic, educational, and environmental conditions that may impact their ability to complete high school. While the literature defines youth at risk in this manner, "youth at promise" connotes a more strength-based definition. With the proper interventions, these once “at-risk” youth can successfully remove their “at-risk” label. Clinicians working with children and adolescents at risk must be aware of the unique historical and contemporary social challenges they face and how this impacts their worldview and the therapeutic relationship. Without understanding the way these challenges affect a child or adolescent positionality, worldview, thoughts, actions, and beliefs, clinicians risk harm to clients. Understanding family dynamics, communication styles, and unique challenges becomes imperative to providing culturally competent counseling.

CHILDREN AND ADOLESCENTS OF POVERTY

According to the U.S. Census Bureau (2018a), 48.5% of racial and ethnic minority families reported living below the poverty line. It remains crucial for clinicians to understand the implications of socioeconomic status on the well-being of children and adolescents by addressing misconceptions. Class and economic status impacts where a family lives, where youth obtain their education, and the family's ability to obtain adequate insurance, thus impacting both the child's physiological and psychological health. Culturally responsive counselors understand how systematic historical oppression, discrimination, and prejudice influence the way at-risk children and adolescents view and interpret life events. These views may be a different perspective from that of the counselor, potentially leaving neither counselor nor client able to understand the other's perspective fully. Taking the time to understand and discuss the cultural aspects of youth and adolescents at risk, along with the class and socioeconomic status of their families, will ensure that the counselors maintain an accurate account of the client's worldview.

Family System

Family dynamics include, but are not limited to, familial socioeconomic status, gender roles, hierarchies, birth order, attachment type (secure vs. insecure), parenting type, religious beliefs, and values, all of which impact the way children and adolescents identify and interact with the world. Family dynamics often carry a strong influence on the way children and adolescents see themselves, their ability to self-advocate, their perception of self-efficacy, and their worldview. These factors influence their relationships, behavior, and well-being. Counselors must understand the cultural aspects of family dynamics and the resulting implications in counseling.

The use of Bowen's family systems theory can be effective when conceptualizing the counseling needs of children and adolescents. Kolbert et al. (2013) states, "The development of the self is not confined within the individual but emerges within the context of the family" (p. 87). Thus, accurately assessing the needs of the child or adolescent cannot be possible without an understanding of the family system. Counselors should explore the client's family system in order to understand the children's or adolescent's self-perception and respond to the foundational needs of the child or adolescent.

Functional family therapy (FFT) can be useful when working with at-risk children and adolescents and their families across cultural, ethnic, racial, and socioeconomic backgrounds. Alexander and Robins (2010) posit, "This framework provides the context for integrating and linking behavioral and cognitive intervention strategies to the specific familial and ecological characteristics of each family" (p. 245). Without the inclusion of pre- and posttreatment activities, FFT consists of five components: (a) engagement in change; (b) motivation to change; (c) relational/interpersonal assessment and change planning; (d) behavior change; and (e) generalization across behavioral domains and multiple systems (Alexander & Robbins, 2010, p. 248). Alexander and Robbins provide a brief synopsis of the ideal FFT intervention (see Tables 10.1 and 10.2).

TABLE 10.1 BRIEF SYNOPSIS OF THE IDEAL FUNCTIONAL FAMILY THERAPY INTERVENTION

Session 1: Engagement, Intake, and Assessment	Between Sessions 1 and 2	Sessions 2 and 3
1. Establish a relationship with the family. 2. Initiate Motivation Phase by using Change Focus and Change Meaning techniques. 3. Begin assessment of Relational Functions and observation of family interaction patterns. 4. End session with assessment protocol and intake documentation.	1. Review each family member's behavior, feelings, and beliefs and consider additional cultural match issues. 2. Identify unclear relationship dynamics within the family and with extended family or other caregivers. 3. Identify resistance patterns of family members/caregivers. 4. Hypothesize Relational Functions for each family member.	1. Repeat techniques from Session 1 and continue to match and build relationships with family members. 2. Continue to use Change Focus and Change Meaning interventions. 3. Continue assessment. 4. If possible, complete Motivation Phase goals.

Source: Alexander, J. F., & Robbins, M. S. (2010). Functional family therapy. In R. C. Murrihy, A. D. Kidman, & T. H. Ollendick (Eds.), *Clinical handbook of assessing and treating conduct problems in youth* (pp. 261–263). Springer International Publishing. https://doi.org/10.1007/978-1-4419-6297-3_10

Unstable Families

Working with youth at risk can be difficult because they may lack support that encourages counseling. Some children and adolescents may be in foster care, child protective custody, living in group homes, or otherwise living with extended family. The instability of their family system may put these children and adolescents at risk of continued abuse (Centers for Disease Control and Prevention, 2020; U.S. Department of Health and Human Services, Administration for Children and Families, Administration on Children, Youth and Families, Children's Bureau, 2004). As a result, they may develop a lack of trust with adults and experience relational difficulties (Centers for Disease Control and Prevention, 2020; U.S. Department of Health and Human Services, Administration for Children and Families, Administration on Children, Youth and Families, Children's Bureau, 2004). Gaining the trust of these youth continues to be imperative to the therapeutic relationship, as youth at risk often seem intuitive and can "read" the adults they encounter. Counselors should appear authentic from the initial interactions in order to foster and establish trust.

COUNSELING IMPLICATIONS FOR CHILDREN AND ADOLESCENTS AT RISK

Brown and Skinner's (2007) model may be useful in gaining youth's trust. The model provides five steps for relational trust building. These steps emphasize the significance of patience, as well as the importance of completing the steps in sequence as youth at risk

TABLE 10.2 BRIEF SYNOPSIS OF THE IDEAL FUNCTIONAL FAMILY THERAPY INTERVENTION CONTINUED

Between Sessions 3 and 4	Middle Sessions	Later Sessions	Termination
1. Develop intermediate and long-term change goals that will address family relational pattern deficits. 2. Establish positive alternatives that provide a rationale and behavioral focus that matches all family members' Relational Functions. 3. Review and develop specific behavior change and educational techniques that will lead to the fulfillment of intermediate and long-term goals.	1. Apply behavior change technology consistent with Relational Functions to family members. 2. Resistance from a family member provides feedback of unsatisfied relational functions. The therapist must then return to motivation and assessment and reevaluate the family member. 3. Develop increased family initiative in behavior change and continue to match Relational Functions. 4. Prompt, look for, and support appropriate family member competence with steadily decreasing assistance from the therapist.	1. Identify relevant systems and specific individual issues (e.g., vocational deficits). 2. Initiation of relapse prevention work. 3. Generalize specific behavior changes to other family situations. 4. Facilitate independence that is consistent with Relational Functions of family members. 5. Maintain and create new links with extrafamilial systems to generalize positive intrafamily changes. 6. Evaluate the quality-of-life issues and plan for future.	1. Problem cessation: determined by verbal report and therapist observation. 2. Spontaneous family process: observation of new interaction styles and attributions for all family members. 3. Primary risk factors, including safety issues, reduced or eliminated; protective factors enhanced.

Source: Alexander, J. F., & Robbins, M. S. (2010). Functional family therapy. In R. C. Murrihy, A. D. Kidman, & T. H. Ollendick (Eds.), *Clinical handbook of assessing and treating conduct problems in youth* (pp. 261–263). Springer International Publishing. https://doi.org/10.1007/978-1-4419-6297-3_10

appear to be cautious in trusting. Counselors should observe the following steps: listen, validate, problem-solve, positive regard, and hope.

LISTEN

Empathic or active listening involves listening and responding in ways that help identify feelings youths may not know existed or may be unwilling to admit. Reflective statements can help identify and name complicated feelings such as "You feel ________ when you are not listened to" (Brown & Skinner, 2007, p. 3).

VALIDATE

Validating makes youths feel heard and allows them to be expressive and transparent. However, it does not support inappropriate behavior. Instead, "validating neutralizes and normalizes a feeling" (Brown & Skinner, 2007, p. 3).

PROBLEM-SOLVE

Helping youth to solve their problems allows them to be active agents of change in their lives. This builds on a strength-based approach that encourages them to utilize already equipped problem-solving skills and demonstrates mutual respect between the counselor and child or adolescent. This leads youth to see the counselor as a caring individual and to actively participate in counseling. Listening and validating must occur before attempting to problem-solve.

POSITIVE REGARD

Positive regard involves taking an interest in the lives of youth at risk, learning about them holistically, and using a strength-based approach to counseling. Life experiences and broken relationships may lead to a reluctance to share personal stories, and some experiences enable these youth to adopt an "I don't care" attitude as a defense mechanism. The clinician must recognize this as such and not take their behavior personally; maintaining positive regard will help encourage a trusting relationship. Working through steps one, two, and three in the Brown–Skinner model will convince youths that their counselor appears to be "real" in their care and concern for them.

HOPE

After the establishment of trust, counselors can assist youth to establish hope that their circumstances can change, establish healthy trusting relationships with adults, and serve as change agents in their lives. The in vivo statement from Roman illustrates the application of the Brown–Skinner model for building trust. Teachers referred Roman, a 15-year-old eighth grader, to counseling due to his consistent class and school disruptions, low grades, and truancy. Although Roman continues to be frequently disruptive or truant in some classes, he attends math, art, and Spanish classes regularly. The school retained Roman in seventh grade and classified him as a student at risk. The system removed him from his home and placed him in foster care for 2 years until his current placement in his aunt's care became possible. The following describes an excerpt from the initial meeting with his school counselor, where she utilizes the Brown–Skinner model to build trust with Roman.

Time-Efficient Situated Client Experience

Roman (R): *Miss, why did you call me down. Why am I in here?*

Counselor (C): *Well, some of your teachers seemed concerned that you miss classes and get into arguments with your teachers.*

R: No response or eye contact.

C: *I am not here to judge or to get you in trouble. Disciplining and punishment does not occur in this office. I just want to know about you. We do not even have to talk about school, just tell me about Roman.*

R: *What is there to tell. I'm here, and I don't like coming here, but it's better than being at home?*

C: *So, school may be the lesser of the two evils?*

R: *Hell Yeah. Y'all don't want me here, and my aunt don't want me at home. But at least here y'all just ignore me instead of yelling and cussin.*

C: *If those represented my only two choices, I'd probably feel frustrated and angry.*

R: *Sh*t, it is what it is.*

C: *True, those represent two things that you do not really hold a lot of control over. But it does matter how you feel about them; because remember, I am trying to know Roman and part of Roman consists of his feelings, even if you try to ignore them.*

R: *I guess, Miss. I mean basically it pisses me off. Everywhere I go somebody got a problem with me.*

C: *So, you feel unwanted at home and school, and that makes you angry?*

R: *Yeah. I gotta deal with bullsh*t at home, and then them teachers try to play me in front of the whole class.*

C: *What do you mean, "play me?"*

R: *You know, like try to embarrass me in front of the whole class. I ain't with that disrespect sh*t, so I embarrass they a** back.*

C: *I hear you saying that when teachers call attention to you in front of the entire class, you feel embarrassed and singled out? Give me an example when a teacher appeared disrespectful.*

R: *Yes, Miss. Okay, so like when I went to English yesterday, Mrs. Head gon' say, "it's nice to see you Roman, long time no see, are you going to actually do work for us today?" Like she didn't have to do all that. Why can't I just come to class and get out? I cussed her a** out and left. She ain't want me there anyway.*

C: *Being called out in class like that would make me feel embarrassed and want to leave too. I don't think I would have cussed her out, though. What do you think?*

R: *Yeah, I guess that was kinda messed up, but she made me so mad, Miss. Like how she gone play me like that?*

C: *I mean, I get being mad, I would have been mad too but sometimes how you display being mad makes a big difference in the results you get.*

R: *What you mean, Miss?*

C: *When you make bad choices out of anger, you usually end up with bad results. What happened after you cussed out Mrs. Head?*

R: *She wrote me up, and Mr. Mosely (assistant principal) overnight suspended me, my aunt had to take off to come up here, and she cussed me out all night about it. She went on and on about how much money I cost. Sh*t was hella annoying, but I didn't say anything back because she take care of me for free, ya know.*

C: *What do you think would have happened if you would have not said anything back to Mrs. Head and just sat down?*

R: *I wouldn't have got written up but I aint going out like that, she played me.*

C: *Okay I understand; you don't like being disrespected. But could there be another way you let her know she disrespected and embarrassed you?*

R: *I guess I could have talked to her at a different time and let her know I don't like it. But won't do sh*t. She still gon' be rude, she just like that.*

C: *Have you ever tried it?*

R: *No.*

C: *So how do you know it won't work?*

R: *I don't know, it's too late now anyway, she hates me.*

C: *You don't know that. She might just be mad at you, just like you seemed to be mad at her.*

R: *Yeah, maybe.*

C: *If you would like, we can work on how to have that conversation with her. And I can even be there to help you.*

R: *For real, Miss?*

C: *Absolutely. Things are not always stuck the way they appear. You can take control over a lot of things in your life. You just need to identify those things and make small changes along the way.*

R: *I don't know about all that.*

C: *You do, but it takes practice to figure out which things you can control and which ones you cannot. But you have already identified what you could do differently in Mrs. Head's class, and made a plan to correct it. That is a start. Give yourself credit for that.*

R: *I guess, Miss. I do like talking to you though. You mad cool and ain't try to make me talk different.*

C: *I'm glad because we've got some work to do.*

ETHNICALLY DIVERSE CHILDREN AND ADOLESCENTS USING SYSTEMIC AND MULTICULTURAL FOCI

AFRICAN AMERICAN CHILDREN AND ADOLESCENTS

The roles that African American youth play within families changed dramatically over generations due to systematic discrimination and oppression. In past generations, African American children played roles "that confirmed their value as important contributors to the welfare of the family and community" (Capuzzi & Gross, 2014, p. 117), such as household chores, attending church services regularly, and working small jobs around the neighborhood (e.g., mowing a neighbor's lawn). Extended family networks and the growing number of women leading single-family households within the African American community resulted in African American children and adolescents experiencing difficulties establishing a sense of self and identity at both school and home (Baruth & Manning, 2016). These youth often perform adult roles at home, caring for younger siblings, cooking, and maintaining household duties at a young age. The transition of roles between home and school can create a confusing sense of self and identity. Often, these adult responsibilities lead the youth to expectations of adult treatment and respect. However, faculty and staff may view students as subordinates who should take directives.

African American children and adolescents seem to be stereotypically perceived as more aggressive than their peers (Skiba et al., 2011). This perceived aggression derives from misunderstandings of cultural norms within the African American community, such as display of distinctive forms of dress and body ornamentation, African American speech styles, playful aggression, and exaggerated forms of bravado (Monroe, 2005). Counselors should be aware of cultural norms and alleviate any bias or prejudice that stems from them. African American children and adolescents may be resistant to counseling because of mistrust and the stigma of therapy within the African American community. Therefore, establishing a trusting relationship remains crucial to success in counseling.

HISPANIC AND LATINX CHILDREN AND ADOLESCENTS

Traditionally, Hispanic American and Latinx families teach children and adolescents about machismo, a term translated as a strong sense of masculine pride (Baruth & Manning, 2016). Machismo encompasses traits of honor and dignity, taking care of and providing for one's family, respect, love, and manhood. Because of the strong sense of masculine pride and manhood, children and adolescents from Hispanic American and Latinx families learn a clear distinction between gender roles. Early in life, children learn that males enjoy rights and privileges traditionally denied to females. Clinicians working with Hispanic American and Latinx youth understand the importance of gender roles within those families. Children and adolescents may struggle with acceptance and their identity within these gender roles. They may also struggle with integrating traditional cultural values and beliefs into contemporary life. Traditional values such as machismo, patriarchy, and noncompetitive behavior within the family conflict with contemporary beliefs and lifestyles such as gender equality, female-led single-parent homes, and the competitive nature of American public schools (Baruth & Manning, 2016). The counselor should conceptualize the youth and acknowledge their values and beliefs in contrast to traditional ones.

AMERICAN INDIAN/NATIVE AMERICAN CHILDREN AND ADOLESCENTS

American Indian/Native American families value extended family and traditional ways of knowing (Lee, 1995). The clinician needs to recognize that these ways of knowing conflict with traditional Western ideas. American Indian children often face difficulties in school due to educators stereotyping and not recognizing the unique learning styles, which contribute to struggles with positive self-concept (Baruth & Manning, 1992). Before working with American Indian/Native American clients, the clinician should seek to learn as much about the specific culture of their client. Cultural traditions, values, and beliefs differ from tribe to tribe, and the clinician should not generalize. Clinicians should also be mindful of the impact of nonverbal communication when working with American Indian/Native American children and adolescents. For instance, while Eurocentric culture values eye contact when speaking, in some American Indian/Native American tribes, this may be viewed as disrespectful (Baruth & Manning, 1992). They may also struggle with finding the place of traditional tribal culture, values, and beliefs and acculturation in mainstream American culture (Baruth & Manning, 2016).

ASIAN AMERICAN CHILDREN AND ADOLESCENTS

When working with Asian American clients, the clinician should recognize that "Asian" does not represent a homogenous group. "Asian refers to people with origins in any of the original peoples of the Far East, Southeast Asia, or the Indian subcontinent, including people from Cambodia, China, India, Japan, Korea, Malaysia, Pakistan, the Philippine Islands, Thailand, and Vietnam" (Baruth & Manning, 2016, p. 159). Each group encompasses different languages, cultures, and beliefs. Family allegiance continues to be of utmost importance for many patriarchal Asian families, where the father maintains absolute authority. Asian American children often do well in school due to the high academic expectations of their parents (Baruth & Manning, 2016). Living up to these expectations can cause high stress and anxiety in Asian youth. Asian American children and adolescents can struggle to find balance with maintaining cultural and family values, bringing honor to their family's names, and acculturating into mainstream American culture. Counselors should be aware that this stereotype does encompass all Asian American groups or individuals and should not generalize.

CHILDREN AND ADOLESCENTS OF LIMITED ENGLISH PROFICIENCY, YOUNG IMMIGRANTS, AND TRANSNATIONALS

Recent immigration data estimate that over five million children aged 18 and under live in an undocumented household. "Undocumented" refers to a person who entered the United States with false documents or who entered legally as a nonimmigrant but violated the terms of their visa and remained in the United States (National Immigration Law Center, 2011). Immigrants refer to people who moved to the United States for more opportunities and a better life. To effectively work with students of undocumented or immigrant status, counselors must understand the importance of the student's life circumstances.

Limited English Proficiency

Counselors play a vital role in addressing the needs of non–English-speaking youth, by being bridge builders for families, the school, and the community. Language barriers may present a major stressor for non–English-language-speaking families. This posits yet another burden for youth, leading to barriers in their education. Counselors should be aware of the barriers that may impede families from feeling welcomed in the United States.

According to the U.S. Department of Education (2002), over six million children and adolescents become diagnosed with LEP. The most significant percentage speak Spanish; however, over 20% represent over 400 other languages.

Youth Immigrants

Immigrant youth may also be undocumented, and "hidden factors" (mentioned earlier in this chapter) may impact the youth socially, emotionally, and academically. Undocumented children and adolescents may feel unsafe and mistrust the U.S. systems. Counselors need to be aware of how immigrant status can affect their life experiences. Children and adolescents who become afraid of deportation will not seek counseling unless they feel safe. Counselors must be aware of the barriers that can impede a youth from being successful and understand the laws, policies, and implications on the lives of youths.

Children and adolescents of immigrant status may need to assist their families due to LEP. They may translate, complete important documents, and attend to their siblings' education needs. Placing children in the position to translate for their parents can have damaging effects on the child, causing additional stress and anxiety (Sue & Sue, 2016). Some of the stressors surrounding child translators may include parent–child conflict, overburdening the child, and an increased sense of responsibility to the family as well as ensuring that children translate parents' intended communication with accuracy. These stressors may lead to an increase in aggressive behaviors, social problems, and risk-taking behaviors, such as drugs and alcohol. On the other hand, there may be some benefits, such as a strengthening of their social, emotional, and interpersonal skills. It continues to be important for counselors to not make assumptions about families; however, they need to have an awareness of how translating for the family could lead to an increase in stress and high-risk behaviors (Sue & Sue, 2016).

During the counseling relationship, counselors should focus on the strengths and cultural capital of the child or adolescent and allow them to tell their stories. Pipher (2002) noted the importance of slowing down, listening, and learning about the child or adolescent through their own words. Failure to do this, however well intended, presents an imposition of personal ideas and cultural practices and, thus, enforces assimilation. Counselors need to use active listening skills and leave their personal views and cultural practices outside of the counseling relationship.

Empowering youth of immigrant status to use their voice and speak up for themselves will help them learn self-advocacy skills. Counseling should be inclusive of all cultures and norms as part of the therapeutic relationship. This can be through books that represent many cultures or multicultural activity interventions such as diversity bingo. In the school setting, the school community plays a vital role in helping the new child and adolescent immigrants experience a positive transition to the new school environment. Counselors can also involve the community by inviting cultural liaisons and community leaders to serve on committees within the school.

Transnationals

Transnational youth differ from immigrant youth in the unique challenge of family separation. Levitt (2001) and Vertovec (2009) describe transnational people as those who live all across the world and travel the world to make the most of their economic, political, educational, and other life opportunities. Coe et al. (2011) estimate that one in four school-age children worldwide get caught up in transnational flows. The system often separates them from their parents or caregivers, leaving them to assume more responsibilities in the home with a lack of support from extended family (Aye & Guerin, 2001). They may be vulnerable to psychosocial adjustments, including cultural conflicts with their parents, grief and loss, extreme pressure from parents to perform well in school, the stress of their parents' marital relationship due to the separation, discrimination, and sense of identity (Creese et al., 1999; Lee & Koo, 2006; Waters, 2002). Despite these barriers, transnational youths come with a breadth of knowledge and cultural wealth. Professional school counselors, who build cultural awareness within their school, can make the climate a more welcoming environment for all youths, especially the marginalized youths not often represented within the school culture.

CASE STUDY 10.1: COUNSELING TRANSNATIONAL YOUTH

Sophia, a 16-year-old high school sophomore, lives with her immigrant mother and father in the home of Sophia's aunt with Sophia's three siblings. Sophia's parents speak limited English. Sophia attends school regularly but reports to school late on many occasions. A few times a year, she travels back home to Mexico to visit her family, causing her to miss a few weeks of school. Sophia, an ELL, speaks fluent Spanish. Sophia struggled to make friends due to language barriers. She earns good grades; however, during the times of her extended visits to Mexico, her grades drop drastically. Her teachers stated, "Sophia's parents must not care about her, why would they take her out of school for weeks at a time? She continues to be late and needs extra time to catch up on her work." You meet with Sophia for the first time, and she seems very shy and quiet.

Activity 10.1: Reflection Questions

1. What theory and techniques can the counselor use when working with Sophia?
2. List some of the cultural considerations the counselor should be aware of.
3. What should be the counselor's response, if any, to the teacher who stated, "Sophia's parents must not care about her, why would they take her out of school for weeks at a time?"
4. How could the counselor implement a partnership approach among Sophia, the teacher, parents, and herself?

COUNSELING IMPLICATIONS FOR ETHNICALLY DIVERSE CHILDREN AND ADOLESCENTS

The historically oppressive and discriminatory treatment of ethnically diverse minorities in the United States caused many to distrust the American systems, including mental health and counseling. As a result, establishing a strong, trusting therapeutic relationship with the child or adolescent will be central to successful counseling. Utilizing Brown and Skinner's model for building trust with at-risk youth will encourage ethnically diverse youth to trust the counseling process and their counselor. The counselor may experience resistance from the family and child or adolescent partially due to distrust of mental health providers due to a history of racist and discriminatory practices in mental healthcare (Wendt et al., 2015) but also the close-knit nature of ethnic minority families (Goodman & Gorski, 2015; Liddle et al., 2001). These families tend to want to keep "family business" in house and discourage disclosing problems to outsiders (Baruth & Manning, 2016; Goodman & Gorski, 2015; Liddle et al., 2001). This further emphasizes the importance of establishing a trusting relationship with the youth and their family.

The counseling field recognizes the importance of the variety of theoretical approaches and strategies, an important factor when working with ethnically diverse children and adolescents. Using culture-centered counseling aids, clinicians correctly conceptualize issues and provide effective interventions for ethnically diverse youth as they seek to understand the client's priorities and behaviors in a cultural context. Culture-centered counseling involves the counselor utilizing basic counseling skills while paying attention to cultural norms, assumptions, and beliefs to gain accurate awareness and meaningful cultural knowledge. This shifts counseling to an "educational" perspective where the child or adolescent becomes a consultant in the counseling process and works together with the clinician (American Psychological Association, 2008). Incorporating creative expression into theory-based interventions creates a cross-cultural aspect that allows children and adolescents to integrate their racial and cultural identity into counseling. Ethnic minorities taking pride in their racial and cultural identities helps them cope with the stressors of discrimination and prejudice and avoid internalizing negative stereotypes (Goicoechea et al., 2014). Resources for creative arts interventions can be found in the section titled Other Helpful Information for Consideration.

LESBIAN, GAY, BISEXUAL, AND TRANSGENDER YOUTH

As mentioned in Chapter 2, lesbian, gay, bisexual, transgender, queer/questioning, intersex, and asexual (LGBTQIA+) children and adolescents continue to be a part of the most vulnerable populations of youth. These youth often suffer from mood and anxiety disorders, depression, suicidal ideations, homelessness, and eating disorders. A report conducted by the Human Rights Campaign Foundation (2018) found that LGBTQIA+ youth appear more likely to experience higher stress levels, be victims of sexual attacks and unwanted sexual advances, experience bullying or harassment, and be homeless than their cisgender peers, persons whose gender identity aligns with that typically associated with the sex assigned to them at birth. The 2017 National School Climate Survey (Kosciw et al., 2018) found that 57.6% of LGBTQIA+ youth felt unsafe at school because of their sexual orientation, 43.3% felt unsafe because of their gender expression, and 85.2% experienced verbal harassment (Kosciw et al., 2018).

Culturally competent counselors should be aware of their biases when counseling LGBTQIA+ youth and seek supervision, as the profession requires counselors to separate their values to foster a safe, nonjudgmental therapeutic environment Counselors experiencing ethical dilemmas regarding counselor values should review the American Counseling Association (ACA) Code of Ethics, specifically sections C.5. Nondiscrimination and E.8. Multicultural Issues/Diversity in Assessment and sections A. 1.f. Supporting Student Development and B.3.i. Responsibilities to Self of the American School Counselor Association (ASCA), with respect to the counseling position (ACA, 2014; ASCA, 2016).

LANGUAGE

Using the correct terminology and pronouns becomes an important aspect of working with LGBTQIA+. It ensures that clinicians communicate in a consistent, respectful, and professional manner. When working with children and adolescents, the counselor should not assume the gender identity or sexual orientation of the youth. Language should be conducive to nongender-specific terms. For example, the question asking a female client "Who is the special boy you are going to prom with?" assumes the child or adolescent to be heterosexual and leaves no room for correction. Questions such as the aforementioned one can be detrimental to the counseling relationship; because after a counselor assumes a client's gender or sexual orientation, the youth may not feel comfortable "outing" themselves to the counselor or continuing with the sessions. Counselors should also recognize that not all children and adolescents identify as cisgender (Human Rights Campaign Foundation, 2018). These youth may desire to be referred to by their identified gender and not their assigned gender, or not to be referred to by a pronoun at all. Instead, they may prefer to be referred to by name. Clinicians should utilize the appropriate noun and pronoun when counseling gender nonconforming youth, a term used to define people's gender expressions that do not fit neatly into male or female categories (Human Rights Campaign Foundation, 2018). Exhibit 10.1 lists frequently used LGBTQIA+ terms. Although not exhaustive, this list provides a foundation of terms counselors need to be familiar with when working with LGBTQIA+ children and adolescents.

EXHIBIT 10.1

Glossary of LGBTQ-Related Terms

Ally: A person who supports and advocates for members of a community other than their own, reaching across differences to achieve mutual goals.

Bisexual: A person who is attracted to and may form emotional, romantic, and/or sexual relationships with both men and women, although not usually equally or simultaneously.

Cisgender: A person who conforms to gender and/or sex-based expectations of society (also referred to as gender normative).

Cisgenderism: Assuming that every person is cisgender, therefore marginalizing people who identify as transgender. Believing cisgender people are superior, holding people to traditional expectations based on gender, and/or excluding people who do not conform to traditional gender expectations.

Disorders/differences of sex development (DSD): Congenital conditions in which development of chromosomal, gonadal, or anatomic sexual organs is atypical.

Gay: A person whose primary sexual orientation is to members of the same sex. "Gay" can refer to men and women, although many gay women prefer the term "lesbian."

Gender-confirming surgeries: Surgical procedures by which a person's physical appearance and function of existing sexual characteristics are altered to resemble those of the sex to which they are transitioning.

Gender expression: The way in which a person expresses gender identity through clothing, behavior, posture, mannerisms, patterns of speech, activities, and more.

Gender identity: Internal and psychological sense of oneself as male, female, both, or neither.

Gender nonconforming: A person who does not conform to society's expectations of gender expression based on the gender binary or expectations of masculinity and femininity.

Heterosexual: A primary sexual orientation toward members of the other sex (also referred to as straight).

Heterosexism: The assumption that everyone is or should be heterosexual and that heterosexuality is inherently superior to and preferable to all other sexual orientations.

(*continued*)

EXHIBIT 10.1

Heterosexual privilege: Benefits derived automatically by being (or being perceived as) heterosexual that are denied to people who identify as having nonheterosexual orientations.

Homosexual: A primary sexual orientation toward members of the same sex or gender. As this term is historically associated with a medical model of homosexuality, most people prefer to self-identify as gay, lesbian, or queer.

Homophobia: The irrational fear or hatred of, aversion to, and discrimination against people who identify as gay, lesbian, or queer.

Internalized homophobia: The experience of guilt, shame, or self-hatred in reaction to one's feelings of attraction for a person of the same sex or gender as a result of societal homophobia and heterosexism.

Intersex: A condition in which sex-related chromosomes, gonads, or anatomy do not develop in a way that is typically male or female. "Intersex" is an umbrella term that includes many different conditions (e.g., disorders and/or differences of sex development).

Lesbian: A woman whose primary sexual orientation is to other women.

Nonbinary: A spectrum of gender identities that are not exclusively masculine or feminine. Nonbinary people may identify as being multigender, having no gender, moving between genders, or having a fluctuating/fluid gender identity, being third gender or other gender (genderqueer is an earlier term with a similar meaning to nonbinary).

Queer: In contemporary usage, "queer" is an inclusive, unifying, sociopolitical and self-affirming umbrella term encompassing a broad range of sexual and gender expression, including people who identify as gay, lesbian, bisexual, transgender, intersex, genderqueer, or any other nonheterosexual sexuality or nonconforming gender identity. "Queer" is a reclaimed term, which was previously seen as derogatory, but many people (though not all people) within the LGBTQ community are comfortable using this term to describe themselves.

Questioning: A self-identification sometimes used by people who are exploring their sexual orientation and/or gender identity.

Sexual orientation: An inherent or immutable enduring emotional, romantic, or sexual attraction to people of the same gender, different gender, or more than one gender.

Transgender or trans: Someone whose gender identity or expression differs from conventional expectations of masculinity or femininity. Often used as an umbrella term that includes people who identify as cross-dressers, transsexuals, two-spirit, intersex, and genderqueer.

Transition: A complicated, multistep process that can take years as transgender people align their anatomy and/or their gender expression with their gender identity.

Transphobia: Irrational fear or hatred of, aversion to, and discrimination against people who identify as transgender.

Two-spirit: A term used by some North American indigenous cultures to describe people in their communities whose nature is composed of both male and female spirits. People who identify as two-spirit may also identify as gay, lesbian, bisexual, transgender, or intersex or have multiple gender identities.

Source: Reproduced with permission from Veltman, A., & Chaimowitz, G. (2014). Mental health care for people who identify as lesbian, gay, bisexual, transgender, and (or) queer. *Canadian Journal of Psychiatry [Revue canadienne de psychiatrie]*, *59*(11), 1–8.

SEX AND GENDER IDENTITY

LGBTQIA+ youth often lack the systematic support of caring adults either by perceived or actual rejection, which leads these youth to suffer alone in silence. Understanding the historical and contemporary harmful, and sometimes deadly, relationships that exist between heteronormative society and the LGBTQIA+ community continues to be integral to clinicians gaining knowledge and strategies useful in working with LGBTQIA+ youth.

On average, LGBTQIA+ youth become aware of their same-sex attraction and gender identity during preteen adolescent years (Gay, Lesbian, and Straight Education Network, 2016a; Institute of Medicine [U.S.] Committee on Lesbian, Gay, Bisexual, and Transgender Health Issues and Research Gaps and Opportunities, 2011; Human Rights Campaign Foundation, 2018; Kosciw & Diaz, 2008; Kosciw et al., 2018; Mallon, 2017). While children and adolescents present with issues or concerns regarding their sexual development or gender identity, it continues to be critical not to assume that this is the only reason for seeking counseling services. Referrals for LGBTQIA+ children and adolescents often occur for reasons with little or nothing to do with sexual orientation and, if so, indirectly. Therefore, sexual orientation should only be considered as contextual information to aid the clinician in conceptualizing the client in order to provide effective counseling interventions. Critical selection of theoretical perspectives is imperative when conceptualizing LGBTQIA+ youth as many traditional theories "are concerned only with heterosexual development and presume heterosexual identity as an eventual outcome" (Mallon, 2017, p. 8).

Coming Out

The use of certain theories and models (e.g., Brofenbrenner's ecologic perspective of human development, a bidirectional model that may be unsupportive of sexual minority youth; Higa et al., 2014) and binary gender and affectional orientation models that do not recognize the fluidity of both gender and affectional orientation (Moe et al., 2017) may be not be appropriate in counseling this population. These models lend themselves to heteronormative human and sexual development, lead to insensitive and unhelpful conceptualization of LGBTQIA+ youth, can damage the therapeutic relationship, and contribute to the child or adolescent feeling alienated and alone. When conceptualizing LGBTQIA+ children and adolescents, counselors should pay special attention to understanding the youth's identity formation, also called the coming-out process, in which people who identify as LGBTQIA+ self-identify and share their sexual orientation or gender identity with others. Models such as the Genderbread Person Version 3.3 and 4.0 (Killermann, 2018; Moe et al., 2017) and the Integrative-Empower Model for Counselors Helping LGBTQIA+ Youth Through the Coming-Out Process (see Figure 10.1 on page 266; Matthews & Salazar, 2012) model constructs such as sex, gender identity, gender presentation, and affectional orientation on a continuum and sexual identity formation as fluid. The identity formation process can be complicated for LGBTQIA+ youth who come out during childhood or adolescence as these youth often navigate the integration of LGBTQIA+ identity development with other aspects of identity development in the context of social stigma and discrimination (Institute of Medicine [U.S.] Committee on Lesbian, Gay, Bisexual, and Transgender Health Issues and Research Gaps and Opportunities, 2011). The counselor must recognize and respect that the child or adolescent may not be ready to self-identify as LGBTQIA+ or "come out," as this denotes a process that can take many years of development and continue through adulthood. Clinicians must recognize that while the coming-out process may be conceptualized as a positive developmental step toward wellness and self-actualization, disclosing oneself may present more significant conflict on the individual, interpersonal, and social levels. Counselors should meet the child or adolescent at their identity level and utilize a positive strength-based approach. Counselors should also discuss safety precautions when counseling youth about the "coming-out" process. "Coming out" can pose safety risks at both home and school for LGBTQIA+ youth as "59.5% of LGBTQ students felt unsafe at school because of their sexual orientation, 44.6% because of their gender expression, and 35.0% because of their gender" (Kosciw et al., 2018, p. 14) and parental response to LGBTQIA+ youth may range from concerns about youth's safety and well-being to abuse and even banishment from the home (Katz-Wise et al., 2016; Linda, 2008). Safety precautions for both home and school need to be established prior to the youth "coming out." Possible precautions include but are not limited to the following: Establish a "safe space" or trust places and adults at school that the youth feels safe and accepted (e.g., a trusted teacher, counselor, or coach); discuss social media and texting security; and provide resources and establish a safety plan for home in the event that their parents are not accepting.

COUNSELING IMPLICATIONS FOR LESBIAN, GAY, BISEXUAL, AND TRANSGENDER CHILDREN AND ADOLESCENTS

In order to fully understand LGBTQIA+ youth, counselors should utilize a holistic and integrative model. The Integrative-Empower Model for Counselors Helping LGBTQIA+ Youth Through the Coming-Out Process (Figure 10.1) serves as a guide to counselors to provide ethical, culturally competent, empowerment and advocacy-oriented support to LGBTQIA+ youth. When shared with clients, the model helps them understand the stages of sexual identity formation; deal with internalized homophobia, self-esteem, and self-acceptance issues; work with the family; and gain awareness of their school and peer environment (Matthews & Salazar, 2012).

ETHNICALLY DIVERSE LGBTQIA+ CHILDREN AND ADOLESCENTS

Ethnically diverse LGBTQIA+ youth also contend with interconnecting systems of discrimination and oppression, such as racism, classism, and sexism, in addition to identifying as a sexual minority. The intersectionality of race and sexual identity can lead to problematic interactions with clinicians when the clinician "frames ethnically diverse LGBT clients within a Eurocentric, heterosexual paradigm that fails to incorporate their ethnocultural worldview or their sociopolitical realities" (Wynn & West-Olatunji, 2009, p. 199). Without accurate contextualization, clinicians risk inaccurate diagnoses and ineffective treatments. Combining culture-centered counseling with the Integrative-Empower Model may be effective in supporting ethnically diverse LGBTQIA+ youth. The integration of culture-centered counseling and the Integrative-Empower Model will ensure appropriate support, with culture being central to creating effective interventions that empower them.

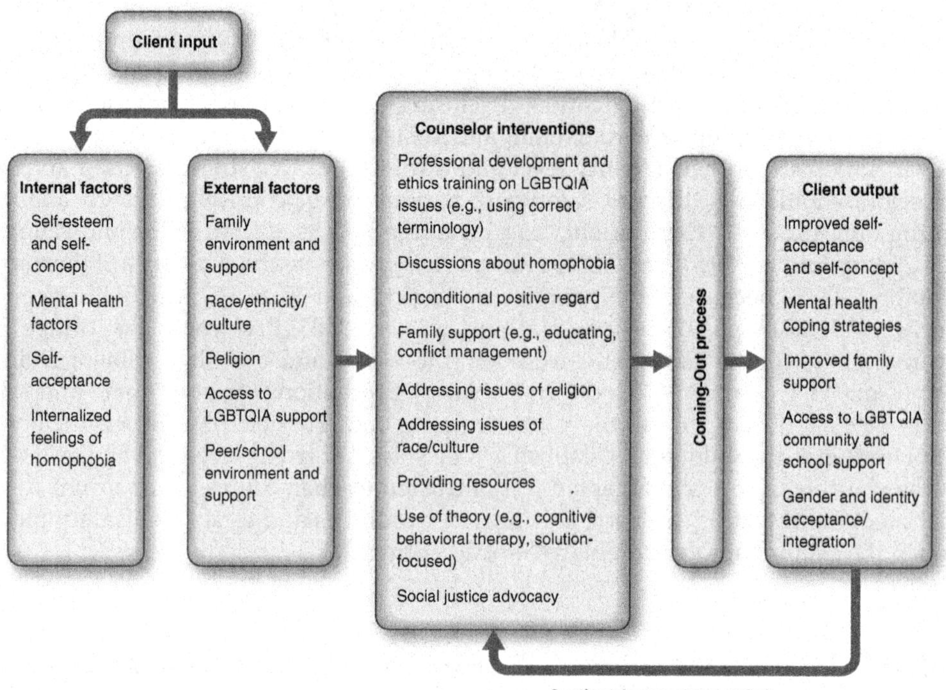

FIGURE 10.1 Counselor strategies and interventions: An Integrative-Empower Model for Counselors Helping LGBTQIA+ Youth Through the Coming-Out Process.

LGBTQIA+, lesbian, gay, bisexual, transgender, queer/questioning, intersex, and asexual.

Source: Matthews, C., & Salazar, C. (2012). An integrative-empower model for counselors helping LGBTQIA+ youth through the coming-out process. *Journal of LGBT Issues in Counseling*, *6*(2), 96–117. https://doi.org/10.1080/15538605.2012.678176. Copyright 2012 by Taylor & Francis.

CASE STUDY 10.2: COUNSELING LGBTQ YOUTH

Sonja, aged 17, enters counseling for anxiety and identifies confusion about her sexual orientation as a major factor. While Sonja reveals her long-standing attraction to men, she also shares that she is sometimes attracted to women. She perceives even considering such thoughts to be a betrayal to her parents, who live by their traditional Catholic Mexican values and beliefs. She continues to be confused about her true orientation. The counselor assures her she need not label herself one way or the other and explores with her, in a neutral, accepting manner, the nature of her attractions, her desires for the future in terms of relationships, and her emotions concerning family and spirituality. After several sessions, Sonja decides she could consider dating women someday and wants to come out to her family but remains fearful of her family's rejection. Her father and mother frequently made disbarring comments about "lesbians and homosexuals going to hell" and "homosexuality being an abomination."

Activity 10.2: Reflection Questions

1. What cultural considerations should be explored before working with Sonja toward coming out to her family?
2. What challenges could heterosexual counselors confront in working with Sonja?
3. What issues would Sonja need to explore regarding her sexual orientation?
4. What unique challenges does Sonja's Catholic upbringing create in the counseling process?

OTHER YOUTH SPECIAL POPULATIONS: CHILDREN AND ADOLESCENTS FROM TRANSIENT FAMILIES

Refugee, migrant, and homeless children and adolescents come from transient families. These children and adolescents encounter unique developmental, systemic, multicultural, and relational experiences that differ from their peers and lead to compounding social, emotional, developmental, and mental health issues. Counselors must understand these youth holistically with consideration for their unique transient experiences and use interventions that integrate multiple approaches, which allows for flexibility in counseling strategies.

REFUGEE CHILDREN AND ADOLESCENTS

Children and adolescents of refugee families often experience a flux of the meaning of home. These youth from families who chose their new country or left their home country because they were forced to do so seek safety, shelter, religious freedom, and freedom to improve their lives. They experience physical and psychological loss of home, which disrupts all systematic aspects of their lives.

Children and adolescent refugees from war-torn countries may experience or witness horrific conditions of violence and murder, causing them to flee with their family or flee alone. They may end up in an unknown country, where they do not speak the language. Besides traumatic experiences, refugee children and adolescents often begin school unsystematically, at different times of the year, and require additional support navigating the school system. Due to the separation of families and structural family changes, supporting refugee children and adolescents often includes supporting the familiar systemic structures in place.

When working with refugee families, counselors should offer community resources that provide basic needs such as food, housing, and language resources. Utilizing Maslow's hierarchy of needs provides efficacy when beginning work with refugee youth as lower-level requirements such as physical safety, food, and shelter needs should be addressed before focusing on higher-level needs such as self-concept and personal changes. The following case study provides an example of a middle school–age adolescent who recently escaped her war-torn country to seek asylum.

CASE STUDY 10.3: COUNSELING REFUGEE YOUTH

Maya, a 10-year-old (soon to be 11) Syrian refugee, came to live with her aunt and uncle in the United States after witnessing rising violence, which forced her family to leave their home. Maya arrived in the United States in 2019 at the age of 9, speaking little English. Since she entered the country with no academic records, the school decided to place her in the second grade. Although she encountered a language barrier, Maya performed well academically and felt unchallenged and bored in school. At home, she experienced trouble adjusting to living in the United States and life without her mother and father. As a result, Maya became increasingly withdrawn and refused to participate in school, causing her grades to drop and her relationship with her aunt and uncle to deteriorate.

Currently, the school has placed Maya in the third grade after she repeated the second grade. Her suicidal ideations and a lack of academic progress leading to another retention sparked a referral to counseling. Maya's aunt and uncle report that Maya routinely wakes up with nightmares and what Maya describes as "bad memories" of her life in Syria. Maya reports, "I hate life in the United States and would have rather died in Syria." She states that she hates school because all of the teachers perceive her to be stupid, and she struggles to make friends.

Maya's counselor begins conceptualizing Maya's needs by utilizing Maslow's hierarchy of needs. Her counselor recognized Maya's immediate need, to feel safe in her new environment followed by the need for belonging and acceptance in her new environment.

Activity 10.3: Reflection Questions

1. What plausible theories or strategies could you utilize to help Maya gain a sense of safety in her new environment?
2. What immediate concerns for Maya would need to be addressed promptly? How should they be addressed?
3. Given Maya's Syrian ethnicity, what potential ethical dilemmas might you encounter while working with Maya?
4. In what ways should you take into consideration Maya's systems (family, friends, religious institutions, schools, and other systemic entities) in your work with Maya?
5. What communication barriers might you experience with Maya, and how can they be resolved?

MIGRANT CHILDREN AND ADOLESCENTS

Two types of migrant families exist. The system characterizes migrant farmers first as families with one or more family members who work temporarily or seasonally in farm fields, orchards, canneries, plant nurseries, fish and seafood packing plants, and other seasonal agriculture jobs. The second includes American workers who work in construction, meatpacking, day laborers, and disaster response and cleanup (Migrant Clinicians

Network, 2014). These families, sometimes designated as immigrants of low socioeconomic status, lack access to healthcare and mental health services. While many children and adolescents from families of migrant farmworkers remain undocumented, some still cross the U.S. border unauthorized to work seasonally and later return to their home country. When working with refugee children, the immediate needs of food, shelter, and safety may need to be addressed before focusing on other social, emotional, and educational needs.

HOMELESS CHILDREN AND ADOLESCENTS

In this chapter, homeless children and adolescents represent youths who share the living space of other persons due to loss of housing, economic hardship, or a similar reason or live in transitional housing (e.g., shelter, car, or tent). These children and adolescents often face safety and physiological challenges such as lack of adequate nutrition, illness, access to health-related resources, and personal hygiene. Homeless children and adolescents often appear reluctant to disclose their homeless status for fear of being reported to Child Protective Services and embarrassment. Clinicians must become aware of any bias they may hold regarding homelessness and refrain from victim blaming or making assumptions about the parents or guardians. Counselors should consider the physical and safety needs of homeless youth and work collaboratively with the family system and social workers when needed. Professional school counselors will often learn of a youth's homeless status first and should be able to recognize the signs of homelessness such as poor and infrequent attendance, poor hygiene, unkempt or dirty clothes, poor academic performance, and lack of contact information for parents or guardians. Once identified, counselors should refer the student to McKinney–Vento services, which can help the family secure adequate transportation, clothes and food, and other resources as needed. The McKinney–Vento Homeless Assistance Act requires that state educational agencies provide all homeless youth with access to the same free, appropriate public education, including a public preschool education, as provided to other children and youths and revise and review barriers that may impede this access (McKinney–Vento Homeless Assistance Act, 2015).

COUNSELING IMPLICATIONS FOR TRANSIENT CHILDREN AND ADOLESCENTS

Counselors should first support transient children and adolescents by working collaboratively with social workers and providing resources and referrals to ensure that physical and safety needs continue to be met before focusing on emotional support. Since the emotional needs of transient children and adolescents will differ significantly, counselors should prepare a variety of counseling interventions, strategies, and theories. Counselors should also prepare for the possibility of language barriers and keep resources or referrals on hand.

As with other youth at risk, trust prevails as the prerequisite for successful counseling. Clinicians should seek parent or guardian approval before referring out for additional services, as outing some transient families (e.g., through college admission, scholarships, and financial aid pursuits) could present unforeseen repercussions such as deportation or loss of a job. Children and adolescents can experience low self-esteem and confidence due to their transient status and will need support in removing the stigma and minimizing the internalization of stereotypes that coincide with their circumstances. They may also be victims of bullying; therefore, counselors should pay special attention and encourage self-advocacy. Interventions should include strength-based strategies that build on the youth's resilience and cultural and social capital.

Multisensory strategies, such as using a coke bottle (Jacobs, 2012) to represent emotional pressure and exploding behaviors to demonstrate the effects of holding in emotions, as used in Ed Jacobs's Impact Therapy (Impact Therapy Associates, 2020), continue to be useful to aid counselor's work with youth who experience language and cultural barriers. Integration of Impact Therapy strategies and culturally responsive theories meets the unique needs of transient children and adolescents.

CHILDREN AND ADOLESCENTS OF MILITARY FAMILIES

Every school district in the nation serves at least one military family, as over 80% of military youths attend public schools (Military Child Education Coalition, 2014). One or more parents of a school-age child may be in the military, requiring many counselors and school staff members to become familiar with the unique nature and challenges of the military in order to maintain optimal student learning. Counselors should explore perceptions and experiences related to the military to become more aware of any biases or preconceptions and may use the following items to reflect on their own biases: (a) discuss your perceptions of war; (b) share your political beliefs regarding the military and war; and (c) discuss who in your family served in the military, and expand on your relationship with this person. Counselors who explore their own biases appear more likely to be reflective and understanding during the counseling process, thus leading to more impactful services for the youth (Hall, 2008).

MILITARY HIERARCHY

The military expects and requires personnel to follow a chain of command. Counselors should be aware of how rank impacts not only the family's income level but also the level of stress a family may be experiencing (Hall, 2008). Hall further indicates that military families of all branches live by a code of ethics that requires families to behave and look a certain way in public. Youths of military parents appear to be always expected to obey authority, be respectful, follow all rules, and not question authority. The military culture represents a unique quality that respects the concept of pride, strength, and a sense of maintaining emotional control. Being diagnosed with a mental illness represents a sign of weakness in the military culture. Counselors must recognize that youths of military families may not seek help in fear of looking weak or getting into trouble for sharing family business (Hall, 2008; Huebner, 2012). The profession recommends that clinicians refrain from using clinical terms and labels when working with children and adolescents and their families. Counselors must recognize the skills and inherent toughness of the adolescent and family. Reviewing the limits of confidentiality and what may or may not be shared with commanding officers remains vital in the therapeutic relationship.

MILITARY LANGUAGE

Since each military branch provides its own unique cultures and languages, and the military expects and requires personnel to follow a chain of command, clinicians should obtain a basic understanding of military culture. Counselors who understand the language of the branches will remove communication barriers and build relationships with the children, adolescents, and families they serve. Military personnel work in fast-paced modes and get their jobs done effectively and efficiently. Utilizing specific language, acronyms, and abbreviations remains crucial for military personnel and allows them to work in a more effective and efficient manner conducive to the fast-paced work they are accustomed to. This language becomes ingrained in the family and how they communicate. By learning the relevant lingo and military culture, clinicians remove barriers to the family (Waldron et al., 1985).

PROMOTING FAMILY RESILIENCY

Self-sufficiency and strength continue to be emphasized within the military culture; therefore, utilizing a strength-based approach to counseling remains critical. Strength-based approaches foster empowerment and promote a positive outlook for the family. When working with families, identifying goals rather than problems promotes a more positive outlook for the family. As part of reducing the stigma of mental health, home visit interventions made by an attendance officer have become increasingly popular. This intervention helps the family members address communication challenges as well as coping with isolation and loneliness during the deployment phase.

PREDEPLOYMENT

The time before the military sends a family member to a new location, often referred to as predeployment, presents a great opportunity for counselors to begin building relationships with families by offering parenting education and providing support. As discussed in Chapter 2, children of military members may experience numerous deployments or may be experiencing the stresses of deployment for the first time. Children and adolescents at different deployment stages present with different needs. The culture of military life may lead to children and adolescents appearing withdrawn and not willing to share information. They may experience sadness, emotional distress, anxiety, and worry as well as experience grief and loss. The counselor must build a relationship with the youth and the youth's family. Every branch develops their own mission and core values; counselors who understand these core values share a willingness to develop a multicultural lens and strategies to work with military families. Counselors who engage in military cultural competences become aware of student's behaviors and understand the values of each branch (Hall, 2008).

Military children and adolescents and their families experience many barriers during preemployment. By providing families with mental health resources and extra counseling support, clinicians can help alleviate barriers and assist families and children develop coping skills. Parent Cafecitos, such as coffee with the counselor and parent nights, serve as opportunities for families to connect. Emotional regulation and mindfulness can also be offered to parents during a parent Cafecito or during a parent night program. Checking in with the family periodically can help build connections and trust between the counselor and family (Warner et al., 2009). Small groups serve as a place for youths to connect, learn about each other, build community, and provide the counselor with an opportunity to learn the distinctive language of military culture. Counselors may also provide families with resources, facilitate parent meetings that allow opportunities for parents to connect as well as serve as an advocate for families.

Once the military family member deploys, the dynamics of the household change. Each family member will perform a new role resulting from the systemic family changes. Discussing and setting goals with parents or guardians around roles and expectations continue to be another strategy counselors can use to help educate on the importance of consistency during the time of deployment. Role-playing with the parent or guardian on their rules and expectations during deployment can be a useful technique (Lapp et al., 2010).

DEPLOYMENT

Deployments, the time away in the military, can last months or years. There are times when soldiers cannot contact their family members for weeks resulting in an increase in worry and anxiety within the family unit. During deployment, children or adolescents may believe they must "take care" of the household, and within the school setting, may want to be "in charge" in the classroom and risk coming across as "bossy" to other youths. They may become withdrawn, distant, and preoccupied with their parent's deployment. Teachers may see a drop in the child's or adolescent's grades and assume distraction and disengagement. Behavior and discipline problems may increase during deployment (Lapp et al., 2010).

School counselors can develop Youth Ambassador Programs to allow children and adolescents to use their leadership skills within the school community. Youth Ambassador Programs provide leadership opportunities as well as sharpen and develop communication, improve interpersonal and conversational skills, and help children feel part of the school community. Counselors who remain proactive and build relationships during the predeployment stages can begin to provide more intense services to the family, such as individual and small-group counseling.

POSTDEPLOYMENT

Postdeployment, the time when the deployed member returns, forces the family to learn and readjust to the change in the family structure and dynamics and reincorporate the returning family member. During this time, children gain a strong sense of independence. Children struggle with giving up this newfound independence. This may cause conflict among the parent and child, leading to further distress in the household. Counselors can continue to be of support to the family during this time by providing resources, continuing youth in a changing family small group, and helping the family to set expectations and normalize the challenges that they may encounter. According to Laser and Stephens (2011), approximately one-third of soldiers returning from deployment come home diagnosed with a posttraumatic stress disorder (PTSD). A diagnosis such as this could possibly lead to physical and emotional abuse of the youth and other forms of domestic violence within the home (Laser & Stephens, 2011). Consequently, counselors must use professional judgment regarding the need to refer a family out for more intense services.

CASE STUDY 10.4: WORKING WITH MILITARY YOUTH

This case study provides an example of a middle school adolescent whose father received orders to deploy to Japan for a minimum of 1 year.

Brandon's father ranks as a general in the Marine Corps. Brandon attended three middle schools over the past 2 years. Brandon typically gets straight As, continues to be a leader on campus, and remains polite and cooperative. Recently, Brandon's grades dropped; he gets distracted easily, and becomes defiant with his teachers on several occasions. Brandon's math teacher referred him to the counselor with concerns about his change in behavior. Brandon tells the counselor all about his father's upcoming deployment and his pride for his father. Brandon expresses that he will be "left in charge" while his dad continues to be deployed and that he "hates math," and "It is not how he learned to do math in his other middle school." When asked what happens when he takes a math test, Brandon states that he gets "pissed off" and throws things because he does not like to feel "dumb" in front of his classmates. Brandon states that he does not ask for help because he does not want his father to consider him to be dumb.

Activity 10.4: Reflection Questions

1. What theories and techniques can be utilized to explore Brandon's' feelings?
2. Given Brandon's family military status, what potential hidden factors may impede Brandon's academic, social, and emotional well-being?
3. How can the counselor work with the teacher and other stakeholders to address Brandon's math concerns?
4. What resources can be offered to the family?
5. What cultural factors affecting Brandon's well-being are related to his family's military lifestyle?

CHANGING FAMILIES

The American family changed drastically over the past 20 years. Many factors led to these changes, including institutionalized racism, socioeconomic factors, as well as many psychosocial factors. Society no longer consider many households to be traditional families (e.g., one that consists of a mother, father, and children). As mentioned in Chapter 2, changing families include grandparents raising grandchildren, incarcerated parents, same-sex parenting, divorced families, and single-mother or single-father families. The counselor plays the role of a caring, trusting adult who can help youths understand that they hold no fault or responsibilities for situations that present struggles for their families. More importantly, the counselor can assist the youth(s) in recognizing their strengths, learn coping strategies to help with emotions, as well as remind youths of the many ways to be a family. Small-group counseling can serve as an effective way to support youths. Participating in a small group provides the youths with a sense of community and normalizes these experiences. Counselors should not get lost in the differences in the type of family a youth comes from. They should, however, focus on the strengths and needs of the youth's family.

GRANDPARENTS RAISING GRANDCHILDREN

More than 10.5% of, or nearly 7.8 million, children under the age of 18 live with their grandparents or other relatives (AARP, 2017). Many factors may be associated with this increase, including incarceration, drug abuse, physical abuse, illness, and death. Extended family plays a major role in many minority families. Kindship care functions as a cultural strength of many minority families. Grandparents become the most common caregivers for children when needed, which causes some added stress to both the child and the grandparent(s). Traditionally grandparents do not serve as the disciplinarian to their grandchildren; this new role may cause adjustment concerns for both the child and the grandparent(s). Support groups for grandparents raising their grandchildren help provide support for the family as well as help to demonstrate the values, strengths, and resiliency that group members bring to the table. Despite the family circumstances, grandparents raising their grandchildren can reflect support and love for their family.

INCARCERATED PARENTS

Mumola (2000), estimates that nearly 3.6 million parents remain under some form of correctional supervision, including parole. Additionally, statistics show that these incarcerated parents bore approximately two million children. Due to the instability of the home, lack of resources, and lack of parent contact, youths may experience an increase in discipline problems, academic problems, and even substance use. Clinicians working with youths of incarcerated parents provide individual and small-group counseling services to meet their social and emotional needs (Mumola, 2000).

Counselors need to understand some of the experiences and emotions that youths may experience. Youths may feel a lack of connection and belonging, abandonment, anger, and grief and loss. A myriad of ways may be used to allow clients to tell their story, which also allows them to express their frustration and anger. Counselors work with youths from a nonjudgmental lens allowing for youth to tell their narrative. Narrative therapy functions as a counseling approach that focuses on the client as the expert. It allows the client to use their voice and tell their story.

Counselors should offer interventions and time for youths to express their emotions in a safe, nurturing environment. The use of play, art, music, and role-playing continue to be useful techniques. In addition to providing services to parents and youths, counselors also advocate for changes in legislation and social programs. Counselors should be aware of current legislative policies, resources, and programs available to assist youths and their families. Working with youths of incarcerated parents requires counselors to understand the incarceration process, to build nurturing and trusting relationships with youths and families as well as utilization of skills and techniques that assist the child in working with their feelings and emotions.

SAME-SEX PARENTS

As mentioned in Chapter 2, same-sex marriages are continuously increasing; many families are conceiving children both biologically or through adoption. Many same-sex couples endure rejection and discrimination not only from the public but often their own families. They often feel isolated or like outsiders to both social and family groups, causing another layer of stress within the partnership, leaving them feeling alone and lost. Many children of same-sex families also experience discrimination and biases, leaving them with the same feelings that their parents may encounter. They may feel a sense of embarrassment and shame, often just wanting to be "normal." Same-sex parents often worry about how their children will be treated in school (Gay, Lesbian and Straight Education Network, 2016b).

Professional school counselors support youths by learning and understanding the diverse structures of an LGBTQIA+ family. Many diverse dynamics of the LGBTQIA+ family system exist to include lesbian mothers who chose to become parents to a child by donor insemination or in vitro fertilization, gay dads who used a surrogate, a mother raising children from a previous marriage with her same-sex partner, or same-sex parents who serve as foster or adoptive parents to children previously in the child protective system. Although not a complete list of family systems, the Glossary of LGBTQ-Related Terms (Exhibit 10.1) serves to assist counselors in understanding the uniqueness of LGBTQIA+ families. Understanding the unique challenges faced by LGBTQIA+ families remains imperative for counselors to provide innovative and strength-based programs that enhance diverse school–family–community relationships (Fisher & Komosa-Hawkins, 2013).

Professional school counselors design classroom guidance lessons around inclusivity, empathy, and encourage conversations that increase acceptance on the school campus. Guidance lessons that teach LGBTQIA+ inclusivity and empathy can be obtained from resources such as the Gay, Lesbian, and Straight Education Network (GLSEN) and Welcoming Schools. The "What Makes a Family?" lesson helps K–2 students learn about diverse family structures (GLSEN, 2016b). These resources can be used to help youths recognize the many ways to define family. Bibliotherapy serves as a technique counselors utilize in individual counseling to assist youths in recognizing and validating the uniqueness of family structures. Professional school counselors can prompt children to draw a picture of their family and follow up with questions, including (a) What title would you give your drawing? (b) Name the members of your family; and (c) What makes your family special? Counselors may also provide families with resources outside of the counseling relationship. PFLAG, an organization that has been serving the LGBTQ+ community since 1972, provides services such as education, advocacy, and support. With over 200,000 plus members across all 50 states, in both large and small cities as well as rural areas, PFLAG advocates and assures that the wider community always hears the voice of the LGBTQ+ communities and makes it part of the conversation when it comes to policies and laws.

Group counseling can be another direct intervention for school counselors. Topics could include stress management, family diversity, and peer support. Group counseling connects youths from other LGBT families and may provide a safe space where youth can process their experiences, challenges, and resiliency with other children. At the end of the group, clinicians may invite parents in for an interactive activity and provide additional LGBTQIA+ family resources.

DIVORCE

The divorce rate in the United States continues to grow each year. According to the U.S. Census Bureau (2018b), 60% of marriages end in divorce. Millions of children continue to be affected by divorce. According to Seltzer (1994), children raised by divorced parents appear more likely to experience problems in school. However, how parents and children respond and react will determine the impact on the child. In other words, divorce does not always present a negative impact on youths. Counselors should not make assumptions about how youths cope with a divorce.

For youths who may need some support, group counseling is an effective approach. It allows counselors to provide services to several youths at a time. Small-group activities represent another way for counselors to help youths learn and express their emotions in a safe space. The group also allows for youth to learn from one another and build community. The counselor facilitates the group by asking open-ended questions that help the group reach impact. Group work with changing families addresses the youth's concerns in a safe, supportive place. Children and adolescents share and exchange ideas and develop an increase in self-awareness and self-esteem. When youths feel connected and understood, they tend to thrive and lead to more positive decision-making. Groups allow for a normalizing experience and peer support with a nurturing and caring counselor.

SUPPORTING CHILDREN AND ADOLESCENTS OF SPECIAL POPULATIONS DURING A NATIONAL OR GLOBAL CRISIS

A national or global crisis, such as the coronavirus disease 2019 (COVID-19) pandemic, can be challenging for all children and adolescents, but may be especially taxing on youth from special populations. The special populations of youth previously mentioned experience preexisting challenges complicated by effects of COVID-19, for example. This pandemic brought about massive school and business closures, layoffs, and furloughs, along with sick and dying family members. This section of the chapter discusses the unique challenges that global and national crises, such as the COVID-19 pandemic, can create and how counselors can support them.

SCHOOL CLOSURES

In the event of large-scale school closures, children and adolescents who depend on schools for food, safety, and support may begin to lack basic needs. Many families receive free or reduced school breakfast and lunch, which helps offset the costs of having to supply food while in school. With schools being closed, youth from these families may no longer be able to access free school breakfast and lunch. The difficult transition from face-to-face to full distance learning can present significant challenges that impede their success, such as having a working computer and internet access or being technologically literate. Families may experience language barriers, as in the case with ELLs. If the parent or guardian works outside of the home, some youth may be responsible for caring for younger siblings and maintaining the home in the adult's absence, leaving little time and support for academics. Although some children may live in a home with an adult, the adult may be working full time, and unavailable for parenting duties. In other cases, the adult may be mentally or emotionally unavailable due to personal struggles caused by the crisis. For many youths, schools represent not just a place they go to learn. For many children and adolescents of special populations, school may be the only source of structure and consistency in their ever-changing lives. In some cases, schools provide a place of physical and emotional safety.

FINANCIAL HARDSHIP AND SAFETY

When businesses feel compelled to close during crises, the family members of children and adolescents may be laid off, furloughed, or otherwise left without livable income. Many of these families already face financial hardship or poverty, therefore creating the additional pressures of unstable income, which increases stress. Those who remain employed do so with increased risks to their personal and to their family's health and safety. For example, during the COVID-19 pandemic, "essential" businesses such as fast-food restaurants and food distribution centers remained open and required employees to continue working despite the significant health risks. According to the U.S. Census Bureau (2018a), over 300 thousand Americans live without health insurance and included many considered to be "essential" workers during the COVID-19 pandemic. "Essential" uninsured workers may be more likely to suffer from preexisting health conditions, increasing their vulnerability. If these workers become sick, many would lose access to or become unable to afford proper treatment. Financial hardship and fear for health and safety may result in some children and adolescents facing abrupt moves with or without their family. The youth of military families may cope with abrupt deployments or assignment to a temporary duty travel (TDY) of the military member, causing compounded fear and concern for health and safety. Unstable finances, poverty, lack of income, and fear for health and safety create additional stressors for children and adolescents from special populations, increasing mental health concerns such as anxiety and depression.

COUNSELING IMPLICATIONS FOR SUPPORTING YOUTH DURING A NATIONAL OR GLOBAL CRISIS

Amid a national or global crisis, counselors should support youth of special populations by first assessing deficits in the child's basic needs and work collaboratively with case managers and social workers in meeting their unique needs. As with other special populations, this may involve supporting the family as well. Families may require resources not previously needed, such as food banks, unemployment, or government assistance contact information. Since counselors may be the only resource the child or adolescent's family can access, they should update themselves on the most accurate information and resources available including work with case managers and social workers. Professional school counselors should work with their district and campus administrators to devise a plan to meet the academic, social, and emotional needs of students from these special populations. Plans may include loaning Chromebooks or laptops to families, providing paper packets for families unable to access online learning, and offering counseling services through online avenues or handouts for strategies to manage stress and anxiety. During these times, it continues to be important for counselors to be creative in the ways they meet the needs of and communicate with families. It becomes even more imperative during a pandemic to keep the lines of communication with families open. Professional school counselors can utilize school-based software such as Schoology or Google Classroom to create an online space or classroom to connect with students. The classroom can include confidential mental health check-ins, guidance lessons that focus on self-care and stress management, mindfulness techniques, and mental health and parenting resources. As a result of the social isolation that occurs when school remains inaccessible, children and adolescents may experience depression or anxiety and lack the motivation to complete academic work. Because of this, professional school counselors should be advocates intervening with school administration when necessary and aiding the child or adolescent in coping skills. Community clinicians and professional school counselors alike should offer multiple options to receive mental health services, including but not limited to video sessions, phone sessions, and in-person options as permitted. Counseling interventions should focus on providing healthy coping skills and working through emotions stemming from the crisis. The effects of global or national crises exacerbate many systemic problems that children and adolescents of special populations face, causing parents or guardians to experience heightened levels of stress and anxiety. With this in mind, counselors must remain vigilant of mental health concerns in youth and their parents, child abuse, neglect, or domestic violence. During a global or national crisis, counselors must review ethical standards for counseling in various settings. They should also consider that the living arrangement of the child or adolescent may not be conducive to receiving counseling services.

CHAPTER SUMMARY

Counselors serve an important role in the lives of youth. They provide safe spaces for children to express their emotions, fears, thoughts, and worries. With our ever-changing world, counselors should be prepared to work with diverse populations in ways that provide them with a sense of self and belonging. Supporting children and adolescents of special populations and marginalized statuses requires that counselors (a) recognize how personal bias may impact the counseling process; (b) utilize culturally competent, theory-based techniques in counseling; (c) understand how socioeconomic status, poverty, race, gender, and sexual orientation impact children and adolescents; and (d) utilize practical, strength-based approaches to counseling. Counselors remain committed to the work of building strength-based, culturally competent, and inclusive practices. The counselor's efforts to provide culturally responsive strategies and interventions will greatly influence the success of counseling diverse populations of children and adolescents. With this in mind, clinicians must remain critically reflective of their worldviews and biases and commit to the lifelong process of cultural competence.

POINTS TO REMEMBER

- Recognize unique cultural, dialectical, language, and other diversities that could lead to clinician mismatch.
- Refrain from victim-blaming.
- Build on and acknowledge strengths.
- Recognize that client failure or reluctance to disclose information during counseling may not be a result of resistance or being uninterested in getting help, but cultural training.
- Aid children and adolescents in the development of self-identity and converging cultural norms with acculturation.
- Incorporate concrete multisensory approaches to counseling.
- Identify hidden factors and integrate them into counseling interventions.

- Develop culturally responsive, strength-based intervention strategies.
- Recognize and acknowledge biases and their impact on the provision of counseling services.
- Support of children and adolescents often involves supporting their families. Be prepared to provide additional community resources as needed.
- Address the basic needs of children, adolescents, and their families as the first priority during global and national crises.
- Recognize that counseling in the wake of global and national crises can continue via creative and innovative means.
- Review ethical and legal standards when counseling in various settings.

OTHER HELPFUL INFORMATION FOR CONSIDERATION

- Impact Therapy: Creative Counseling Techniques: http://impacttherapy.com/PDF/ImpTherapyFullset.pdf
- Dulwich Centre (https://dulwichcentre.com.au/): Established by Michael White and David Epston, the Dulwich Centre provides information, workshops, and trainings.
- Malchiodi, C. (2015). *Creative interventions with traumatized children* (2nd ed.). Guilford.
- Testa, R. J., Coolhart, D., & Peta, J. (2015). *The gender quest workbook: A guide for teens and young adults exploring gender identity*. New Harbinger. https://timetothrivetherapy.com/wp-content/uploads/2018/01/Gender-Quest-Workbook.pdf
- Working Effectively With Military Families: 10 Key Concepts All Providers Should Know: https://www.nctsn.org/resources/working-effectively-military-families-10-key-concepts-all-providers-should-know
- The National Child Traumatic Stress Network: www.NCTSN.org
- The National Resource Center for Healthy Marriage and Families. (2013). A support and resource guide for working with military families: https://www.acf.hhs.gov/sites/default/files/ofa/msp.pdf
- Killermann, S. (2018). The Genderbread Person v4. It's Pronounced Metrosexual: https://www.itspronouncedmetrosexual.com/2018/10/the-genderbread-person-v4

QUESTIONS FOR FURTHER DISCUSSION

- What information should counselors be aware of when working with military families?
- How do counselors go about identifying hidden factors that may affect youth at risk?
- What considerations should counselors bear in mind when planning individual, group, and family counseling for youth at risk?
- How do the counseling needs of children and adolescents differ across cultures?

- What experiences in your life helped you gain awareness of your cultural identity? Reflect on how your cultural identity can create biases that negatively impact the therapeutic relationship.
- What challenges confront counselors of LGBTQIA+ children and adolescents?
- How can counselors affirm the social capital of immigrant, refugee, and transnational children and adolescents?
- Discuss the importance of counselors coordinating a variety of community resources for counseling children and adolescents of special populations. What resources should counselors make readily available?
- What approaches and strategies can community clinicians use to meet the needs of youth from special populations during a global or national crisis?

KEY REFERENCES

Only key references appear in the print edition. The full reference list appears in the digital product on Springer Publishing Connect: connect.springerpub.com/content/book/978-0-8261-4764-6/part/part03/chapter/ch10

Baruth, L. G., & Manning, M. L. (1992). Understanding and counseling Hispanic American children. *Elementary School Guidance & Counseling, 27*(2), 113–122.

Baruth, L. G., & Manning, M. L. (2016). *Multicultural counseling and psychotherapy: A lifespan approach* (pp. 1–364). https://doi.org/10.4324/9781315659961

Capuzzi, D., & Gross, D. (2014). *Youth at risk: A prevention resource for counselors, teachers, and parents*. American Counseling Association. https://ebookcentral-proquest-com.libweb.lib.utsa.edu/lib/utsa/detail.action?docID=1866802#

Gay, Lesbian, and Straight Education Network. (2016b). *Ready, set, respect! GLSEN's elementary school toolkit*. https://www.glsen.org/sites/default/files/GLSEN%20Ready%20Set%20Respect.pdf

Hall, L. K. (2008). *Counseling military families: What mental health professionals need to know*. Routledge.

Impact Therapy Associates. (2020). Impact therapy: Putting theories into practice. http://impacttherapy.com/PDF/TheoriesIntoPracticeHandouts-2.pdf

Laser, J. A., & Stephens, P. (2011). Working with military families through deployment and beyond. *Clinical Social Work Journal, 39*(1), 28–38. https://doi.org/10.1007/s10615-010-0310-5

Luby, C. D. (2012). Promoting military cultural awareness in an off-post community of behavioral health and social support service providers. *Advances in Social Work, 13*, 67–82.

U.S. Census Bureau. (2018a). People in poverty by selected characteristics: 2017 and 2018. https://www.census.gov/content/dam/Census/library/visualizations/2019/demo/p60-266/Figure8.pdf

PART IV

Clinical Applications for Working With Minors

CHAPTER 11

Child and Adolescent Maltreatment

Jane M. Webber and Carol M. Smith

LEARNING OBJECTIVES

After completing this chapter, the reader should be able to:

- Identify procedures for mandated reporting to Child Protective Services.
- Describe signs and symptoms for child abuse and neglect.
- Explain counseling strategies for abused children and adolescents.

CACREP STANDARDS FOR THIS CHAPTER

- CACREP 2016: 2.F.1.b., i.; 2.F.3.g.; 2.F.5.h.; 2.F.7.d.; School Counseling, 5.G.2.g., 5.G.2.n.; 5.G.3.f.; Clinical Mental Health Counseling, 5.C.2.i., l.
- CACREP 2009: School Counseling, III.A.2.; B.1.; C.3., C.6.; G.1.; Clinical Mental Health Counseling, III.A.2., 9.; E.3.

INTRODUCTION

Every child's rights include good health, learning, and a family free of violence and abuse. Yet child maltreatment occurs in all cultures and societies and across socioeconomic levels. Child abuse and neglect, as mentioned in Chapter 1, damage the development of children, who also suffer serious physical and mental health problems later in life. Even with anonymous reporting and immunity, mandated reporting of child abuse remains a daunting responsibility for counselors (Kenny et al., 2018). Prevention and early intervention reduce the incidence of child abuse and neglect, and integrated counseling interventions, grounded in play therapy and family therapy, show treatment efficacy. Family support remains the most significant single factor in the abused child's recovery from trauma, and psychoeducational programs strengthen parent–child relationships, promote positive discipline, and connect families with community support (National Scientific Council on the Developing Child, 2015).

ADVERSE CHILDHOOD EXPERIENCES

As mentioned in Chapter 2, adverse childhood experiences (ACEs) dramatically changed our knowledge of immediate- and long-term negative effects of maltreatment and transformed the way counselors and mental health professionals viewed the impact of maltreatment on children's development. Adults with traumatic childhood experiences endured subsequent health risks, chronic illnesses, and mental health problems. Pregnancy, sexually transmitted diseases, fractures, smoking, substance abuse, and suicide ideation occurred at substantially higher rates and more frequently in teens with higher ACE scores (Felitti et al., 1998). ACEs in the home and family include parent separation or divorce, an incarcerated parent or one with mental illness or substance abuse, and a child witnessing domestic violence. About 67% of adults reported at least one ACE, and 12.5% reported four or more (Felitti et al., 1998). Adults with six or more ACEs appear to be 4.5 times more likely to experience depression; those with four ACEs evidence 11 times the use of intravenous substance abuse, 3 times more smoking-related lung disease, and 14 times the number of suicides than adults with no ACEs (Felitti et al., 1998).

CHILD ABUSE AND NEGLECT

In the United States, the confirmed abuse or neglect of a child occurs every 47 seconds (Children's Defense Fund, 2018). Each day, four children die by abuse or neglect, and violence injures or kills a child or teen every 32 minutes (Children's Defense Fund, 2018). One in four adults experience physical abuse during childhood, and each year, one in 20 children experience physical abuse before the age of 18 (World Health Organization [WHO], 2020). One in 5 girls and 1 in 13 boys worldwide experience sexual abuse before they reach the age of 18 (WHO, 2020).

The most heinous crime against children may be sexual betrayal by a trusted adult. Perpetrators of abuse come from all socioeconomic levels, and a child's parent or guardian appears to be responsible for more than nine tenths of children's deaths from abuse or neglect (Child Welfare Information Gateway, 2019a). The most vulnerable victims include infants and young children who remain at highest risk because of their relative invisibility at home and dependence on caregivers.

The Convention on the Rights of the Child (United Nations [UN], Human Rights Office of the High Commissioner, 1989), the most widely adopted international convention, binds countries globally to use all measures to address child maltreatment so that "the child is protected against all forms of discrimination and punishment" (Article 2.2). To date, the United States stands only as a signatory of the Convention and not a party to its duties.

FORMS OF CHILD ABUSE

In the United States, the federal Child Abuse Prevention and Treatment Act (CAPTA, 1974), the Reauthorization Act of 2010, and succeeding amendments provide funding and support to states and a national clearinghouse for information. CAPTA (2010) set the federal definition of maltreatment as follows:

> Any recent act or failure to act on the part of a parent or caretaker which results in death, serious physical or emotional or harm, sexual abuse or exploitation, or an act or failure to act, which presents an imminent risk of serious harm. (p. 102)

An important CAPTA amendment in 2015 incorporates the inclusion of sexual exploitation and trafficking. In 2018, CAPTA expanded immunity from civil and criminal liability for good faith reporting of child abuse and neglect (Child Welfare Information Gateway, 2019b).

Child maltreatment includes four categories: physical abuse, sexual abuse, psychological abuse, and neglect. Incidents can be intentional or unintentional acts; fatal or nonfatal; singular, chronic, or long term; or of commission or omission. The *International Classification of Diseases*, Tenth Revision, Procedure Coding System (*ICD-10-PCS*; American Medical Association, 2020) lists neglect, abandonment, or negligent treatment; sexual abuse, physical, and emotional mistreatment and abuse; exploitation; and other maltreatment syndromes. The *Diagnostic and Statistical Manual of Mental Disorders*, Fifth Edition (*DSM-5*; American Psychiatric Association [APA], 2013) cites child maltreatment and neglect problems as "Other Conditions That May Be a Focus of Clinical Attention" and added psychological abuse in 2013 (APA, 2013).

Physical Abuse

Physical abuse continues to be the most frequent type of abuse (17.6%), including paddling, hitting, burning, shaking, throwing, choking, slapping, and kicking with the intent of hurting or threatening to hurt the child (Estroff et al., 2015). Most physical abuse appears to be nonaccidental, inflicted with the intent to discipline or punish, such as spanking or hitting with a belt, strap, or yardstick, which results in injuries, bruises, fractures, or welts. However, spanking for discipline without intentional physical injury may not automatically be considered abuse (Kenny et al., 2018). The American Professional Society on the Abuse of Children (APSAC, 2018) advocates for the "elimination of all forms of corporal punishment and physical discipline of children in all environments including in schools and at home" (p. 1). Yet, 19 states still permit spanking or paddling of children, although Head Start programs, juvenile detention centers, and military training facilities prohibit corporal punishment (Caron, 2018).

Psychological Abuse

Psychological or emotional abuse damages children and deeply affects the quality of the relationship and attachment between the child and parent or caregiver. Children typically experience psychological abuse concurrently with physical or sexual abuse or neglect. The *DSM-5* describes psychological abuse as "nonaccidental verbal or symbolic acts by a child's parent or caregiver that result, or indicate reasonable potential to result, in significant psychological harm to the child" (APA, 2013, p. 719). The APSAC defined psychological maltreatment as "a repeated pattern of caregiver behavior or extreme incident(s) that convey to children that they are worthless, flawed, unloved, unwanted, endangered, or only of value in meetings another's needs" (APSAC, 1995, p. 2). APSAC guidelines group psychological maltreatments into (a) spurning; (b) terrorizing; (c), isolating; (d) exploiting/corrupting; (e) denying emotional responsiveness; and (f) mental health, medical, and educational neglect. Examples include nonphysical threats or ridicule, such as constant criticizing, humiliating, bullying, restricting, belittling, name-calling, harassing, scaring, scapegoating, or acts of discrimination. Psychological abuse also includes children's experiences of confinement, restriction, or isolation from others; threats of harm or abandonment; or witnessing domestic violence or criminal activity (Hart et al., 2018). As parents or caregivers inflict most abuse and neglect, helping parents change their behavior, parenting, and discipline reduces child maltreatment. Teaching parents and caregivers how to listen and respond to their children provides practical ways to reduce the potential for psychological abuse.

Both adults and teenagers embed emotional and psychological abuse in cyberbullying, sexual harassment, and sexting, which resulted in children running away or attempting suicide. The Netflix series *13 Reasons Why,* based on the novel, chronicled the experiences leading up to the suicide of a high school student and evoked strong concerns among educators and counselors about the graphic presentation of sexual assaults, rape, bullying, and suicide (Yorke, 2017). In a study of high school students in four areas of the world, nearly 80% of the students reported the series accurately reflected high school life and helped them understand victims' problems (Northwestern School of Communication, Center on Media and Human Development, 2018).

Sexual Abuse

Sexual abuse remains the most abhorrent violation, where an older and more powerful person deliberately uses "force, coercion, or manipulation" with a younger and less powerful child for their own sexual gratification, a victimization that may continue through the child's development (Conte & Vaughan-Eden, 2018, p. 144). Female teens and children experience more sexual abuse than males, and the frequency of sexual abuse increases with the age of the child (Finkelhor, 2012; WHO, 2020). Many incidents of abuse and neglect occur in homes cloaked in secrecy, fear, and guilt so that no one reports these events to Child Protective Services (CPS). Young victims of sexual abuse cannot developmentally understand the physical and psychological trauma and violation of trust committed by a caregiver even if the child gave consent.

Perpetrators of child maltreatment, especially sexual abuse, most often include parents or family members whom the victim loves and may not want to betray. Nearly all (90%) sexual perpetrators know their victims, and the majority of offenders sexually abuse children in their own family or extended family (Finkelhor, 2012; Whealin & Barnette, 2007). Abusers can be other persons of responsibility or authority, including teachers, coaches, clergy, police, physicians, caregivers, and healthcare workers, and can also be friends, acquaintances, strangers, or other children. Sexual predators use the internet to entice minors into meeting "in real life" by posing as adolescents or trusted, sympathetic friends.

Neglect

Failure to provide for a child's physical and psychological well-being, health, safe living, nutrition, and education denotes neglect whether intentionally, recklessly, or with disregard, including withholding love and affection, or by being unavailable (Erickson et al., 2018). Maltreatment by neglect includes placing a child in serious risk of imminent harm because of poor care, lack of supervision, or caregiver's use of drugs or alcohol. Neglect also represents abuse by omission by failing to consider, provide for, or respond to a child's emotional, physical, social, or psychological needs (Erickson et al., 2018). The Children's Bureau identified neglect (78.3%) as the most frequent category of maltreatment (U.S. Department of Health and Human Services, Children's Bureau, 2019a).

Most countries agree on what constitutes child sexual maltreatment (Fontes, 2018). However, since many view countries as individually autonomous, there can be less agreement with other countries to define child neglect or physical abuse in areas such as discipline for misbehavior, child rearing, lack of adult supervision, household responsibilities, child labor, and the care of younger children at home.

IMPACT OF CHILD ABUSE ON DEVELOPMENT

Children become "victims of violations of human connection" (Herman, 2015, p. 54). For an abused child, normalcy represents life in an unsafe world, a world in which people, including family members, likely betray one another and act in hurtful and unpredictable ways. Abused children do not experience healthy attachments during developmentally sensitive periods, and normal development and attachment remain blocked (Siegel, 2015). In therapy, sexually abused children experience feelings of anxiety, shame, or fear of betrayal with their counselor. Abused children appear literally "scared speechless," unable to use their words or feelings to help them escape from the abuser. Van der Kolk (2005) and others proposed that "developmental trauma" represents a new *DSM* diagnosis for children suffering from complex trauma.

Complex trauma or repeated sexual abuse shatters children's natural sense of safety and attachment to a caregiver (Kinsler et al., 2009; van der Kolk, 2005). Youth abused at an early age may demonstrate no internalized feeling or concept of safety (Schore, 2013). Their home or the homes of relatives may not be safe places. Following repeated abuse, many victimized children do not maintain a sense of the extreme abusiveness or abnormality of their situation. They seem surprised to learn that this behavior does not happen to all children in all families.

Children who experience horrific abuse will frequently "play it out or act it out" (Terr, 1994). Counselors should be alert to children in repetitive posttraumatic play, where they enact the same play behaviors over and over. Such posttraumatic play does not heal, and the child may be stuck repeating the traumatic experience without a therapeutic intervention. Posttraumatic play represents a symptom of complex trauma requiring a measured response through trauma-informed therapy.

PROTECTIVE FACTORS

As mentioned in Chapter 1, successful prevention and intervention programs focus on *protective factors* that include family functioning and resilience, social support, concrete supports, nurturing and attachment, and the caregiver and practitioner relationship (Friends National Center for Community-Based Child Abuse Prevention, 2018a, 2018b). Protective factors go hand in hand with caregiver *protective capacities* (U.S. Department of Health and Human Services, Children's Bureau, 2019b). Protective factors buffer and safeguard parents at risk with coping skills, authoritative and caring parenting, positive discipline, and social support to prevent abuse. While protective factors enhance child and family development and well-being, caregiver protective capacities comprise individual qualities of parents and caregivers that promote child safety and prevent maltreatment and harm. With the development of protective capacities, parents gain knowledge of child development to recognize signs of maltreatment and empower themselves to stop child abuse and utilize community resources. Family support remains essential to the child's treatment, and counselors cannot effectively do child therapy without parent therapy (Cohen et al., 2006).

FACTORS AFFECTING MALTREATMENT

Child maltreatment varies by age, gender, severity, situation, community, relationships with intimate partners and whether other forms of violence remain present in the child's environment. Younger children more likely suffer from neglect, and children with disabilities appear more vulnerable to physical victimization (Finkelhor, 2012). Parents with an authoritarian parenting style or who use harsh or punitive discipline appear to be more likely to hurt or physically abuse their children (WHO, 2020). The parents' or caregivers' lack of knowledge of normal child development and behavioral milestones may be associated with unrealistic and rigid expectations of their children's behavior and increased use of corporal punishment. Higher rates of child maltreatment occur in homes with substance or alcohol abuse, depression, attempted suicide, or domestic violence. These variables tend to increase isolation from the outside world and prevent or discourage access to community support and resources.

Unfortunate events or circumstances that affect families and day-to-day stressors appear related to higher rates and increased severity of neglect. These stressors include providing food, shelter, or childcare; loss of employment; illness; emotional and marital distress and conflict; or child misbehavior (Knapp et al., 2019; WHO, 2020). Unemployment, illness, and a lack of financial resources may pressure parents into working multiple shifts without adequate childcare or leaving young children to take care of each other, sometimes with tragic consequences (Knapp et al., 2019).

IMPACT OF DISASTERS AND PANDEMICS

In the aftermath of a disaster or pandemic (e.g., tornado, hurricane, school shooting, coronavirus disease 2019 [COVID-19]), families struggle to cope with loss, devastation, and emotional distress. With the rapid spread of the COVID-19 pandemic, "new methods of delivering disaster first aid and general social support to victims and survivors will be needed. . . . People will need help in other ways as social distancing, isolation, quarantine, and travel restrictions occur" (Mascari & Webber, 2010). Parents may experience confusion, fear, and shock and react in neglectful or harmful ways to their children as they try to manage throughout the day. Families at home many react with frustration and constant fear of infection. Tempers quickly flare up, leading to rigid discipline and physical punishment as maladaptive ways of coping in closed-in spaces. Loss of jobs, income, and day care;

lack of access to basic needs; closed schools; and separation from relatives and friends, especially those in hospitals, contribute to extreme distress and anxiety. Youngsters remain home without a way to escape their abusers. Infected parents in self-quarantine remain emotionally and physically unavailable to their children. For example, in a 19th-floor apartment building, a mother and child both sick with COVID-19 self-quarantined in one room while two children fended for themselves after their grandmother had died in the hospital.

SIGNS AND SYMPTOMS OF MALTREATMENT

New counselors may struggle with recognizing signs of maltreatment. Experienced counselors report more confidence-recognizing symptoms, especially overt signs of physical abuse, than new counselors (Tuttle et al., 2019). Signs of emotional or sexual abuse may be less visible than bruises or welts from physical abuse (Table 11.1). Knowing one's counselees and seeing them often provide a baseline for counselors to notice changing behaviors. In addition to physical signs, such as a black eye or abrasion, common signs of abuse include bedwetting and excessive crying. Signs also may overlap in different types of abuse, and verbal or nonverbal psychological abuse continues to be an integral part of most physical and sexual abuse (APSAC, 2018).

Adolescents may suddenly change their clothing, hair color, or style. They also change behaviors, cut class or run away, engage in risky behaviors, or become rebellious or distant. Children may stop paying attention or doing their homework or respond inappropriately to teacher's questions. Children and teens may avoid friends and common social places like the school bus or lunchroom or quit sports teams and clubs. Younger children often seek excessive attention and affection from significant adults; observing parent and child behaviors when together during school arrival and departure can illuminate potential relationship problems. For example, does the parent criticize, belittle, or blame the child for little or no reason? Does the parent threaten to smack the child for slight misbehaviors? Does there appear to be excessive conflict or tension between them? Does the child appear to be afraid of the parent or caregiver? Does the parent ignore the child around other people?

WHEN CHILDREN DISCLOSE ABUSE

Mental health and medical professionals need to remain calm and supportive of children or teenagers who disclose abuse. Counselors should assess the environment and find a safe, confidential space away from other children and adults, suggesting a move to a more discrete location before speaking by saying, for example, "Let's walk to my office and talk there." Respect and privacy remain critically important when observing injuries or bruises. The school nurse typically remains the designated school professional to examine a child's injuries, and asking for the child's consent for the nurse to observe, especially in private areas of their body, affirms respect for the child.

Fearing a rupture in the therapeutic relationship, a counselor might inappropriately assure the child that "everything we say is confidential" or "I promise to keep a secret," which complicates reporting sexual abuse. When confidentiality must be breached, a teenager may angrily say, "You told me you were not going to tell anyone. You lied, and I'm never talking to you again!" Explaining confidentiality clearly to a distressed and

TABLE 11.1 SIGNS OF CHILD MALTREATMENT BY TYPE

Physical Abuse	Sexual Abuse	Psychological Abuse	Neglect
Bruises	Torn or bloody underwear	Passive or compliant behavior	Excessive crying or crying when other children cry
Abrasions	Cuts, abrasions, or itching on or around genital area	Aggressive, rebellious, destructive, or risky behavior	Unusual moodiness
Bedwetting	Bedwetting	Bedwetting	Inappropriate dress or clothing for seasonal weather
Excessive crying	Venereal disease	Rocking	Change in hygiene or poor hygiene
Complaints of soreness	Frequent trips to the bathroom	Sucking	Lack of supervision
Worried when others cry or are hurt	Touching others inappropriately	Biting	Taking or hiding food
Unexplained bruises or welts on face, hands, neck, buttocks, or back	Using inappropriate sexual terms	Inappropriate adult or infant behavior	Reluctance to leave school or rushing to leave school
Unexplained cigarette or rope burns, or burn marks from an electric cord or iron	Walking or sitting with visible difficulty and discomfort	Seeking excessive attention and affection from significant adults	Clinging to or studiously avoiding trusted adults
Abrasions or cuts on lips, face, or gums	Changed behavior	Quitting sports teams or clubs	Separating and isolating oneself from friends
Appearing afraid of parent or caregiver	Appearing afraid of parent or caregiver	Running away	Increased school absences or tardies
Wounds in different stages of healing	Touching their private areas	Avoiding friends or common places like bus or lunchroom	Changes in eating or sleeping or consistent hunger
Wounds or bruises that appear after a weekend, holiday, or vacation	Rebellious, withdrawn, or distant behavior	Rebellious, withdrawn, or distant behavior	Skipping school study hall or extracurricular activities

(*continued*)

TABLE 11.1 SIGNS OF CHILD MALTREATMENT BY TYPE (*CONTINUED*)

Physical Abuse	Sexual Abuse	Psychological Abuse	Neglect
Talking about abuse or being abused	Engaging in risky behaviors	Unusual fears	Frequent visits to the nurse without reason
Reluctance to change clothes for or participate in gym class	Unusual knowledge or preoccupation with sex	Decrease in school participation, achievement, or homework	Sudden decrease in academic performance
Sudden broken nose or bone injury without explanation	Changed clothing style	Repetitive play	Excuses that do not match the seriousness of the situation
		Responding differently or inappropriately to teacher's questions	Not attending school or receiving education

Source: Data from Klika, J. B., & Conte, J. R. (Eds.). (2018). *The APSA handbook on child maltreatment* (4th ed., pp. 219–242). Sage; Mayo Clinic Staff. (2020). *Child abuse*. Mayo Clinic. https://www.mayoclinic.org/diseases-conditions/child-abuse/symptoms-causes/syc-20370864; State of New Jersey, Department of Education. (2019). Reporting child abuse and neglect: What school personnel need to know. https://www.state.nj.us/education/students/safety/socservices/abuse/training; World Health Organization. (2020). Child maltreatment: A guide to taking action and generating evidence. https://www.who.int/news-room/fact-sheets/detail/child-maltreatment

frightened youngster requires developmentally and culturally appropriate language. Following is an example:

> What we say here stays here. But there are times when we need to get more help if you may hurt yourself or someone else or if you have been abused or you know someone who has been abused. Then I need to tell adults who can help you and keep you safe. That's my job. (Mascari & Webber, 2017, slide 12)

When the situation mandates reporting, the counselor reminds the child or teenager:

> Remember I said what we say here stays here except for those times? This is one of those times we need to tell others because someone abused you. You are not to blame, and it is not your fault. I need to tell adults who will help you be safe. (Mascari & Webber, 2017, slide 13)

In clear, developmentally appropriate language, the counselor asks an open-ended question, such as "What happened to you?" Basic counseling skills, such as listening, reflection, and paraphrasing, contribute to keeping a calm, empathic stance without expressing discomfort about the child's disclosure. Counselors avoid shifting to an investigative role and do not press for details; rather, they affirm the youngster's courage, saying, "Telling me was the right thing to do. I am very proud of you" (Mascari & Webber, 2017, slide 14).

When abused children and adolescents express fear or guilt that they caused the abuse or put loved ones at risk by their disclosures, counselors unequivocally assure them that "No one will blame or fault you." For example, 15-year-old Angel blamed herself repeatedly for not fighting back hard enough to stop the abuse because the abuser threatened to hurt her mom if she reported him. The counselor responded, "Angel, it's not your fault. You are not the problem. The abuse is the problem" (Webber, 2007, p. 6). This narrative approach helps survivors separate from both the problem and their self-blame.

REPORTING ABUSE AND NEGLECT

Professional school and clinical mental health counselors often report feeling anxious and uncomfortable when reporting suspected or known child sexual abuse (Lambie, 2005; Tuttle et al., 2019). Weighing the decision whether to report child abuse constitutes a serious legal concern for counselors (Herman, 2002). Counselors stay alert to the tendency to shift from a therapeutic role to an investigative role, which could interfere with the child's testimony. Further, forensic investigators must follow specific, highly structured protocols when working with minor children who disclose abuse. Counselors avoid taking on an investigative role that could, paradoxically, influence the legal investigation. The counselor conducts a "minimal facts" interview and does not press for details. The counselor sits or kneels at the child's eye level, speaks in developmentally appropriate language, and maintains a nonjudgmental and accepting voice. Mandated reporters base their decision to report on reasonable suspicion. States and territories do not require reporters to present proof or to investigate (Henderson, 2013). Even though all states provide "good faith" regulations for immunity and protection, reporting may strain working relationships with parents and families who may conclude that the counselor likely reported the abuse. Reporting the sexual abuse of a teenager depends on the age of consent. For example, the states of New York and Texas consider 17 as the age of consent, meaning youth 16 and under cannot give consent. New Jersey considers 16 as the age of consent, meaning youth 15 and under cannot give consent. However, minors who are 16 but younger than 18 years old can legally consent to sexual activity. To avoid prosecuting youth, some states allow *close-in-age consent* when both partners under the age of consent agree consensually to sexual activity (ageofconsent.net, 2020). Inability to give consent includes those with a physical or mental impairment or who are unconscious, sleeping, or "voluntarily or involuntarily under the influence of alcohol or other substance" (NJSA 2C:14.2).

Every state mandates reporting suspected child abuse and neglect by medical, mental health, and school personnel, and some states require anyone to report. The timeline to report abuse varies by state. For example, New York also requires an investigation within 24 hours, which expedites determining the safety of the child and risk in the home. The State of New Jersey requires immediate reporting, meaning within 30 minutes (State of New Jersey, Department of Children and Families [NJDCF], 2020). Professionals in the state of Texas must make a report within 48 hours after first suspecting child abuse or neglect. A professional may not delegate to or rely on another person to make the report (Texas Family Code, 2020). Mandated reporters in a school should make the call from school; and to protect the child, counselors do not delay calling until after school.

In some abuse situations, reporters must notify both CPS and law enforcement. An example in New Jersey indicates that reporters must also call police or sheriffs in the following incidents: (a) child's death, (b) sexual abuse by parent or caregiver, (c) injury requiring treatment in the ED or hospital, (d) injury requiring more than superficial treatment, (e) repeated violence to a child, and/or (f) child abandonment. Coordination remains critically important so that the child does not encounter multiple interviews (State of New Jersey, Department of Education, 2019). Reporters give information in the familiar "who, what, when, where, how" order, although state and individual school protocols may vary. See Table 11.2.

TABLE 11.2 REPORTING CHILD ABUSE OR NEGLECT INFORMATION

	Information Requested
Who	Child's name Parent/caregiver's name, Child's age Child's last known address Siblings or other family members Name of the alleged perpetrator Alleged perpetrator's relationship to the child
What	Type and frequency of alleged abuse/neglect Current or previous injuries to the child Reasons for current concern School nurse examined or treated the child Medical treatment needed
When	When the alleged abuse/neglect occurred When you learned of alleged abuse
Where	Where the alleged incident occurred Immediate location of the child Whether the alleged perpetrator can access the child Date child will be released from school or agency How the child will be released from school or agency
How	Determine whether the situation presents imminent danger for the child Assess the urgency of the need for intervention

Source: Adapted from State of New Jersey, Department of Children and Families. (2020). When and how to report child abuse/neglect. https://nj.gov.def.reporting/how

CHILD PROTECTIVE SERVICES

The counselor stays with the child until a credentialed CPS worker arrives. Children may want to run away or immediately go home without knowing the location of the perpetrator. If the student worries about what will happen next, the counselor should reassure the student that "a special person who can help will come soon, and I will stay with you."

Counselors and school personnel must understand state procedures as well as recommended best practices. School administrators should verify the credentials of unfamiliar people who claim official roles or if CPS personnel say that they need to interview a child alone. Using New Jersey procedures as an example, an adult (e.g., counselor, teacher, or nurse) familiar with the child may remain in the room during the interview. Counselors do not answer for the child or provide their own opinion. Remaining calm models coping skills for the youngster and provides a comforting physical presence. Depending on state procedures, CPS can interview other students about the situation without parental or guardian consent.

When making a CPS report, mandated reporters do not need to inform parents. This disclosure could put the child at further risk or lead to the loss of evidence. Counselors should consider the child's best interests, safety, and well-being and consult with supervisors. Speaking in a respectful, compassionate way promotes a working relationship with parents and invites collaboration. Pietrantonio et al. (2013) recommend that counselors acknowledge the parents' strong emotions and validate their concern for the child's welfare. Counselors affirm their own mandated reporting responsibilities clearly and compassionately to the parents in order to maintain focus on the best interests of their child.

AFTER REPORTING

After reporting presents a difficult time for counselors if CPS removes the child from their home and family; conversely, in potentially dangerous situations, counselors may fear that CPS will not act fast enough. CPS responds to every report and generally conducts an investigation to decide the level of risk to the child and the next steps. The CPS interviewer holds the right in New Jersey, for example, to access the child's records, copy them, and remove the child from school. Rather than make a determination of maltreatment, CPS may design an alternative response to focus on the immediate physical or emotional needs of the family or contact counselors for more information or an update. School records and attendance reports might suggest that the family of the abused child moves frequently or can possibly move again after a mandated report. Many states offer online training to learn the signs of abuse, and, as an example, New Jersey provides an online course with four modules that address (a) policy requirements, (b) what to look for, (c) how to report, and (d) what happens after reporting (State of New Jersey, Department of Education, 2019).

When a parent or primary caregiver abuses, counselors can provide family counseling to help the nonoffending parent and family members cope with their reactions of shame, guilt, denial, confusion, or anger and potential housing or financial distress. CPS could place the family in a safety plan with the intention of keeping the child in the family, and the counselor may provide individual counseling, play therapy, or in-home therapy for the child. When a sibling or child member of the extended family perpetrates, the counselor may support family members to cope with the removal of the perpetrator from the home and changes in the family system.

Community volunteers and resources include Court-Appointed Special Advocates (CASA) trained to advocate for abused and neglected children in the juvenile court process. Big Brothers and Big Sisters represent volunteer role models who connect with students needing another caring adult figure in their life. The big–little team (big brother/sister and little brother/sister) gets together regularly for activities and companionship.

After reporting abuse, the professional school and clinical mental health counselor continues to maintain a working relationship with the child and family. Talking with parents after mandated reporting can challenge school, mental health, and medical professionals. Speaking in a caring, respectful way preserves the working relationship with caregivers and invites collaboration as they anticipate future steps (e.g., court appearances, testimony, and moving).

COUNSELING STRATEGIES

MULTIMODAL COUNSELING

Survivors of maltreatment need the unconditional support and love of parents or caregivers and a physically and emotionally safe home. Each maltreated youngster will respond to trauma in different ways and evidence unique needs. Counselors benefit from a framework to conceptualize with the child or teen what they need to work on and how they would like to do so. The multimodal HELPING model provides a simple structure for the counselor and the child when establishing needs and goals according to each modality: **h**ealth, **e**motions, **l**earning, **p**eople (**p**arent, **p**eer, **p**artner, **p**erpetrator), "**I**" image, **n**eed to know (**n**ew information), and **g**uidance of actions, behaviors, and consequences (**g**ood decisions)—adapted from Keat (1979); Webber (2007). Counselors integrate trauma-informed coping skills including (a) developing a sense of safety; (b) learning self-stabilization and emotional regulation skills; and (c) establishing safe communication channels with the counselor, family, teachers, and others (Webber et al., 2015). Treatment plans address the developmental levels of each child, as well as their therapeutic needs. For example, preschool children can learn to self-regulate by belly breathing like a balloon slowly letting air in and out. Choosing what toy to play with or whether to play first and then talk or vice versa, youngsters rebuild a sense of control and mastery over their world. Children and teens learn how to self-regulate by checking on any increases in their subjective units of distress (SUD) levels, which then alert the counselor that they need to bring their SUD back into the window of tolerance (Hinkle & Perjessy, 2018; Wolpe, 1992). Youngsters of all ages can nonverbally communicate the level of their distress to the counselor by holding up their fingers to represent their SUD or pointing to the traffic light color (e.g., green, orange, or red). When teenagers appear unable to talk, they may communicate more comfortably by texting the counselor in the session, even though they seem physically close to the counselor.

COGNITIVE BEHAVIORAL THERAPY

Originally developed for youth who experienced sexual abuse, trauma-focused cognitive behavioral therapy (TF-CBT) works well with children and teens comfortable with structure (Cohen et al., 2006; Feather & Ronan, 2009). This evidence-based treatment incorporates relaxation training, trauma psychoeducation, in vivo trauma exposure, cognitive reprocessing of maladaptive beliefs about abuse, and support from the nonabusing parent or caregiver. The TF-CBT case conceptualization model, CRAFTS, provides a direct skills approach to addressing types of problems: **c**ognitive problems, **r**elationship problems, **a**ffective problems, **f**amily problems, **t**raumatic behavior problems, and **s**omatic problems (Cohen et al., 2006). The PRACTICE protocol sequences the treatment plan and prepares the parent and child for conjoint sessions at home using "(a) psychoeducation, (b) relaxation, (c) affective modulation, (d) cognitive coping and processing, (e) trauma narrative, (f) in vivo mastery of trauma reminders, (g) conjoint parent–child sessions, (h) and enhancing future safety and development" (Cohen et al., 2006, p. 45). Game-based CBT incorporates TF-CBT, play therapy, and group therapy using developmentally appropriate therapeutic games and techniques focusing on the strengths of communal sharing for African American and Latinx youth (Hinkle & Perjessy, 2018; Misurell & Springer, 2013).

NARRATIVE- AND SOLUTION-FOCUSED COUNSELING

The narrative therapy approach to having "conversations" rather than therapy sessions promotes a nonthreatening, egalitarian environment that fosters multiple ways to share the abuse experiences of youth. Thus, counselors facilitate multiple possibilities for solutions and new stories. By externalizing and distancing themselves from the problem, survivors no longer see themselves as the problem and understand that the problem (i.e., the abuser and the abuse) controlled their stories. Survivors can now imagine future possibilities and stories that do not include the problem (White & Epston, 1990). Remembering exceptions or "sparkling moments," when the survivor avoided or outwitted the perpetrator, strengthens their innate power and creativity and fosters the survivor's unique hopes and wishes for a future healthy life (Winslade & Monk, 2007). The counselor can memorialize their sparkling moments with awards and certificates and collaboration on a new story ending with the survivor (White & Epston, 1990).

The solution-focused miracle question promotes future-oriented thinking and unique solutions rather than problem-focused talk. The counselor asks, "Suppose that one night, while you were asleep, a miracle happened, and this problem of remembering the abuse was solved. How would you know it was solved? What would I see you doing differently?" (adapted from de Shazer, 1988, p. 5; Webber, 2007, p. 13). For example, tech-savvy teenagers use "videotalk" to narrate what actions the first author (J.W.) would see them doing differently and showed the videos in their counseling group. Both narrative- and solution-focused counselors write letters or emails to their young clients in between sessions, drawing on ideas shared in conversations, "sparkling moments," and successes, as well as questions raised. These letters provide a bridge between sessions to continue the conversation and strengthen therapeutic growth.

MOTIVATIONAL INTERVIEWING

Motivational interviewing (MI) approaches appeal to teenagers who experienced sexual abuse from a parent or trusted adult (e.g., athletic coach, priest or cleric, boy scout leader) and who may believe a parent pushes counseling for a quick fix. Using MI strengthens an adolescent's own power for decision-making rather than that of a parent, caregiver, or therapist who might shift from support to pressure and threats when a teenager challenges their authority. Like narrative therapy, MI's egalitarian approach to conversations strengthens a teenager's motivation to change and resolve their ambivalence (Naar-King & Suarez, 2011). The counselor evokes and increases the teenage client's "change talk" and diminishes "sustain talk" to support their capacity to make good decisions. Responding to change talk uses core empathic counseling skills or OARS: open questions, affirmation, reflection, and summary. Many teenagers support change more comfortably when they hear themselves say it rather than others.

EXPRESSIVE MODALITIES

Integrating expressive modalities (e.g., art, clay, music, sand tray, photography, drama) into individual and group counseling gives children and teens a voice without needing words. Survivors can more easily express themselves in a small group through multimedia and multisensory materials. Sharing a sand tray scene, painting, photo story, or items that teenagers created can "resolve the paradox of engaging adolescents in group therapy, despite it being potentially triggering" (Haen, 2015, p. 243).

Books written for children and teens about abuse help to start conversations, especially when they think they stand alone in their experience of abuse. *Brave Bart: A Story for Traumatized and Grieving Children* connects us with a kitten "who had something very bad, sad and scary happen" and finds help and healing through a feline counselor (Sheppard, 1998, p. 1). In the children's book *Please Tell! A Child's Story About Sexual Abuse*, Jesse, the author and survivor, tells us her story: "Dear friends everywhere, I was hurt by someone I loved and trusted when I was four. He was my uncle and my godfather" (Jesse, 1991, p. 3). As they progress through therapy, youngsters may create a book, play, or photo story about their experience. Cohen et al. (2006) provide a protocol for story writing in TF-CBT. Many child therapists use narratives and child-centered story boards, stories with puppets, or sand tray stories as developmentally appropriate ways for children to express themselves.

SAFE TOUCH AND PET THERAPY

Pet therapy provides a natural extension to child-centered play therapy. Therapy dogs provide unconditional attention, empathy, and acceptance as an animal ally and a "cotherapist" with abused children who talk naturally with the dog. The play therapist carefully integrates the therapy dog to actively participate in the therapeutic relationship and facilitate disclosure and communication. Learning to trust good touch by loved ones and feel safe remains the responsibility of child, parent, counselor, and, in many cases, the therapy dog. Neglected or abused children often hug or snuggle with a therapy dog while rejecting the touch of parents or caregivers.

A trip to a petting zoo can jump-start therapy by providing contact with domesticated animals. Reaching out to a lamb through the fence represents a safe way to begin to experience what safe connections feel like. Neglected or abused children often welcome a trusted grandparent's comfortable lap and the soothing movement of a rocking chair. Learning safe touch with pets exemplifies an important therapeutic tool (Association for Play Therapy, 2019). Trained therapy dogs comprised an integral part of children and family counseling and support in Newtown, Connecticut, after the Sandy Hook School tragedy. Like the life-size puppets in Child Assault Prevention (CAP) programs, "a lot of times, kids talk directly to the dog. They're kind of like counselors with fur. They have excellent listening skills, and they demonstrate unconditional love. They don't judge you or talk back" (Hetzner as cited in Fiegl, 2012).

CHILD-CENTERED PLAY THERAPY

Experiencing a safe, trusted adult and environment in child-centered play therapy remains a critically important part of healing from abuse. Kinsler et al. (2009) observed that "victimized children are hurt in relationships, yet, paradoxically, relationships can be the core component of healing from these injuries" (p. 183). The very elements that present the most damage—trust and relationships—may unavoidably also serve as the vehicles for healing. The youngster who experiences sexual abuse will likely need time and patience to realize this. Abused children may act out aggressively in play as they cope with emotional dysregulation, somatization, disorganized attachment, and relational dysfunction caused by sexual abuse and interpersonal betrayal. While play represents a natural vehicle for children to express their feelings and ideas, rigid *repetitive play* of maltreated children reflects unresolved trauma (Gil, 2017).

Play therapists must balance building a trusting relationship early with enforcing clear limits in the playroom so that the child learns that therapists do not expect them to perform the same sexual abuse that perpetrators demanded. Drawing pictures, telling a story, or describing feelings can provide a safe distance between the child and a strange new adult. As children establish a safe relationship with the therapist, they may play with baby bottles, dolls, and blankets to develop a realistic attachment to the therapist.

PERCEPTIONS OF PLAY THERAPY

Counselors must assess any personal values or feelings of shame, disgust, or dread about child or teen sexual victimization that convey to the survivor a sense of being bad or contaminated and interfere with their ability to fully experience their present world. Affirming the young client as a "survivor" and "hero" rather than as a victim helps parents understand that play therapy provides a different experience than courts and social services. Touring the play therapy room with parents and sharing handouts acclimates them to play therapy as a process that unfolds over time and centralizes the importance of play and expressive activities and corrects their misperceptions about what happens in play sessions. For example, counselors can share the following with parents of young children:

> Children communicate and resolve problems through play, and they heal through play therapy. This is a child's developmental way to work through their abuse. Your daughter is five years old and needs special child-size counseling tools so she can feel safe and play as a child again. As parents and adults, you would likely find it easier to talk with me than to play with me. Children often find it easier to play first and talk later. As we move through therapy, your daughter and I will invite you to our special play therapy room. (Webber, 2007)

Providing a brief general summary to parents at the end of a session tends to reduce their anxiety and expectation that the counselor can fix the problem quickly. Through parent–child relationship training and filial therapy, parents learn how to play with their children, attend, and respond. Since children naturally play with other children, group play promotes a sense of safety within a trusting group experience.

POSTTRAUMATIC PLAY

The play therapy room should display diverse miniature figures, as well as dolls and stuffed animals so that youngsters can choose figures that look like them, as well as generic figures (e.g., Playmobil) that they can use as symbols. Children may represent a perpetrator with an emotionally evocative figure or puppet, such as an alligator, dragon, three-headed dinosaur, shark, witch, space alien, or a villainous movie character such as Darth Vader, Lord Voldemort, or the Joker. Self-symbols range from vulnerable toy figures like a smaller doll, infant, lamb, or piglet early in the play and shift to invincible figures with special powers or magic like a lion, tiger, gladiator, superhero, king or queen, Wonder

Woman, or Harry Potter later in the resolution narrative. Children with interpersonal trauma play out symbolic solutions to dangers. For example, Devon triumphed over a scary alligator in the play therapy room.

> Devon hit the bop bag repeatedly. Then he grabbed a stuffed alligator and ran, pointing its jaws close to the therapist's face. Devon turned around suddenly, jumped into the sand box and buried the alligator in the sand as he shouted, "Bad gator. Bad gator!" He curled up with an infant doll in a corner, rocked, and sucked his thumb. (Webber et al., 2015, p. 5)

A child may point a monster puppet dangerously close to the therapist until they move an animal protector or superhero to destroy the attacker and save the therapist from harm. As children transform their role from victim to victor, they might bury the predator in sand. Devon learned to trust the safety of the play and he triumphed by burying the alligator in the sandbox. As children regain control over their lives, they may change their self-representation to a disproportionately large, powerful figure and reconstruct the trauma story ending.

> When she could not find a miniature large enough to symbolize her new courage, a seven-year-old girl who experienced sexual abuse by her stepfather for two years, replaced a small self-symbol figure in the sand tray with an oversized superhero action figure from the playroom. She then replaced the perpetrator figure with a tiny two-inch miniature figure, turning him upside and burying him in the sand. (Webber & Mascari, 2008, p. 7)

During posttraumatic play, children may express their need for more distance from the abuser through protective actions. For example, in a play therapy session with the first author (J.W.), when Katy's distress increased, the preschooler hid behind a life-size stuffed turtle for protection. In another session, Jorge frequently repeated a series of actions. He hid his self-symbol in the playhouse and placed a gladiator's shield over the figure for protection. Then Jorge stuffed the "bad soldiers" into the toy chest, shut the lid, locked the chest, and then hid the large key in the sandbox. A 15-year-old whose mother's boyfriend sexually abused her painted a pair of enormous life-size red high heels "big enough to stuff everything in" and taped the drawing to the door, symbolically declaring her safety in the room from her perpetrator (Webber, 2007).

Symbolic play provides reparative attachment and mastery experiences for children who missed critical developmental stages. Children treat animals' symbolic injuries, parent the dolls, or ask the therapist to feed baby dolls with a bottle. Children also enact regressive play behaviors as nurturing experiences that facilitate the development of more secure attachments. Puppets and stuffed animals represent important multisensory props for conversations in that they provide children tools to externalize their actions, feelings, and thoughts. A youngster who seems reluctant to talk may respond easily to an animal puppet who "talks" to the child through the therapist's voice. For instance, a turtle puppet can pull its head inside and hide in its protected shell, or a lion puppet can roar. Children who suffered from physical abuse may reenact ED trauma with an "injured" stuffed animal using miniature hospital sets, ambulances, stretchers, and bandages. Children traumatized by chronic domestic and community violence may engage in repetitive play with police cars and fire trucks, a jail, or a miniature courtroom.

PARENT AND FAMILY THERAPY

Child therapy efficacy significantly increases with the involvement of parents or guardians in play therapy treatment, and family support remains the most significant single predictor of the child's healing and recovery from trauma (Cohen et al., 2006). Child therapy requires parent therapy, especially with externalizing problems. Perry (2019) found that the distance a family traveled to therapy represented the strongest predictor of success in their therapy. The time a family spent in the car traveling to the session and talking together significantly predicted progress in both therapy and developmental milestones. Family involvement in treatment remains essential to the child's reintegration into the family, school, and neighborhood.

Several parent and family therapy programs combine cognitive restructuring with other components, such as parent–child communication skills, positive discipline, and emotion regulation. Empirically supported programs include Positive Parenting Program (Triple P), Alternatives for Families-Cognitive Behavioral Therapy (AF-CBT), Multisystemic Therapy for Children and Adolescents (MST-C), Nurse–Family Partnership, parent–child interaction therapy (P-CIT), and TF-CBT (Merritt et al., 2018; Rubin, 2012).

When a parent enacted the abuse, the participation of the nonabusive parent and the extended family remains critical to the child's healing process. Religious beliefs and cultural traditions can influence parents' reactions to physical, sexual, and psychological abuse, and the therapist's sensitivity to cultural issues that arise in family play therapy sessions promotes greater participation by nonoffending members. Family issues may include discipline, corporal punishment, domestic violence, shaming, and ostracizing. As the child's play therapy moves toward reconnection with family members and reintegration into the family, Gil (2006) encourages everyone to share their feelings and reactions using genogram and circle outlines. Using a large genogram of the family, Gil invites the child to place a figure representing each family member on their respective circle or square and then asks family members to place an object symbolizing their own feelings about the child's abuse next to the figure selected by the child. Using a circle within a circle, she invites families to select a figure that shows their feelings about the sexual abuse on the small circle. In the larger outer circle, family members place miniature figures representing how they dealt with the abuse and what helped them process the events as a family (Gil, 2006).

Filial therapy trains parents to lead play sessions with their children. In the sixties, Louise and Bernard Guerney found that parents could be more effective than therapists when helping their own child (Guerney & Ryan, 2013). Training parents in play techniques enhances the parent–child relationship, increases parental confidence and their understanding of their child's feelings and behaviors, and improves communication. The use of filial therapy proves effective between nonoffending parents and their sexually abused children (Costas & Landreth, 1999) and parents of children who witnessed domestic violence (Smith & Landreth, 2003).

In dynamic play therapy, families with domestic violence or separations engage in collaborative interactive family play, storytelling, and video making (Harvey, 2008). Family play activities at home, such as drawing the family, playing "follow the leader," or creating a family story with stuffed animals strengthened and enhanced the quality of their playtime. P-CIT showed strong improvements in parent–child relationships (Merritt et al., 2018; Timmer et al., 2005).

COUNSELING ADOLESCENTS

Preteens and teens may perceive a therapy room as "childish" or "too adult." A blended environment of adult and youthful materials affirms an older teen's needs including a laptop or tablet, basketball hoop and Nerf balls, games (*Battleship, Clue*), action figures, miniatures, art supplies, and videos or TV series (e.g., Harry Potter, *Lord of the Rings, Star Wars, black-ish, Big Bang Theory*). Parents may express discomfort with the ideas that teens "play" or assume the lead in the session. For example, the counselor may reframe their concern this way:

> It was very important for you to find a good counselor for your son. He has suffered through a terrible experience, and I know you want him to feel better. It will take some time for him to get to know and trust me, just as you and I have done together in our meetings here. . . . Teenagers often like to do something while they talk and I have some of the video games and *Stars Wars* figures he likes, along with other hands-on activities. He will be more comfortable if he can choose what he would like to do while we talk together. (Webber, 2007, p. 4)

In the initial sessions, teenagers can show "attitude," arrogance, and resistance, complaining that their parents forced them to go to counseling with a stranger when they would rather be anywhere else. MI responses emphasize the teenager's power to decide and to commit to counseling. Other teens present as depressed, sad, or fearful, facing the wall silently ignoring the counselor for much of the session. Cajoling and pleading only intensify the tension and distance between the client and counselor but acknowledging their intense negative feelings shows that the counselor accepts the client unconditionally.

Inviting teens to the session and touring the therapy room sets the tone that the older teenager remains free to make choices. Offering teens the same control as in child-centered play therapy fosters remarkable results, and the attitude and rudeness or distance begins to diminish. Gil (1996) encouraged teens in the same freeing way: "You can say as much or as little as you want in here. . . . You'll be the judge of when you feel comfortable enough to say whatever you want. . . . Tell me what you think I need to know about you" (p. 163).

When abused adolescents experience difficulty with risk taking, impulsivity, and assessing danger, counselors can use technology and neuroscience metaphors in conversations about how they respond to trauma. Useful neurometaphors include the *snooze alarm* that rings repeatedly no matter how many times they try to stop it. The symbolic trauma *smoke alarm* goes off even when no danger occurs but may also fail to sound in the presence of real danger (Webber & Mascari, 2015).

When the first author (J.W.) played *Battleship* with Tony, a 14-year-old teenager whose uncle molested him, Tony challenged her to guess which battleship represented the perpetrator. They played his version of the game over and over, changing the location of the perpetrator's ship and then sinking it. Group sand tray also represents a powerful experience that promotes teens' natural desire for exploration and connection with their peers. Shy or cautious teens may find a group adventure trip or outdoor meeting, or virtual scavenger hunt an inviting escape from school, home, and the counselor's office (Webber et al., 2015).

Around the age of 14, the risk of sexual abuse by a peer or nonfamily adult increases (WHO, 2020). Engagement by a perpetrator online acting as a teenager or friend increases the risk of abuse of lonely or isolated teens. Group counseling and group sand tray represent modalities for teenagers who isolated themselves from friends after sexual abuse. Group counseling provides social engagement in a safe, protected space with new opportunities to expand their connections with other teens. After her mother's boyfriend sexually abused her, 15-year-old Angel joined a support group of abused students, who accepted and supported her.

> I couldn't even talk to my best friends who stuck with me through it all. I hid from them. And then the support group. . . . I felt I was safe here, and my group members understood what happened to me. (Webber, 2007)

When abused teens begin group counseling, they may react with resistance or hostility. Doing something different and unexpected exemplifies a time-efficient counseling technique that melts their reluctance. Schimmel and Jacobs (2011) used a large metal trash can in the middle of a group session with teens and instructed them to "bitch" and "trash-talk" by speaking or yelling simultaneously into the trash can for a period of about 10 minutes, before getting "down to business." The group leader then "ceremoniously put the lid on and removed the can from the middle and said, 'Let's begin. I'm going to tell you how this group can be valuable'" (p. 4).

RISK OF RETRAUMATIZATION

Retelling experiences of abuse and trauma can retraumatize youngsters. Addressing the client as a survivor, not a victim, promotes present and future-focused action and validates their natural capacity to heal and move forward. Although some survivors may want to retell their story, counselors must first check themselves and their personal beliefs to assure that the client, not the counselor, wants to hear their abuse story. Conventional talk therapy does not work with all children, who naturally and developmentally play to communicate and work through their problems. In child-centered play, counselors accept children just the way they reveal themselves to be and not as miniature adults. Showing relevant clips from *Mr. Rogers's Neighborhood* affirms and validates the child and provides a model for parent–child communication. Talking to an animal puppet or a therapy dog provides total safety and unconditional acceptance without judgment.

Each child survivor in a safe relationship with a trained play therapist will find their unique ways to heal. However, abused children can literally find themselves "tongue-tied" and "scared speechless." Child survivors may not want to or need to retell and revisit their abuse to experience a healthy future (Rothschild, 2017; Webber et al., 2019). Having to retell their story of abuse can terrify and retraumatize children and teenagers (Webber & Mascari, 2008, 2018). In place of talk treatment, multisensory play and expressive arts become the child's way to express, communicate, and heal with or without words. Counselors should help youngsters learn to manage emotional dysregulation and hyperarousal by pressing the "brakes" to keep themselves within their window of tolerance (Rothschild, 2000, 2017). Rothschild's metaphor of learning to brake before accelerating especially resonates with teenagers. She taught her teenage friends how to "drive" by insisting that they learn how to use their "emotional" brake and practice slowing down or stopping altogether before learning to press down on the gas. Pressing prematurely on the emotional gas pedal often leads to moving too fast in the counseling process, resulting in problematic emotional hyperarousal for the teen.

PREVENTION AND EARLY INTERVENTION

Reducing the incidence of child abuse remains a high priority for all counseling and mental health professionals, policy makers, and world leaders. A common misbelief about child sexual abuse is that most children do not know their predator. In fact, the child's parent represents about 90% of predators. Parents caution children to beware of strangers; yet many parents do not inform their children about good touch and bad touch that could lead to sexual abuse in a family. Religious, societal, and cultural stigmas also increase the silence about sexual abuse. Counselors should understand the cultural perspectives and experiences of the family as well as the family's own culture in caring for children and how the home and the family protect the child or expose the child to risk (Fontes, 2018). Parent education and support groups play an essential role in reducing child abuse and increasing early intervention, understanding what ways the family and the home environment protect the child or expose the child to risk. The Texas Help and Hope program provides information and videos to guide parents in improving relationships with their children.

Several community prevention programs combine cognitive restructuring with parent–child communication and problem-solving skills, safe and positive discipline, modeling nurturing behavior, peer support, psychoeducation about maltreatment, home visits, and emotion regulation. Empirically supported programs include Triple P, AF-CBT, Nurse–Family Partnership, Strengthening Family Programs (SFP), and Darkness to Light (D2L) (Fitzgerald & Berliner, 2018; Merritt et al., 2018; Rubin, 2012).

CHILD ABUSE PREVENTION PROGRAMS

School sexual abuse prevention programs significantly increase children's protective knowledge and behavior regardless of the program type (Walsh et al., 2015). State, agency, and school programs provide multiple projects and performances, such as the Child Abuse Prevention Program (CPP; New York Foundling Hospital, 2019), or similar programs with life-size puppets, such as Kids on the Block that "talk" to children about safety and abuse. At the end of the programs, counselors present children with the opportunity to talk to puppets and also to counselors. After a school puppet performance, 6-year-old Devon walked up to the life-size puppet and, for the first time, shared his secret that his stepfather had sexually abused him repeatedly since kindergarten (adapted from Webber, 2007, p. 8).

INTERVENTION DURING THE PANDEMIC

The COVID-19 pandemic caused a crisis in mental health and the delivery of counseling interventions. Virtual classes place greater stress on teachers and school counselors to recognize signs of maltreatment and to notice when students at risk become absent themselves online. The lack of laptops and tablets reduces students' capacity to connect with significant adults. Social distancing, sheltering at home, quarantines, and school closures break connections with relatives and caring adults and loved ones and need novel ways to remain in touch (Webber as cited in LaMotte, 2020). Isolation from caring adults increases fear, anxiety, and uncertainty and can lead to anxiety, depression, and regressive behaviors (Mascari & Webber, 2010). Using puppets and therapy dogs in online sessions, class meetings, and birthday celebrations in group online chats increase children's sense of safety and engagement. Online parent psychoeducation groups provide information and practice for caregivers to learn to recognize signs of abuse and understand that they can access services even while physically isolated.

HANDLE WITH CARE: A STATEWIDE ADVOCACY EXEMPLAR

The second author (C.S.) remains involved in programs that reflect the child abuse prevention advocacy initiatives in West Virginia. Handle With Care exemplifies a simple but highly effective trauma-informed initiative that communicates serious needs for children affected by family traumas that interfere with the child's ability to learn (West Virginia Center for Children's Justice, 2020a). When a police officer responds to a call that involves children (e.g., arrest of a parent, death notification, fire, accident, criminal incident), the officer notes the children present and the school(s) the children attend. The officer uses a private encrypted mobile phone app created for the police to securely notify the child's school to "handle with care" in the subsequent days. The school does not need to know the details; they only need to know to "handle with care." A child whose parent faced arrest for drug use or domestic violence almost certainly experiences a state of traumatic stress, which will interfere substantially with the child's ability to pay attention and possibly even stay awake (due to sleep and location disruptions) in class. Because of the school alert by the police, the child's teacher knows to respond supportively rather than punitively.

Schools throughout West Virginia receive Handle with Care training as their school transitions to a trauma-informed school. Basic responses include allowing a child to go to the school nurse's clinic to take a nap or provide an extra textbook or a change of clothes. Other examples of responses include excused time to receive support from the school counselor or more intensive therapy from a trauma-informed clinical counselor from the community who offers contract services at the schools. Schools institute trauma-informed rituals (such as handshakes, high fives, fist bumps, or hug greetings) by teachers at the classroom door. Stress-level indicators like green glass gems for "okay" and red glass gems for "not okay" dropped into a dish at the teacher's desk indicate the general "temperature" of a classroom as the day starts. If the teacher sees numerous red gems, the teacher knows to start the day with some grounding or self-regulation exercises before moving forward with the day's lessons. The creators of the Handle with Care program provide a tool kit ready for export to other states (West Virginia Center for Children's Justice, 2020b).

STATEWIDE ADVERSE CHILDHOOD EXPERIENCES COALITION

West Virginia created the statewide interprofessional ACEs Coalition of stakeholders, who tear down silos and increase communication and collaboration among all professionals who work with children affected by traumatic stress (ACEs Coalition of West Virginia, 2020). Representatives from K–12 public education, higher education (public and private), medicine, public health, public policy, private insurers, social work, counseling, psychology, social justice, first responders, nonprofit agencies, and researchers meet to describe programs, breakthroughs, needs regarding responding to trauma, and fostering resilience among children in a state heavily hit by the opioid crisis. The Coalition focuses on both the seriousness of trauma and what to *do* about the trauma. Current efforts include statewide training through a "Connections Matter" initiative to foster posttraumatic growth and resilience throughout systems that interact with and support a developing child. The Coalition provides no-cost memberships and bimonthly meetings (both virtually and in person) to facilitate connection across a state with difficult topography and variable weather.

CASE STUDY 11.1: KENNY'S INVISIBLE ILLNESS

After their mother died, 12-year-old Kevin and his 8-year-old brother, Kenny, walked to school every day with their dad on his way to work until he suddenly lost his job in town. Their dad found a temporary job that required leaving for work early while the children slept. Dad often worked late, arriving home after the boys went to bed. When Kenny became sick, Kevin stayed home from school to care for him, watching TV while Kenny slept.

With his dad already at work, Kevin left the house for soccer practice one Saturday morning. Kevin returned from practice to find Kenny still sleeping. When their father came home that night, he could not wake up little Kenny who had died in his sleep of undiagnosed diabetes. Consumed with grief over the loss of their mother, combined with financial and household stress, no one in the family or at school noticed Kenny's loss of 28 pounds over the past 5 months.

Activity 11.1

With students in small groups, each group role-plays various individuals affected by Kenny's illness and death in sessions with the counselor: his brother Kevin, his father, Kenny's classroom teacher, Kenny's best friends who played on his soccer team and were in his class, parents of Kenny's friends worried about what to say to their children who feel guilty about his death, and the school nurse who examined Kenny and did not notice his weight loss and weakness. Two students serve as process observers in each group. The small groups return to the class and share their reactions and feelings. The class brainstorms ways to provide support for those affected.

Activity 11.2

Form groups of five to six students. As future mental health professionals, consider the clinical priorities if you were working with either Kevin or Kevin's dad. Clinical priorities are the issues or problems that are most pressing and most likely to cause difficulty in a given client's return to health and wellness. Based on the case description, what are the top two potential clinical concerns you identify for Kevin and the top two potential clinical concerns you identify for Kevin's dad? Be able to defend your reasoning for why the two issues you selected were most clinically pressing. Compare your priorities to those identified by others in your group. Did others identify concerns that were different? Did your priorities change? Did your reasoning for your clinical priorities influence others to change or rearrange their priorities? What did the discussion reveal to you about different approaches to providing care for the same case?

CHAPTER SUMMARY

The prevalence of child maltreatment impacts all countries and cultural and social groups. Children hold no responsibility for the abuse, and telling a caring adult about abuse represents a positive action. Counselors and mental health, educational, and medical professionals serve as mandated reporters who can report child abuse anonymously with federal law offering immunity from civil and criminal suits. Treatment efficacy for child abuse increases significantly with family support and when parents participate in child-centered play therapy or filial therapy. A multimodal counseling model includes play therapy, MI, TF-CBT, and narrative- and solution-focused counseling. Play therapy provides a developmentally appropriate modality for counseling abused children. Adventure therapy, sand tray therapy, games, and group counseling represent effective strategies that provide safety, support, and mastery for adolescents.

POINTS TO REMEMBER

- All children deserve the right to a safe and healthy life free of abuse.
- ACEs lead to physical and mental health problems later in life.
- A parent or caregiver perpetrates most abuse.
- States provide for anonymous reporting, good faith reporting, immunity, and protection.
- Children must know they never hold fault or responsibility for abuse.
- Counselors report suspected child abuse; they do not investigate it.
- Child survivors may benefit more from play and expressive modalities than from talk therapy.
- Protective factors include secure attachment; authoritative, caring parenting; positive discipline; knowledge of child development; family connections; community support; and resources.
- Group counseling provides peer support to children and adolescents.
- Family support stands as the significant single predictor of the abused child's healing.
- Treatment efficacy for child abuse increases significantly with parent involvement in play therapy.
- When a parent perpetrates, the participation of the nonabusive parent continues to be critical to healing.
- Child survivors benefit from play, sand tray, and filial therapy. Teen survivors benefit from adventure therapy, activity counseling, sand tray therapy, games, and group counseling.
- CPS and law enforcement must be notified in cases of sexual abuse by a parent or caregiver, child's death, injury requiring treatment, repeated violence to a child, and an abandoned child (according to the state).

OTHER HELPFUL INFORMATION FOR CONSIDERATION

- Child Welfare Information Gateway. (2019). State guides and manuals search. https://www.childwelfare.gov/topics/systemwide/sgm
- Children's Bureau. (2020). Tip sheets (for parents in English and Spanish). https://www.childwelfare.gov/topics/preventing/preventionmonth/resources/tip-sheets
- Darkness to Light. (n.d.). Resources. https://www.d2l.org/resources
- Darkness to Light. (n.d.). Stewards of children. https://www.d2l.org/education/stewards-of-children
- Klika, J. B., & Conte, J. R. (Eds.). (2018). *The APSA handbook on child maltreatment* (4th ed., pp. 219–242). Sage.
- National Child Traumatic Stress Network. (2020). Trauma types. https://www.nctsn.org/what-is-child-trauma/trauma-types

QUESTIONS FOR FURTHER DISCUSSION

- Discipline methods may be influenced by culture, society, or religious values or parental style. How would you approach a family who maintains the right to discipline as they wish, including harsh or rigid physical punishment?
- How can we better protect children and teens from internet predators?
- Physical and emotional abuse declines when parents receive education about healthy child development, authoritative parenting, and positive discipline. How can communities and schools advocate for prevention programs and reach out to parents at risk?
- How can school and community mental health professions increase skills and confidence for mandated reporting?

KEY REFERENCES

Only key references appear in the print edition. The full reference list appears in the digital product on Springer Publishing Connect: connect.springerpub.com/content/book/978-0-8261-4764-6/part/part04/chapter/ch11

Conte, J. R., & Vaughan-Eden, V. (2018). Child sexual abuse. In J. Klika & J. Conte (Eds.), *The APSAC handbook on child maltreatment* (4th ed., pp. 143–166). Sage.

Gil, E. (2006). *Helping abused and traumatized children: Integrated directive and nondirective approaches*. Guilford Press.

Hart, S. N., Brassard, M. R., Baker, A. J. L., & Chiel, Z. O. (2018). Psychological maltreatment of children. In J. B. Klika & J. R. Conte (Eds.). *The APSA handbook on child maltreatment* (4th ed., pp. 219–242). Sage.

Henderson, K. L. (2013). Mandated reporting of child abuse: Considerations and guidelines for mental health counselors. *Journal of Mental Health Counseling, 35*(4), 296–309.

Kenny, M. C., Abreu, R., Helpingstine, C., Lopez, A., & Matthews, B. (2018). Counselors' mandated responsibility to report child maltreatment: A review of U. S. laws. *Journal of Counseling & Development, 96*, 372–397. https://www.10.1002/jcad.12220

Pietrantonio, A. M., Wright, E., Gibson, K. N., Alldred, T., Jacobson, D., & Niec, A. (2013). Mandatory reporting of child abuse and neglect: Crafting a positive process for health professionals and caregivers. *Child Abuse & Neglect, 37*, 102–109. https://www.doi:10.1016/j.chiabu.2012.12.007

Sheppard, C. A. (1998). *Brave Bart: A story for traumatized and grieving children.* Institute for Trauma and Loss for Children. Magination Press.

Tuttle, M., Ricks, L., & Taylor, M. (2019). A child abuse reporting framework for early career school counselors. *The Professional Counselor, 9*(3), 238–251.

U.S. Department of Health and Human Services, Children's Bureau. (2019a). Child maltreatment 2018. https://www.acf.hhs.gov/cb/research-data-technology/statistics-research/child-maltreatment

Webber, J., & Mascari, J. B. (2018). Re-storying the survivor narrative with sexually abused adolescents. In M. Scholl & J. Hansen (Eds.), *Postmodern perspectives on contemporary counseling issues* (pp. 122–143). Oxford.

CHAPTER 12

Addressing Trauma With Child and Adolescent Clients

Claudia G. Interiano-Shiverdecker, Devon E. Romero, and Brenda Jones

LEARNING OBJECTIVES

After completing this chapter, the reader should be able to:

- Distinguish the complexity and range of trauma experienced by children.
- Identify the neurobiological, social, psychological, and academic impacts of trauma-causing events on children.
- Recognize various trauma-informed and creative interventions when working with child and adolescent clients, as well as important considerations for school counselors.

CACREP STANDARDS FOR THIS CHAPTER

- CACREP 2016: 2F. 2. a., f; 3. e, f, g, i; 5. h, j, m; School Counseling: 5.G.2.a.b.d.e.f.g.j.k.; Clinical Mental Health Counseling: C. 2. f, g, j, C. 3. b.
- CACREP 2009: 2. B. 1; G. 2. a, e; 3. c, f; School Counseling: A.6.,7; C. 1.,3.,6; D.1,3.; E.1,2,3,4; F.2,3,4; G.1; H.2,4,5; K.1; L.1,3; M.1,2,3; N. 3,5; and O.2,4; Clinical Mental Health Counseling: A. 9; C. 6, 8, 9; D. 3; E. 1.

INTRODUCTION

This chapter explores the nature of trauma among child and adolescent clients. Critical incidences and traumatic events occur daily in the lives of children. They can be experienced individually or be shared through generations. Therefore, understanding the complexity and range of trauma experienced by children remains essential. When trauma occurs, certain factors aggravate or alleviate the repercussions of trauma. The authors discuss biological, social, and cultural factors known to delineate the process of recovery as well as address the neurobiological, social, psychological, and academic impacts of trauma on children. This chapter concludes by offering a discussion of assessment and a variety of child- and adolescent-centered trauma interventions for clinical mental health and professional school counselors.

DEFINING TRAUMA IN CHILDREN AND ADOLESCENTS

The pervasiveness of mental health issues among school-age children and adolescents endures as a serious matter. The U.S. Department of Education (2014) states that "no student or adult should feel unsafe or unable to focus in school" (p. i), yet unimaginable tragedies persist in the reality of today's youth. Nearly half of the nation's population experiences at least one type of abuse, neglect, or other potentially traumatic experience before the age of 18 (Centers for Disease Control and Prevention [CDC], 2019). Therefore, childhood and adolescent trauma remains one of the most discussed topics in the scholarly literature, with significant attention given to (a) the prevalence of trauma in childhood (McCormack & Thompson, 2016; van der Kolk, 2005); (b) psychological, physical, and neurobiological effects of trauma (Bremner, 2006; Delima & Vimpani, 2011); and (c) age-appropriate, evidence-based interventions (Briere & Scott, 2014; Courtois & Ford, 2013).

The *Diagnostic and Statistical Manual of Mental Disorders, Fifth Edition* (*DSM-5*; American Psychiatric Association [APA], 2013) defines trauma as a direct experience of "actual or threatened death, serious injury, or sexual violence"; witnessing these events as they occur to others; learning that these events occurred to a close family member or close friend; and/or experiencing repeated or extreme exposure to aversive details of the traumatic event (APA, 2013, p. 271).

Despite its extensive description, the *DSM-5* definition posits certain limitations on our understanding of trauma among children and adolescents. For example, perception remains excluded from this definition. Children and adolescents may perceive an event as traumatic without actual or threatened death, serious injury, or sexual violence to oneself or others, as in the case of bullying explained in more detail further in this chapter. The definition of trauma extends beyond the *DSM-5* definition in the literature to also include emotional harm that overwhelms the individual's internal coping resources and produces lasting psychological impact (Briere & Scott, 2014). Other forms of distress such as emotional abuse and neglect, discrimination, and oppression can also create similar responses to trauma as exposure to actual or threatened death, serious injury, or sexual abuse (Myers et al., 2015; van der Kolk, 2014). It is for this reason that throughout this chapter, we explore different categories of trauma and consider the child's emotional, mental, and physical response to an experience or series of situations.

CATEGORIES OF TRAUMA

A single incident or multiple occurrences can create traumatic symptoms (Briere & Scott, 2014). In some situations, children may resolve their response to trauma, while others may continually experience physical, emotional, spiritual, and social concerns. Factors such as frequency, longevity, and the nature of trauma remain critical components. We provide a breakdown of categories of trauma based on these considerations and further discuss prevalence and symptomology.

Acute Trauma

Acute trauma refers to a one-time event, such as natural disasters, assault, or a car accident. A range of reactions can follow acute trauma exposure, including transient distress, pathology (Miron et al., 2014), and resilience (van der Kolk, 2014). In instances of transient distress, oftentimes counselors make a diagnosis of acute stress disorder (ASD), a posttraumatic stress (PTS) reaction that occurs within a month following a traumatic event (APA, 2013). A child or adolescent experiencing ASD can present with a variety of symptoms, such as panic or extreme anxiety, confusion or irritation, feeling disconnected from self and one's surroundings, eating or sleeping difficulties, poor grooming habits or a lack of self-care, and academic or occupational difficulties (APA, 2013). Although experiencing acute trauma may lead to functional impairment in the immediate aftermath of trauma exposure, several studies attest to considerable natural recovery in youth within 2 to 3 months posttrauma (McLaughlin et al., 2013). However, several studies also documented that youth reporting ASD symptoms in the immediate aftermath can also develop more chronic psychiatric disorders, like posttraumatic stress disorder (PTSD), anxiety, depression, somatic reactions, dissociation, among others (Miron et al., 2014). Generally, risk factors such as the severity of the traumatic event and available support systems predict the development of chronic PTS symptoms (Miron et al., 2014).

Chronic Trauma

Chronic trauma occurs when traumatic experiences ensue as repeated and prolonged (e.g., ongoing family or community violence, chronic bullying) or when children and adolescents become exposed to multiple traumatic events in a specific time frame (Finkelhor et al., 2009). Children continue to be a population vulnerable to multiple and co-occurring types of trauma (Finkelhor et al., 2009, 2015). Finkelhor et al. (2015) found that among a sample of 4,000 children 0 to 17 years old, more than 50% experienced two or more kinds of violent trauma in a single year. Victimized youth also remain two to seven times more likely than nonvictimized youth to experience revictimization in the following year (Finkelhor et al., 2009). Chronic trauma during childhood significantly increases the risk for a variety of short- and long-term negative mental health symptoms and academic outcomes (Finkelhor et al., 2015). However, a more powerful predictor of youth outcomes appears to be the frequency of exposure, regardless of similar or different experience. In one of the largest studies (n = 8,667) to examine the additive effects of negative childhood experiences, the number of experiences endorsed appeared to be inversely related to mental health functioning (Chapman et al., 2007).

Complex Trauma

Van der Kolk (2005) defines complex trauma in childhood (as mentioned in Chapter 11) as "the experience of multiple, chronic and prolonged, developmentally adverse traumatic events, most often of an interpersonal nature, often within the child's caregiving system" (p. 2). These events may include sexual, physical, or emotional abuse, neglect, or the witnessing of violence within the family system (van der Kolk, 2005, 2014). Complex traumatic events in childhood and their potential for negative outcomes in adult life differ from chronic trauma in that early caregiving relationships underpin children's development of self, others, and the world (Cook et al., 2005). By repeatedly attending to a child's needs, caregivers foster a sense of safety that allows the child to develop appropriate emotional regulation. In contrast, repetitive and various forms of maltreatment negatively impact a child's developing sense of self, impairing crucial domains of development such as attachment, biological or physical functioning, emotional regulation, dissociation, behavioral control, cognition, and self-concept (Cook et al., 2005; McCormack & Thompson, 2016). Chronic trauma appears correlated to depression, anxiety, PTSD, somatization disorder, and borderline personality disorder in early years of development as well as adulthood (van der Kolk, 2005). Complex PTSD, a diagnostic criterion not currently included in the *DSM-5*, is typically associated with experiences of complex trauma (Courtois & Ford, 2013). Complex PTSD transcends the PTSD criteria by presenting significant impairment in emotion dysregulation, loss of self-integrity, and disturbances in the ability to relate to and be intimate with others (Courtois & Ford, 2013).

Historical Trauma

Originally introduced to describe persistent trauma among Holocaust survivors and their children after World War II, historical trauma is now understood as cumulative psychological wounding *resulting* from group traumatic experiences transmitted across generations within a community (Mohatt et al., 2014). Examples of historical trauma include experiences of colonialism; systematic discrimination based on race, gender, sexual orientation, or country of origin; years of political violence; genocide; and generations of structural inequality such as poverty (Crawford, 2014). As a result of historical trauma, the oppressed group may internalize oppressive prejudices and biases about their own group identity, known as internalized oppression (David, 2014). Internalized oppression can trickle down from parent–child relationships in a variety of ways that impact young, developing children (e.g., eating or sleeping disruptions, low self-worth and self-esteem, feelings of shame and helplessness; David, 2014). In addition, historical trauma appears to be associated with an array of psychological problems such as denial, isolation, nightmares, substance abuse, fixation on trauma, identification with death, and unresolved grief (Crawford, 2014; Mohatt et al., 2014). In recent history, many groups face historical trauma. Examples include recent shootings and social injustices targeting marginalized minorities such as the Black, Hispanic, LGBTQ, or Muslim communities.

CASE STUDY 12.1: FAMILY SYSTEM: A FAMILY'S EXPERIENCE OF TRAUMA

Chelsea, a 14-year-old African American girl and a recent addition to your case load, came to the intake accompanied by her mother, Rita. Chelsea reports experiencing symptoms of depression due to constant bullying at school for the past 2 years.

(*continued*)

CASE STUDY 12.1 (*continued*)

Chelsea briefly opens up about detesting school—not because of the academics, but because of her peers. She explains further, highlighting that every day that she attends school, her peers say terrible things to her. They call her "ugly" and "fat." Recently, the harassment escalated and became physical. Chelsea's peers shoved her into her locker and shoulder-checked her intentionally in the halls. Chelsea also explains that she cannot escape because of the constant bullying through Instagram, and she keeps comparing herself with models.

Her mother continues to be extremely concerned about Chelsea. Chelsea reports suicidal ideation. Her mother provides additional information about Chelsea and her family. Chelsea is the youngest of two in the family. However, someone killed her older brother 2 years ago in a church shooting. David, Chelsea's father, who is a military veteran, took it the hardest. At the age of 18, he attended a renowned military school, and accordingly became a high-ranking officer at a young age. He did two tours, where he led groups of young men and women through dangerous circumstances. In doing so, David lost several dear friends, people that he supervised in his platoon. Rita explains that he became increasingly angry since the death of their son. Rita adds that she became overly protective of Chelsea since the death of her son. She explains, "She is all I have left." Chelsea, however, feels like she cannot talk to anyone; "Everything makes my dad angry," she states, and "my mom gets anxious about everything."

Activity 12.1: Reflection Questions

1. What types of trauma appear present within Chelsea's family?
2. How do individual and shared experiences of trauma impact Chelsea's path to recovery?

IMPACT OF TRAUMA ON CHILDREN AND ADOLESCENTS

Exposure to trauma, even as a witness, persists as a large problem and remains a significant impact on the development and social-emotional health of youth. These experiences frequently result in physiologic reactions that overwhelm a child's capacity to cope (National Children's Traumatic Stress Network, n.d.). Childhood exposure to trauma maintains significant effects on long-term development, as evidenced by current knowledge regarding brain development and negative associations with attachment, learning, and academic achievement.

SYMPTOMS OF TRAUMA IN CHILDREN

Despite the manifestation of trauma symptoms particular to each category of trauma, traumatic stress in children differs from reactions experienced in adults, even more so for those with exposure to repeated or multiple traumatic events (van der Kolk, 2003). The manifestation of traumatic stress in children varies and will depend on the child's age and developmental level. These traumatic stress reactions may interfere with the child's daily life and their ability to function and interact with others. For instance, traumatized youth often experience strong cognitive (e.g., nightmares, intrusive thoughts, loss of memory or concentration, mood swings, disorientation), behavioral (e.g., internalizing and externalizing behavior problems, antisocial behaviors), physical (e.g., tachycardia, sleep problems, sexual dysfunction, easily startled, change in eating patterns, aches, pains), and psychological (e.g., depressive symptoms, fear, compulsive behaviors, shock, anger, anxiety) reactions immediately following exposure to a traumatic event (Delima & Vimpani, 2011; van der Kolk, 2003). In addition to the effects on a child's ability to regulate, identify, and express emotions, exposure to trauma may also negatively impact the child's ability to relate to others (Delima & Vimpani, 2011). These reactions to traumatic stress begin to mirror those of adults as children get older. For instance, older children may engage in drug or alcohol use, risky behaviors, or unhealthy sexual activity. For some, these symptoms may not dissipate and instead become increasingly severe and result in long-lasting effects (Cook et al., 2005) such as substance use and abuse, violence, risky behaviors, depression, suicidal ideation, suicide, school disengagement, and intergenerational perpetrating (McCormack & Thomspon, 2016). When professionals fail to identify trauma symptoms in children, such children may experience a misdiagnosis of depression, attention deficit hyperactivity disorder (ADHD), anxiety disorders, conduct disorder, or even psychosis.

NEUROSCIENCE AND TRAUMA

Traumatic events can negatively affect children and adolescents in the form of traumatic stress reactions and alter how the brain assesses threat and how youth respond. These experiences during the early developmental years cultivate an especially high potential to impact all aspects of present and future neural functioning, including the cognitive, affective, relational, and somatic domains. As such, psychotherapeutic approaches for the treatment of traumatic stress conditions must address the neurodevelopmental changes to brain anatomy and functioning produced by exposure to trauma and violence. Effective treatments must also consider the age and developmental level at which the child suffered the insults to normal brain development.

Unique phases of brain development referred to as sensitive periods become exceptionally susceptible to experiences that may alter future brain function or structure (Knudsen, 2004). At birth, the brain reflects an immature state and will not reach its maturity until the second decade of life (Mundkur, 2005). Throughout this extended period of neurodevelopment, the human brain appears highly dependent on and shaped by experience. The first 2 years of life involves a period of robust growth that likely represents a critical period of development and vulnerability for neurodevelopmental disorders (Gilmore et al., 2011). In contrast to the evidence of sensitive periods for brain development, neuroscience also points to the brain's ability to change through neuroplasticity (Andersen et al., 2008). Notable, however, is that trauma experienced in early periods of one's life does not always result in later life psychopathology. Other variables may contribute to later life resilience (e.g., secure attachment).

The Stress Response System

Innovations in the field of neuroscience shed light on the impact of traumatic stress on the brain's functions. Mechanisms of the stress response system include the sympathetic–adrenal–medullary (SAM) axis, the limbic system, and the hypothalamic–pituitary–adrenal (HPA) axis. These neuromechanisms serve essential roles for the regulation of body systems deemed important for the maintenance of an individual's well-being in the face of a threat. They also ensure a return to homeostasis upon removal of the threat. All of these remain significant for the maintenance of mental health (Shea et al., 2004).

The Sympathetic–Adrenal–Medullary Axis

The SAM axis embodies the importance of maintaining and reinstalling homeostasis after the presence of a stressor. Activation of the SAM system represents the classic "fight or flight" response. Upon introduction of a stressor, secretion of catecholamine becomes activated, including adrenaline (epinephrine) and to a lesser extent noradrenaline (norepinephrine). Adrenaline often becomes associated with an acute stress response and reactivity, whereas the release of noradrenaline balances or downregulates the stress response (Beijers et al., 2014).

The Limbic System

The limbic system contains the hypothalamus, the amygdala, and the hippocampus. The hypothalamus, responsible for maintaining homeostasis within the body, also carries out an essential function for outputting information to the cardiovascular system and in maintaining body temperature (Bremner, 2006). The amygdala processes and then helps to store emotions and reactions to emotionally charged events. Lastly, the hippocampus remains essential both in learning and in helping to put emotionally charged events and emotions in a life timeline of past, present, and future. Proper functioning of the limbic system remains vital for sufficient processing of life's events, especially those that seem to be stressful (Shea et al., 2004). Though the hippocampus matures between the ages of 3 and 4, children do not generally remember facts or events before that time (Andersen et al., 2008; Grosjean, 2005). However, the amygdala appears near full maturation after birth and becomes immediately ready to process emotions and sensory experience. This means that although young children may be too young to store a specific event in cognitive memory they can implicitly store the emotions and sensations associated with that event (Grosjean, 2005).

Dysregulation of the Stress Response System

The biological stress response system activates a physiologic and behavioral change within the body in response to a mild stressor. From this normal process, emotional and intellectual growth and development become enabled. The biological stress response becomes regulated through the HPA system and the sympathetic nervous system. When a stressor appears, the HPA axis releases corticotropin releasing factor, which stimulates the pituitary gland to release adrenocorticotropic hormone (ACTH). ACTH then stimulates the adrenal gland to produce glucocorticoid cortisol (Bremner, 2006). Cortisol, important for smooth functioning as well as for facilitating survival, can present negative effects on learning, memory, and other cognitive functions, particularly if the individual experiences chronic stress (Bremner, 2006). The literature pertaining to the effects of stress, and in particular, high levels of cortisol on the brain's development of specific regions (e.g., corpus callosum, hippocampus, amygdala) provides evidence that PTSD symptoms and trauma characteristics significantly correlate with size reduction, poor connection, communication, and overall functionality of specific brain regions (Andersen et al., 2008).

TRAUMA, ATTACHMENT, AND INTERPERSONAL RELATIONS

Broadly speaking, attachment refers to the tendency of a child to rely on a parent figure for comfort, support, and protection when frightened, stressed, or ill. The field of attachment owes much to John Bowlby, who articulated an evolutionary account of attachment, and Mary Ainsworth, who pioneered its study in naturalistic contexts. Ainsworth originally proposed that the extent to which the parent remained sensitive and responsive to the child's attachment signals appeared to be the critical determinant of attachment security (Ainsworth et al., 1978). Trauma that affects the safety of attachment security interferes with the youth's ability to integrate sensory, emotional, and cognitive information (van der Kolk, 2003).

Under typical rearing conditions and through learned experiences, human infants form attachments to caregivers who appear available and dependable. Variations in the quality of attachments, particularly whether or not they form, generate important implications for development in the young child. Trauma, especially of the sort arising from interpersonal violence and exploitation, can take on a highly negative impact on a youth's capacity to develop and maintain relationships. Lieberman (2004) noted that young children's ability to recover from the damaging effect of traumatic events appears deeply influenced by the quality of the child's attachments and by the parent's ability to respond sensitively to the child's traumatic responses.

IMPACT OF TRAUMA ON LEARNING

Diagnosticians use the term "developmental trauma" to describe when children and adolescents get identified and diagnosed with critical mental health concerns (van der Kolk, 2005). During this state, traumatized students struggle to cope; and, many times, their reactions to trauma transmute into serious behavior problems. Current research points to an assortment of adverse experiences that impact and alter brain development (Fecser, 2015). As described earlier in this chapter, exposure to trauma can affect cognitive, behavioral, physical, and psychological functioning in children. These symptoms also appear likely to impact learning. A study conducted by Goodman et al. (2012), who examined the relationship between socioeconomic status, trauma, and academic achievement, found an association between trauma and school performance. The study found that students with histories of trauma presented significantly lower standardized test scores and appeared more likely to need an Individualized Education Plan (IEP). Children exposed to trauma experience cognitive difficulties in abstract reasoning, executive functioning, attention, memory, concentration, verbal processing, and comprehension (van der Kolk, 2003), which can in turn affect learning. For example, preoccupation with worries about immediate safety or feelings of guilt may interfere with their ability to focus in the academic setting and their motivation to engage in schoolwork. Trauma can also occur in the school setting. In these instances, the environment itself can be a reminder of the primary trauma and make it difficult for the child to concentrate.

In a quest for survival during a traumatized state, youth, many times, may operate in hypervigilance and hyperarousal modes (i.e., similar to an emotional state of walking down a dark and terrifying street). The individual's level of awareness becomes heightened with anticipation that something bad could happen. This leaves the individual under continuous pressure to remain safe, even with no knowledge of what will happen next and when. Performing during a state of hypervigilance while in the classroom inhibits the ability to concentrate, usually leading to attention and learning difficulties. Trauma-impacted students may enter a hyperarousal state, lose their ability to focus on the learning tasks at hand, embark on a continual scanning of their environment, and become distracted by the slightest incitements. Behavioral problems may result, especially if the traumatized student perceives a particular stimulus to be threatening (i.e., a teacher pointing out that a student's assignment seems incomplete when the student feels targeted unfairly; Fecser, 2015). Threat responses ensue as the amygdala (the emotional side of the brain) sends messages of impending danger to the prefrontal lobe (the cognitive sides of the brain) resulting in possible experiences where the individual feels weak, exposed, or defenseless. This could spark a fight or flight reaction leaving students unable to control their responses during this hyperarousal state. Reflexes, not logic, drive students' actions in this state (Fecser, 2015).

Trauma-exposed students may also experience an overwhelming feeling of loss of control (Perry & Szalavitz, 2006). During this state, students' choices of behavior depict a sense of self-protection and a quest to maintain control. A student may exhibit a need to remain in control even with a simple correction or command made by a teacher. A simple instruction by a teacher to sit down can call forth the need to stay in control. Students sometimes demonstrate this quest for control through oppositional behavior due to their level of discomfort when the teacher's correction or command, for example, occurs in a large-group situation. Trauma-exposed students may sometimes perceive force from the teacher, and overt resistance may occur to exert some sense of control. This can be problematic for some teachers in that the students' behaviors may appear calculating and domineering (Fecser, 2015).

PSYCHOLOGICAL, SOCIAL, PHYSICAL, CULTURAL, AND SYSTEMIC FACTORS AFFECTING TRAUMA

Conceptualizing the impact of trauma appears to be complicated for two people can encounter a similar event and yet experience different responses. Trauma can impact anyone, causing disequilibrium and taxing resources (James & Gilliland, 2017), yet the impression of a traumatic experience depends on different elements. For example, as described earlier in the chapter, different types of trauma (i.e., acute vs. complex) may present unique impacts on individuals' psychological, social, physical, and emotional well-being. Yet other significant factors require attention. The biopsychosocial approach, introduced by the Substance Abuse and Mental Health Services Administration (SAMHSA, 2014a), highlights interactions among personal, genetic, and demographic factors with psychological and social influences. For example, factors that occur before trauma may directly or indirectly affect a youth's vulnerability to traumatic stress and risk for disorder, and later factors may exacerbate or alleviate negative emotional responses to extreme stress. In addition, trauma literature frequently mentions demographic variables—particularly gender, race/ethnicity, education, and socioeconomic status (Carlson et al., 2016).

PROTECTIVE AND RISK FACTORS

Risk factors occur with decreased availability of internal and external resources, thus aggravating prevalence and severity of symptoms following traumatic stress (Trickey et al., 2012). Pretrauma risk factors include adverse childhood environment, psychopathology in the individual and parent, and pretrauma life stress (Trickey et al., 2012). Posttrauma risk factors include reminders that evoke early responses of reexperiencing, cognitive and behavioral avoidance, depression, negative thinking, and dissociation (Trickey et al., 2012). Depression symptoms such as hopelessness and negative thinking about oneself, others, and the world may also impede behaviors that could foster recovery, such as seeking social support. In addition, coping with alcohol and substance abuse, cutting, or other unhealthy behaviors can debilitate the individual's natural coping abilities and disrupt their recovery (Briere & Scott, 2014).

Protective factors refer to conditions or attributes that shield or help youth deal more effectively with the impact of trauma. Risk and protective factors operate in combination and at different times, and their relative contribution and interaction vary across individuals to either aggravate or alleviate the psychological pain of trauma. Protective factors presented across social, emotional, and neurobiological domains may buffer children either from enhanced threat processing or from further exposure to trauma (McLaughlin & Lambert, 2017). The most frequently studied factors in trauma literature include social support, family cohesion, and resilience. Through meta-analytic studies, evidence indicated that children who receive social support, especially from caregivers, appear less likely to develop psychopathology following trauma exposure (Trickey et al., 2012). Social support negatively associates with psychopathology because social connections contribute to well-being and can foster cognitive and emotional processing of traumatic events (Trickey et al., 2012). Interaction with consistent, emotionally responsive caregivers during infancy can facilitate social, emotional, and cognitive development. Children learn to calm themselves when emotionally threatened, think about others' and one's own emotional states, or create and maintain relationships that can provide emotional comfort when needed (Carlson et al., 2016). Subsequent to social support, Meng et al. (2018) found that resilient children and adolescents displayed a lower risk for mental health problems (e.g., depression, PTSD, alcohol abuse, illicit drug use, interpersonal and psychological distress).

GENDER AND AGE DIFFERENCES

Many studies examined child gender as a potential moderator of the relationship between the onset of trauma and the development of symptomatic distress. Researchers propose that males face greater odds at experiencing traumatic stressful events related to violence and crime victimization, whereas females experience physical and sexual assault more frequently (SAMHSA, 2014a). Regarding symptoms, females exhibit more extreme acute reactions, which may lead to increased risk of later PTSD and also appear most likely to ruminate leading to depressive symptoms (Du Plessis et al., 2015). Moreover, males tend to show greater externalizing behaviors while females tend to display more internalizing behaviors (Du Plessis et al., 2015).

Age also plays a factor in how a crisis or traumatic event interacts with developmental and situational variables. For example, trauma experienced at younger ages can affect development, connection, and beliefs about trust and safety (SAMHSA, 2014a). Younger children also possess less prior knowledge and less language, which affects their understanding and appraisal of the event. Similarly, younger children appear less able to regulate their emotions, which will also affect the way in which they process the event (van der Kolk, 2003).

MULTICULTURAL CONSIDERATIONS

It is important to keep in mind that the experience of trauma occurs within the context of social and cultural systems that can either hinder or support recovery. Systems of power and privilege continuously oppress economic, racial, ethnic, gender, and sexual minority experiences and limit their access to much needed resources, social support, and opportunities for healing (Mohatt et al., 2014). Minoritized groups experience several overt acts of oppression such as harassment, verbal or physical attacks, threats to livelihood, social avoidance, exclusion, and discrimination (Myers et al., 2015). Minority youth groups also experience an array of covert acts of oppression, such as microaggressions, racial profiling, institutional racism, racial ambivalence, and racist beliefs, behaviors, and attitudes (Hirschberger, 2018; Mohatt et al., 2014). Experiencing oppression as children can lead to long-term consequences in self-confidence and identity, internalization of discriminatory messages and internalized voicelessness, and poor access and quality of mental healthcare (Mohatt et al., 2014). More extreme reactions to oppression result in maladaptive coping strategies, including suicide, displaced hostility or aggression, domestic violence, substance abuse, or sexual promiscuity (Myers et al., 2015). Experiences of discrimination and prejudice can also result in race-based trauma (Hirschberger, 2018). Race-based trauma can result in denigration of one's sociocultural in-groups, feelings of helplessness, numbing, paranoid-like guardedness, medical illnesses, anxiety, fear, and the development of PTSD (Myers et al., 2015).

SYSTEMIC FACTORS

The adapted Social–Ecological Model (SEM) used by SAMHSA (2014b) illustrates systemic factors that impact trauma among children and adolescents (see Figure 12.1). Applying the SEM to trauma work with youth involves conceptualizing traumatic events among many interwoven social systems that interact with and influence one another (SAMHSA, 2014b). The SEM allows counselors to address the factors that put people at risk or protect them from experiencing or perpetrating violence. It also helps counselors determine prevention strategies at different levels. At the core of this model, we find the child's individual characteristics (e.g., sex, age, gender). This makeup continues to be affected and modified by the child's interpersonal relationships with their immediate physical and social environment including family, peers, and school. The "Community/Organizational" circle represents social support networks, neighborhoods, and institutions that directly influence the individual's relationships. Broader social, political, and economic conditions (e.g., laws, state policies) influence the structure and availability of resources for the child. Finally, the outermost ring, "Period of Time in History," reflects the significance of the period of time during which the event occurred. Society's attitudes to a particular event (e.g., teenage pregnancy, rape) change over time and can dictate the overall response and support the child receives (SAMHSA, 2014b). The thicker arrows in the figure represent the key influences of cultural and development factors, and the type of trauma experienced previously discussed in this chapter.

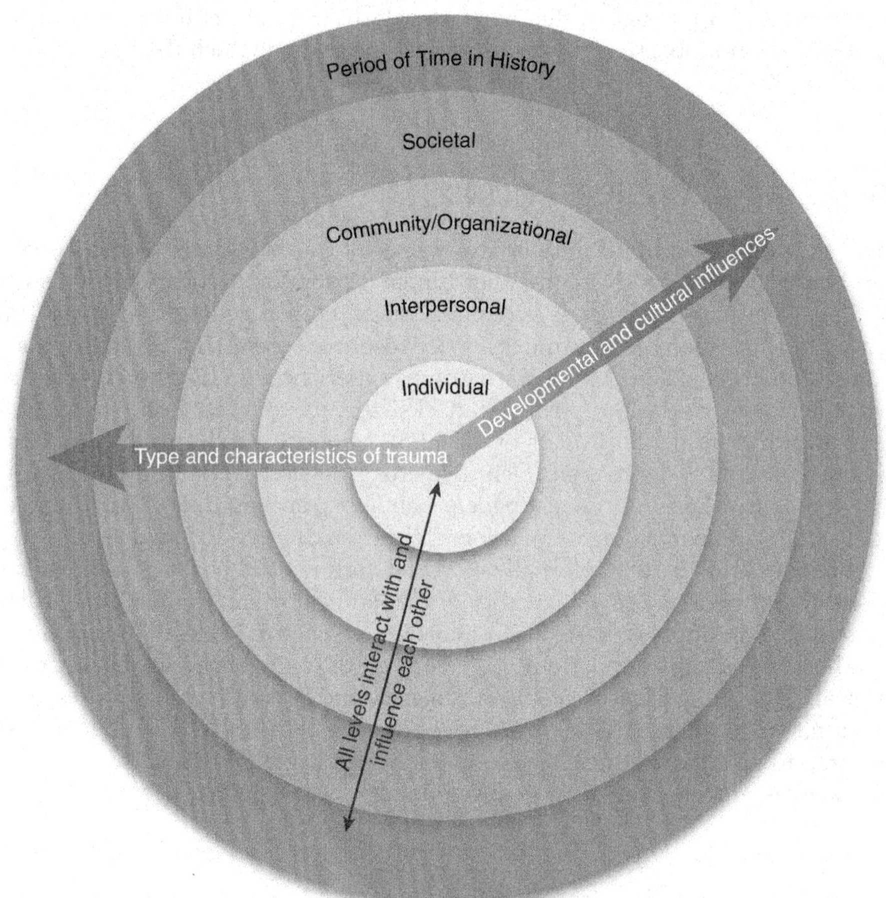

FIGURE 12.1 Substance Abuse and Mental Health Services Administration's (2014) Social–Ecological Model.

Source: Substance Abuse and Mental Health Services Administration. (2014b). *Trauma-informed care in behavioral health services. Treatment Improvement Protocol (TIP) Series 57.* HHS Publication No. (SMA) 13-4801. Substance Abuse and Mental Health Services Administration.

TRAUMA-CAUSING EVENTS IN CHILDHOOD AND ADOLESCENCE

A discussion of child and adolescent trauma requires special attention to prevalent horrors affecting girls and boys across the nation. The following sections discuss the most prevalent and concerning forms of traumatic events pertinent to today's youth.

CHILD ABUSE

Previously discussed in Chapter 11, professionals consider child abuse as a common form of child maltreatment. The authors provide a short summary echoing concerns of child abuse pertinent to counselors. Professionals consider the continued prevalence of child abuse to be one of the major concerns regarding child maltreatment. In the 2017 Child Maltreatment Report, 674,000 children were confirmed as victims of abuse and neglect by Child Protective Services (CPS) systems, of which 74.9% were designated as neglected, 18.3% as physically abused, and 8.6% as sexually abused (U.S. Department of Health and Human Services [U.S. HHS], 2017). Furthermore, much violence against children remains largely hidden and unreported because of fear, stigma, and the societal acceptance of this type of violence. Parents or parental guardians constitute the alarming majority of 91.6% of perpetrators (U.S. HHS, 2017). Poverty, mental health problems, low educational achievement, alcohol and drug misuse, history of abuse, and family breakdown of violence between other family members persist as important risk factors for parents abusing their children (Institute of Medicine and National Research Council, 2014). In children, the consequences of abuse and neglect can vary widely. Physical injuries and, in extreme cases, death present direct consequences (U.S. HHS, 2017). In nonfatal cases, invisible wounds lead to significant impairment in multiple domains of functioning such as self-regulation, attachment, and social helplessness (Cook et al., 2005). McCormack and Thompson (2016) found severe child abuse to be highly correlated with depressive and anxiety disorders, eating disorders, conduct and oppositional defiant disorder, substance and alcohol abuse, somatoform disorders, suicidal behavior, and PTSD.

CYBERBULLYING

Previously discussed in Chapter 8, bullying continues as a contemporary issue among children and adolescents. For today's youth, cyberbullying includes bullying through email, instant messaging, chat rooms, websites, or messages or images sent to cell phones (Schneider et al., 2012). Anonymous identities of bullies complicate and set back the identification and prevention of bullying behaviors among children (Schneider et al., 2012). The anonymity provided by online platforms compared with face-to-face situations also reduces responsibility and accountability of bullies (Schneider et al., 2012). In addition, cyberbullying exposes children to a wider audience. Social media platforms such as Facebook, Instagram, Snapchat, and Twitter make it easier for lies and rumors to quickly spread over the internet and through digital devices (Schneider et al., 2012). For these reasons, cyberbullying can present short- and long-term repercussions on academic, social, and psychological domains. For example, youth harassed online seem more likely to report two or more detentions or suspensions, skip school, and appear eight times more likely than other youth to report carrying a weapon to school (Schneider et al., 2012). As a result of repeated cyberbullying, children can often feel ashamed, embarrassed, insecure, and can develop low self-esteem and school phobia (Schneider et al., 2012). Long-term effects of any type of bullying, including cyberbullying, can *consist* of aggressive or criminal behavior, social phobia, depression and substance abuse, self-harm, and suicide (Hinduja & Patchin, 2010).

COMMUNITY VIOLENCE

Many children around the world continuously witness violence within their community, fall victim to violent acts, or continue to be subjected to a combination of both experiences (Finkelhor et al., 2015). Community violence persists as a major public health problem in the United States despite considerable attention from researchers, policy makers, law enforcement officials, and community-based organizations. Community violence includes exposure to violent crimes, terroristic acts of violence, mass shootings, natural disasters, displacement due to war and conflict, and other violently abusive acts.

Exposure to Violent Crimes

According to the Bureau of Justice Statistics (BJS, 2019), the number of violent-crime victims aged 12 or older rose from 2.7 million in 2015 to 3.3 million in 2018, an increase of 604,000 victims. In the National Survey of Children's Exposure to Violence (NatSCEV), Finkelhor et al. (2015) found that among a representative sample of 4,000 children aged 17 and younger, nearly two fifths (38%) reported being a witness to violence in their lifetimes, with almost twice as much reported among children aged 14 to 17 (68%). In this study, male children (56%) appeared more likely than females (47%) to be victims of assault. Males (31%) also appeared more likely than females (25%) to witness violence in the community. Risk of exposure may also vary as a function of age, with older youth more vulnerable than younger youth (Finkelhor et al., 2015). For example, in 2014, all types of exposure to violence, except for physical assault, occurred more frequently among younger children (ages 6–9), while physical assault appeared to be more common among children aged 14 to 17 (Finkelhor et al., 2015). Class and race also appear to positively correlate with violence exposure. For example, exposure to community violence is disproportionately higher among the poor, children of color, and those who live in urban areas (Turner et al., 2013).

A vast body of work exists identifying exposure to community violence as a major risk factor for the development of emotional and behavioral problems among young people. Studies on harmful mental health effects of pervasive youth violence predominantly focus on the development of PTSD symptomatology as an outcome (Turner et al., 2013). Adolescents exposed to community violence manifest a higher risk for depressed mood, anxiety, self-harm, and other mental health disorders (Astell-Burt et al., 2015). In addition, violence-exposed youth appear to present with a significantly higher risk for developing school problems including lower grade point averages, decreased standardized test scores in reading and math, and poor school attendance (Turner et al., 2013). Children who frequently witnessed violence in their neighborhoods also appear more likely to engage in delinquency and criminal activities during adolescence and adulthood (e.g., assaultive behavior, weapon carrying; Hong et al., 2014).

Mass Shootings

The Federal Bureau of Investigation defined mass shootings as an incident in which an individual or group kills four or more people during one event or in multiple places in close proximity to each other (Krouse & Richardson, 2015). These violent acts invade K–12 schools and institutions of higher education, causing significant emotional, physical, and psychological distress (Katsiyannis et al., 2018). Throughout recent years, rampage shootings took place on school premises or at functions connected with schools carried out by a current or former student or employee. From 2018 to 2019, at least 177 of America's schools experienced a school shooting, with 114 killed and 242 injured (National Council for Behavioral Health, 2019).

These events can greatly affect individuals' sense of safety, actual safety, and connection to others. Research indicates that children's exposure to assaultive violence, or learning that a close friend or loved one faced such exposure, is associated with an increased incidence of a range of negative mental health outcomes, among them PTSD, major depression, disenfranchised grief, and existential crisis (Katsiyannis et al., 2018). Mass shootings not only exert a psychological toll on their direct victims, but also affect members of the communities in which they took place, known as collective or shared trauma (Hirschberger, 2018).

Global Crisis: Refugees and Asylum Seekers

According to the United Nations High Commissioner for Refugees (UNHCR, 2019), an estimated 70.8 million persons worldwide became forcibly displaced by war or persecution in 2018, of which officials formally designated 25.9 million as refugees and 3.5 million as asylum seekers. The United Nations (2019) defines refugees as "persons who are outside their country of origin for reasons of feared persecution, conflict, generalized violence, or other circumstances that have seriously disturbed public order and, as a result, require international protection" (2019, para. 1). An asylum seeker refers to someone pursuing refuge for similar reasons. However, an asylum seeker applies for refugee status after entering the host country, whereas the U.S. government stamps acceptance on a refugee's asylum application. Children constituted about 50% of the refugee population in 2018 (UNHCR, 2019). Also, 138,600 unaccompanied or separated children sought asylum that year, with 27,600 applying on an individual basis (UNHCR, 2019).

Refugee children and asylum seekers experience trauma and psychological distress through three distinct, yet summative, phases of migration: premigration, migration, and postmigration. Premigration war experiences of children transpire as highly variable. While not all refugee children undergo traumatic experiences, others witness war atrocities and become victims of torture or intimidation, separated from family, deprived of water and food, and experience disruption of schooling (Pacione et al., 2013). Unaccompanied minors appear to be particularly at risk (Jensen et al., 2014). Migration experiences of children may also be traumatic and include separation from caregivers, exposure to violence and harsh living conditions, poor nutrition, and uncertainty about the future (Interiano-Shiverdecker et al., 2019). Recent policies in the United States, for example, led to fairly routine separation of children from parents. Finally, postmigration experiences for children may add stress related to their family's adaptation, difficulties with education in a new language, acculturation, shifts in ethnic and religious identity, gender role conflicts, intergenerational conflict within the family, and the experiences of discrimination and social exclusion (Pacione et al., 2013). In addition, refugee or asylum seeker claimants may be involved in lengthy negotiations with the legal system to avoid rejection of their claim and forced repatriation (Steel et al., 2011). However, the sad reality is that most child refugees and asylum seekers do not obtain asylum, remaining in refugee camps or their countries of origin (Feseha et al., 2012).

HUMAN TRAFFICKING

The Trafficking Victims Violence Prevention Act (TVPA, 2000) describes human trafficking as a form of modern-day slavery, "the act of recruitment, harboring, transportation, provision, or obtaining of a person for the purpose of a commercial sex act" (§ 103). The International Labour Organization (ILO, 2014) highlights human trafficking as the world's third most profitable criminal enterprise, with annual profits estimated at $150 billion. Economic marginalization and poverty, social isolation, social services breakdown, political instability, educational inopportunity, and rampant violence throughout different nations create a readily available supply of victims (U.S. Department of State, 2019). Forced labor, prostitution, and other forms of sexual exploitation, slavery, and organ removal ensue as forms of exploitation for which persons may be trafficked. Each of these categories involves the use of force, fraud, or coercion. Figure 12.2 illustrates the Human Trafficking Power and Control Wheel developed by the Polaris Project (2010).

The U.S. Department of State (2019) Trafficking in Persons Report estimated a global 24.9 million victims of trafficking, with 5.5 million of them reported as children under the age of 18. Although the average age falls between 11 and 14 years of age, traffickers continue to prey on victims as young as 9 (U.S. Department of State, 2019). Minor victims appear to be trafficked through social media websites, telephone chat lines, and after-school programs; at shopping malls and bus stops; in clubs; or through friends or acquaintances who recruit students on school campuses. Unfortunately, these numbers may be inexact since obtaining accurate estimates of prevalence and trends of human trafficking among children remain challenging. The main problem with human trafficking appears to be its

Sex Trafficking
street/online prostitution, residential/commercial-front brothels, truck stops
Labor Trafficking
businesses, farms, domestic work, begging/peddling, stripping
COERCION and THREATS
Threatens to harm victim or family • Threatens to expose or shame victim • Threatens to report to police or immigration
INTIMIDATION
Harms other victims, children or pets • Displays or uses weapons • Destroys property • Lies about police involvement in trafficking situation
EMOTIONAL ABUSE
Humiliates in front of others • Calls names • Plays mind games • Makes victim feel guilt/blame for situation • Convinces victim they're the only one that cares about them
ISOLATION
Keeps confined • Accompanies to public places • Creates distrust of police/others • Moves victims to different locations • Doesn't allow victim to learn English or to go to school • Denies access to children, family and friends
DENYING, BLAMING, MINIMIZING,
Makes light of abuse or exploitation • Denies that anything illegal or exploitative is occurring • Places blame on the victim for the trafficking situation
SEXUAL ABUSE
Uses sexual assault as punishment or means of control • Forces victim to have sex multiple times a day with strangers • Treats victim as an object for monetary gain • Normalizes sexual violence and selling sex
PHYSICAL ABUSE
Shoves, slaps, hits, punches, kicks, strangles • Burns, brands, tattoos • Denies food/water • Exposes to harmful chemicals • Forces pregnancy termination • Induces drug addiction as means of control
USING PRIVILEGE
Treats victim like a servant • Uses gender, age or nationality to suggest superiority • Uses certain victims to control others • Hides or destroys important documents
ECONOMIC ABUSE
Creates debt that can never be repaid • Takes money earned • Prohibits access to finances • Limits resources to a small allowance
POWER & CONTROL

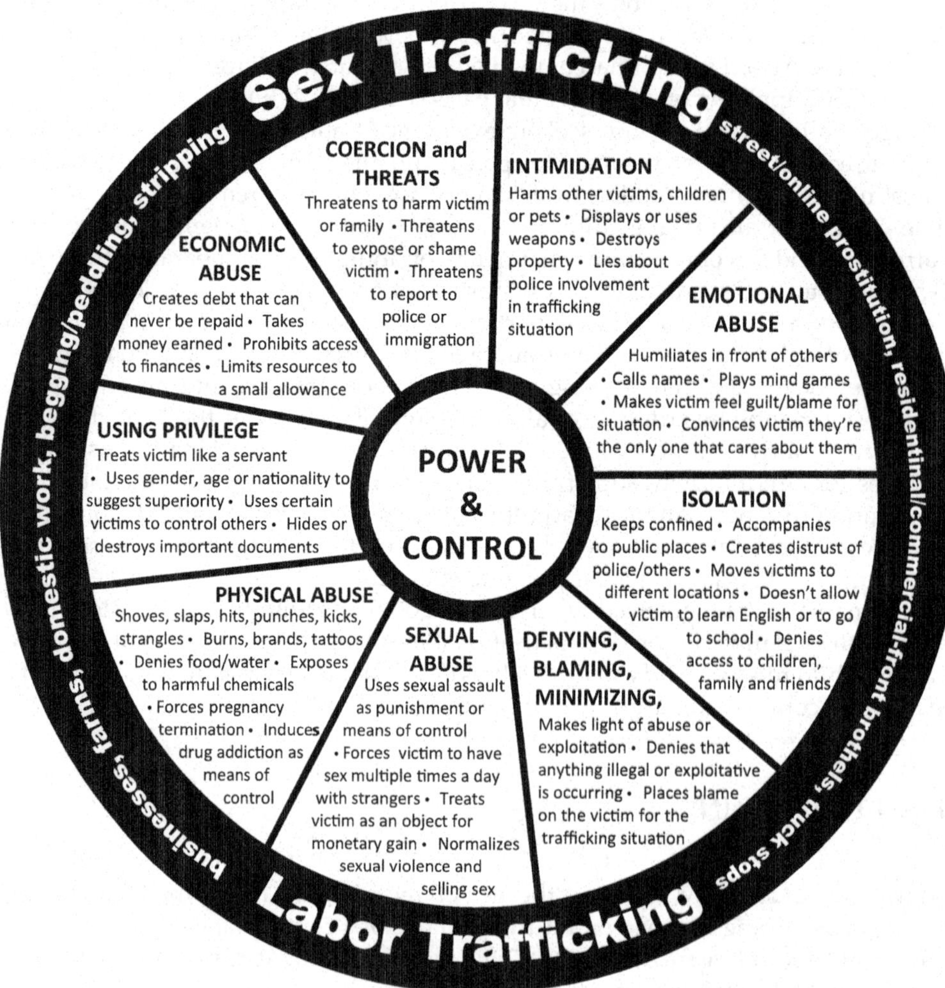

FIGURE 12.2 Human Trafficking Power and Control Wheel.

Source: Reproduced with permission from Polaris Project. (2010). Human trafficking power and control wheel. https://humantraffickinghotline.org/sites/default/files/HT%20Power%26Control%20Wheel%20NEW.pdf

invisible nature. Tactics of coercion and force prevent victims from coming forward based on fear, safety, participation in illegal activities (e.g., underage drinking, prostitution, or drug use), and necessity to meet their basic needs. Human trafficking results in profound adverse effects on trafficked youth's well-being. Trafficked individuals can experience multiple types of violence and abuse (e.g., sexual, physical, and emotional), unsafe living and work conditions, isolation, and malnutrition, substance use, legal and immigration issues, economic and housing challenges, and difficulties reintegrating into society (Ottisova et al., 2016). We further discuss two of the most common and concerning issues affecting today's youth: labor and child sex trafficking.

Labor Trafficking

Labor trafficking refers to the use of force, fraud, or coercion to induce an individual into one of many forms of forced labor situations, including involuntary servitude and debt bondage (U.S. Department of State, 2019). *Involuntary servitude* refers to a condition of servitude induced by one of two types of threats. In the first type, a trafficker threatens to harm an individual, or one or more members of their family, if the victim does not provide some form of work. In the second type, the trafficker threatens to report the victim to legal authorities (U.S. Department of State, 2019). Most trafficked laborers within the United States appear to be undocumented workers. Estimation statistics for labor-trafficked victims appear to be around 16 million, with 7.5 million (47%) forced to work in construction, manufacturing, mining, or hospitality (e.g., food or hotel service, tourist work); 3.8 million (24%) forced into domestic servitude situations, such as maids and nannies; and 1.7 million (11%) forced to work in agriculture (ILO, 2014). Such operations tend to thrive in states where large immigrant communities and populations exist, such as Florida, New York, California, and Texas (ILO, 2014).

Sex Trafficking

The TVPA (2000) defines sex trafficking among youth as "a commercial sex act induced by force, fraud, or coercion, or in which the person induced to perform such an act has not attained 18 years of age" (§ 103). Although the extent of this epidemic problem remains unknown, 67.3% of the United States and U.S. territories charged at least one human trafficking case in 2018, of which over half (51.6%) categorized as sex trafficking cases involved only child victims (Human Trafficking Institute, 2018). Types of sex trafficking among youth include commercial sexual exploitation, pimp-controlled trafficking, gang-related trafficking, survival sex, familial trafficking, and forced marriages. Populations at risk include children and adolescents who come from racial and ethnic minorities, part of the LGBTQ community, lower socioeconomic status, foster care, and those with cognitive and physical disabilities, or foreign-born (Human Trafficking Institute, 2018). Sex trafficked youth may experience untreated wounds, scars, and bruises on their bodies. They sometimes present with complex physical health problems that appear to be dermatologic, neurologic, musculoskeletal, gastrointestinal, and/or gynecologic in nature (Oram et al., 2012). Limited precautions to engage in safe sexual practices leave sex trafficked youth exposed to unwanted pregnancies, sexually transmitted disease, and infections including HIV/AIDS, chlamydia, genital warts, genital herpes, urinary tract infections, scabies, gonorrhea, syphilis, human papillomavirus (which causes cervical cancer), and hepatitis

A, B, and C (Banović & Bjelajac, 2012). Sex trafficking also correlates highly with different forms of substance use, mental health diagnosis, and suicidal behavior (Cole et al., 2016).

ASSESSMENT OF TRAUMA AMONG CHILDREN AND ADOLESCENTS

Early identification and assessment of PTSD or other trauma-related symptoms in children and adolescents remain extremely important. As previously discussed, untreated trauma symptoms can lead to many poor social, behavioral, cognitive, physical, and psychological outcomes. Assessment in counseling remains an objective and systematic ongoing process that involves some type of measurement, the gathering of samples of behavior, and the integration and interpretation of information. Counselors can obtain such information through a variety of methods, measures, and sources. Assessment is an ongoing process that remains integral to the counseling process as it helps determine presenting concern(s), enables us to conceptualize and define the problem, aids the development of the treatment plan, and affords an opportunity to evaluate change over time.

THREAT ASSESSMENT VERSUS MENTAL HEALTH ASSESSMENT

Threat assessment addresses a communicated threat made to determine the lethality of the threat and apply interventions to mitigate the risk to person, school, and community. Threat assessment promotes a fact-based problem-solving approach to violence prevention that uses a set of investigative and operational activities that focuses on threats and other forms of conflict before escalation into violent behavior (Fein et al., 1995). This includes three essential steps: identify, assess, and manage individuals who appear to be at risk for violence (e.g., self-harm, assault, risk-taking behaviors, suicide, substance abuse, other aggressive or dangerous behaviors) against themselves or others. The goal of the threat assessment process transpires as preventive, not punitive. However, mental health assessments focus on evaluating mental health concerns and providing a differential diagnosis and treatment recommendations. When used in conjunction with a threat assessment, the mental health assessment identifies any mental health needs, identifies reasons for the threat, and proposes strategies for reducing risk.

TRAUMA ASSESSMENTS: THE SIGNALING OF SOMETHING WRONG

Though more specific assessments for various populations, contexts, and identified types of trauma that an individual may experience (e.g., domestic violence, sex trafficking) exist, more general trauma assessments can be found. This section provides a brief review of standardized instruments appropriate for assessing PTSD and other trauma-related symptoms in children and adolescents. Table 12.1 presents a listing of select child and adolescent trauma instruments counselors may use in the assessment process. It is important to mention that this is not a comprehensive review and counselors should review other available measures and use clinical judgment when selecting an appropriate assessment. Also, when selecting a suitable instrument, the assessment should be both reliable and valid. Thus, this section also highlights psychometric properties for each instrument reviewed.

TABLE 12.1 TRAUMA ASSESSMENT TOOLS FOR CHILDREN AND ADOLESCENTS

Assessment	Reference
Adolescent Dissociative Experiences Scale	Armstrong et al. (1997)
Child Dissociative Checklist	Putnam et al. (1993)
Child PTSD Symptom Scale	Foa et al. (2001)
Clinician-Administered PTSD Scale for *DSM-5* Child/ Adolescent Version	Pynoos et al. (2015)
Posttraumatic Stress Symptoms in Children	Ahmad et al. (2000)
PTSD Symptoms in Preschool-Age Children	Levendosky et al. (2002)
Trauma System Checklist for Children	Briere (1996)
Trauma Symptom Inventory	Briere et al. (1995)
UCLA Child/Adolescent PTSD Reaction Index for *DSM-5*	Elhai et al. (2013); Steinberg et al. (2013)

DSM-5, Diagnostic and Statistical Manual of Mental Disorders, Fifth Edition; PTSD, posttraumatic stress disorder; UCLA, University of California at Los Angeles.

University of California at Los Angeles Child/Adolescent Posttraumatic Stress Disorder Reaction Index for *DSM-5*

The University of California at Los Angeles (UCLA) Child/Adolescent PTSD Reaction Index for *DSM-5* (PTSD-RI-5; Elhai et al., 2013; Steinberg et al., 2013) can be used as a diagnostic tool and to monitor client progress. The PTSD-RI-5 assesses posttrauma symptoms and the *DSM-5* PTSD diagnostic criteria in youth aged 6 to 17. This instrument consists of a comprehensive trauma history section, 27-item PTSD symptom scale with an additional four items to assess the Dissociative Subtype of PTSD, frequency rating sheet, and a distress and impairment functioning section. Doric et al. (2019) studied psychometric properties of translated versions of the PTSD-RI-5 with adolescents from 11 countries. Alternate versions consist of the UCLA PTSD-RI-5 for Children Age 6 and Younger and the UCLA Brief Screen for Child/Adolescent Trauma and PTSD.

Clinician-Administered Posttraumatic Stress Disorder Scale for *DSM-5* Child/ Adolescent Version

The Clinician-Administered PTSD Scale for *DSM-5* Child/Adolescent Version (CAPS-CA-5; Pynoos et al., 2015) contains a semistructured, 30-item, clinician administered assessment. This instrument assesses *DSM-5* PTSD and associated symptoms in children and adolescents aged seven and older. The CAPS-CA-5 consists of an administration time of 45 minutes and includes standardized questions and probes for each PTSD symptom. The CAPS-CA-5 demonstrates adequate internal consistency (r = .89), interrater reliability (r = .80), and convergent validity (r = .51) with the PTSD-RI-5.

Trauma Symptom Checklist for Children

The Trauma System Checklist for Children (TSCC; Briere, 1996) consists of a self-report instrument developed for children aged 7 to 16 years. While the TSCC is not designed for use as a diagnostic tool, it measures trauma-related symptoms using 54 items rated on a four-point Likert-type scale (0 = never to 3 = almost all of the time). The TSCC contains a 15- to 20-minute administration time and consists of six clinical scales (Anxiety, Depression, Anger, PTS, Dissociation, and Sexual Concerns), four subscales (Overt Dissociation, Fantasy Dissociation, Sexual Preoccupation, and Sexual Distress), and two validity scales. Counselors use the TSCC in assessing symptoms after sexual abuse. The TSCC demonstrates alpha coefficients ranging from .77 to .89 in the standardization sample, and normative and clinical samples demonstrate adequate convergent, divergent, and predictive validity (Briere, 1996).

Alternate forms of the TSCC can be found. For example, the Trauma Symptom Checklist for Young Children (TSCYC; Briere, 2005), a 90-item caretaker report, measures PTSD and other trauma-related symptoms in children aged 3 to 12 years. The TSCYC contains eight clinical subscales (PTS-Intrusion, PTS-Avoidance, PTS-Arousal, Sexual Concerns, Anxiety, Depression, Dissociation, Anger), a summary PTS scale, PTS total, and validity scales to measure reliability of responses. The TSCYC demonstrates good reliability, with alpha coefficients ranging from .81 to .93, as well as adequate convergent validity and predictive validity for childhood trauma (Briere, 2005).

Moreover, the profession provides a Trauma Symptom Checklist for Young Children Screening Form (TSCYC-SF) and Trauma System Checklist for Children Screening Form (TSCC-SF). Diagnosticians consider both to be screening tools with a 5-minute administration time. These screening forms identify young children aged 3 to 12 (TSCYC-SF) and children aged 8 to 16 (TSCC-SF) who experienced trauma. Derived from the TSCC and TSCYC, the screening forms consist of 20-item instruments with two subscales—general trauma (12 items) and sexual concerns (eight items).

ADDRESSING TRAUMA USING TRAUMA-INFORMED INTERVENTIONS

TRAUMA-INFORMED CARE

Early identification, remediation, education, and intervention remain essential in alleviating and preventing the negative symptoms associated with trauma exposure in youth. Professionals characterize approaches such as medication, psychological first aid, cognitive behavioral therapy, and eye movement desensitization and reprocessing (EMDR) as effective in promoting healthy recovery from traumatic stress. Common elements of trauma-informed interventions include emotion awareness and regulation strategies in addition to skills training and practice. The following section discusses teaching youth to recognize physiologic cues to enhance self-awareness, activities for teaching self-regulation, and teaching mindfulness skills for self-regulation.

Teaching Self-Awareness

Teaching children to recognize physiologic cues creates opportunity for youth to utilize a range of coping skills to manage feelings and emotions more successfully. Counselors can achieve this by teaching children to identify the behavioral (e.g., easily distracted; throws tantrums), cognitive (e.g., "I will never be safe"; "I hate them"), and physiologic (e.g., shortness of breath; face gets hot) components of various types of emotions (e.g., disgust; joy; fear), especially their own. For example, using a thermometer analogy, one can teach youth to assess various levels of emotion intensity they may experience (e.g., disappointed [very low level of sadness], defeated [medium level of sadness], hopeless [very high level of sadness]) and different types of problems that trigger these different levels of intensity (e.g., *"when other children make fun of me,"* "when my dad yells at me for doing something wrong"; Lochman et al., 2008). After achieving a basic introduction and review of physiologic cues, emotions, and triggers, children then practice noticing and describing situational triggers and intensities (e.g., "I felt a little cheerful when my mom packed my favorite snack for lunch"; "I felt medium happy when my big sister let me borrow her necklace"). Counselors can also assign homework for practice and reinforcement of skills learned.

Teaching Emotional Regulation

Self-regulation targets youth's ability to identify, modulate, and express internal experiences. Individual and group counseling strategies for emotion regulation include distraction techniques, relaxation exercises, and coping self-statements. Counselors teach distraction techniques as means to divert attention away from triggering situations. Guided imagery, deep breathing, and progressive muscle relaxation techniques promote regulation of physiologic responses and prevent escalation. Finally, coping self-statements (e.g., "I can handle this. I just need to cool off first"; "Slow down and focus on breathing") can be taught through a series of in vivo activities designed to be increasingly more realistic. Coping statements consist of those things that we say to ourselves (i.e., thoughts that we think to ourselves) that help us stay calm or calm down (Stromeyer et al., 2020). Counselors may use individual and group role plays in a safe and controlled environment to practice these emotional regulation strategies. Improving youth's ability to effectively communicate emotional experiences will enable the formation and maintenance of healthy relationships and attachments.

Teaching Mindfulness

Exposure to traumatic events at a young age can lead to negative developmental effects including maladaptive coping strategies to manage the negative affective experiences (Perry-Parrish & Sibinga, 2014). As mentioned in Chapter 6, mindfulness interventions can target regulation of emotion and coping processes associated with stress (Perry-Parrish & Sibinga, 2014). Research on mindfulness interventions with children shows effects in reducing anxiety, rumination, depression, stress, and emotional arousal, increasing self-efficacy in emotional regulation (Metz et al., 2013), and PTSD and other trauma-related symptoms (Gordon et al., 2008).

Generally speaking, mindfulness practice (e.g., breath awareness, yoga) may be appropriate for children as young as kindergarten and appears to be associated with improvement in attention, emotion regulation, self-awareness, and behavior resulting in structural changes in several brain regions (Holzel et al., 2010). Mindfulness practice can be integrated into existing counseling processes (Miller et al., 2020) and entails a range of techniques that help foster an intentional focusing of attention on one's present-moment experience while letting go of negative, counterproductive thought processes (Kabat-Zinn, 2015). Counselors might consider integrating activities from the following categories into their counseling process: (a) sensory experiences (e.g., mindful eating, guided imagery); (b) body awareness (e.g., walking meditation, simple yoga poses); (c) breath awareness (e.g., belly breathing, timed breath awareness); and (d) mindfulness of thoughts and nonjudgmental acceptance of feelings. One suggestion for the integration of mindfulness into one's work with children and adolescents is to be habitual and consistent in both language and practice.

CREATIVE INTERVENTIONS

Following a traumatically stressful experience, children may experience trouble understanding and expressing their thoughts and feelings. Counselors may find the integration and use of more creative interventions beneficial in increasing youths' self-awareness and need for self-expression. The Association for Creativity in Counseling (ACC) defines creativity in counseling as the "shared counseling process involving growth-promoting shifts that occur from an intentional focus on the therapeutic relationship and the inherent human creative capacity to affect change" (Duffey et al., 2016, p. 448). Creativity in counseling makes use of the full range of human expression, imagination, and resourcefulness to help clients address issues. Different mediums may facilitate conversations about trauma when verbal expression may be difficult. Creative methods include, but are not limited to, dance movement therapy, music therapy, play activity, animal-assisted therapy, bibliotherapy, using a sand tray, and art therapy. Creative approaches can be used to complement and enhance other theoretical approaches and may assist in helping a "stuck" client move forward (Duffey et al., 2016).

SUPPORT GROUPS

Support groups or group therapy appear to be helpful interventions when working with youth, particularly adolescents. The benefits of a group format include the contention that groups reduce social isolation (Hoskins et al., 2018). By sharing personal stories, support group members validate each other's understanding of and reactions to the abuse (Hoskins et al., 2018). Deblinger et al. (2001) indicated that group formats can also help destigmatize therapy. Across several studies on support groups, group therapy improved self-esteem, anger levels, anxiety, and depression (Abel, 2000). Furthermore, ethnic minority youth report statistically significant improvements between PTSD symptoms, depressed mood, and anxiety symptoms and share positive experiences in group formats because students share similar cultural values, traditions, and the same language as the other group members (Hoskins et al., 2018). Notwithstanding these advantages, school settings lack clearly delineated procedures for referring, assessing, and conducting support groups for children and adolescents. Given the sensitive nature of traumatic and bereavement experiences, a one-on-one interview with the school counselor before joining a group format can be advantageous. However, we recognize that conducting an in-depth individual assessment with all referred youth can be impractical given competing demands and funding resources for school counselors. In addition, many groups and online relationships also serve as means for communication, support, information, and targeted interventions to help youth in crisis. Numerous websites allow children and adolescents to connect with each other and obtain information that will help them during crises, stressors, suicidal thoughts, and disasters. The National Suicide Hotline, the National Child Traumatic Stress Network, and the Red Cross serve as examples of sites that provide information online to help those in crisis.

PROVIDING REFERRALS

Being mindful that each individual's trauma will appear unique and recovery takes time, school personnel must also know when and how to seek professional assistance. If after an extended time (3–6 months) prolonged reactions that inhibit effective functioning persist, professional attention may be warranted. Professional school counselors do not diagnose students from a *DSM-5* type perspective. Professional school counselors may extend referrals to clinical mental health counselors, school psychologists, psychiatrists, and other outside mental health professionals if needed. Parents and teachers need to know the school's referral process: how to report their concerns, whom to turn to, and how to access support.

ADDITIONAL CONSIDERATIONS FOR SCHOOL COUNSELORS

SOCIAL–EMOTIONAL HEALTH AND ACADEMIC SUCCESS

The link between social–emotional health and academic success remains strong in American schools (Guzman et al., 2011). Children and adolescents' social and emotional development occurs in environmental or systemic contexts and schools rank high as major systemic, multicultural, relational, and developmental influences on students. Schools provide students an opportunity to not only grow academically; they also strive to prepare students to grow in life. As stated earlier in this chapter, trauma exposure produces far-reaching impacts and presents immediate and long-term difficulties for school-age children and adolescents. At school, the harmful impacts of trauma serve as impediments to academic and career success in the school setting. Considering this strong correlation between mental health and academic achievement, the finding appears predictable that mental health disorders account for as much as 46% of school dropouts (Guzman et al., 2011). Constant attempts to transform schools into emotionally responsive environments remain imperative.

THE ROLE OF PROFESSIONAL SCHOOL COUNSELORS

Schools throughout America recognize the importance of providing school-based mental health support for identified students at risk; and professional school counselors play an increasingly important role in creating developmental, systemic, multicultural, and relational contexts to help youth cope with the challenges of growing up. Students benefit in a variety of ways from the guidance and counseling services provided by professional school counselors. As mentioned in Chapter 9, professional school counselors assess students academically, socially, and emotionally; obtain an adequate understanding of this assessment; monitor trauma symptoms and functioning; make appropriate clinical decisions about guidance and counseling; and connect students with appropriate therapeutic treatments and resources (American School Counselor Association [ASCA], 2019; Gysbers & Henderson, 2013; Texas Education Agency [TEA], 2018). Professional school counselors' ability to organize, lead, and implement mental health screening in schools remains consistent with many of the School Counselor Competencies put forth by ASCA (2019).

Optimistically, brain research highlights practical strategies that can assist educators in working with students in regulating their behavior and fostering success at school. Trauma-exposed students need a sense of immediate safety, and positive relationships remain imperative to restore the students' path to effective goals for learning. As previously stated in this chapter, neuroplasticity research highlights the fact that the brain can rewire itself and cultivate new ways of coping. When dealing with trauma-reactive behavior, educators should seldom start with logical reasoning. Innovative strategies must work from the bottom up, addressing the emotional side of the brain first—the amygdala, and then progressing to the higher brain—the prefrontal lobe. Adults around trauma-exposed students can foster this rewiring by implementing simple but often overlooked interventions designed to change neural pathways (e.g., remaining patient, consistent, and very much in control of their own emotions). Adults' calmness restores a sense of safety in students. With this, counselors can form effective workable relationships and reason with traumatized students (Gysbers & Henderson, 2013). Again, tangible changes become possible when students feel safe enough to develop these relationships, which promotes their ability to process situations in the prefrontal lobe brain using language (Fecser, 2015).

WHAT SCHOOLS CAN DO TO HELP TRAUMATIZED STUDENTS

School culture sets the tone for many interactions (ASCA, 2019). Osher and Fleishman (2005) presented key factors necessary for positive school culture: (a) connectedness; (b) behavioral support; and (c) social and emotional skills. Additionally, ASCA listed strong leadership, high expectations, collaborative decision-making, order and discipline, parent/community involvement, and careful and continuous evaluation as central factors for focused school culture improvements.

School crises that evoke trauma (e.g., death of a student or teacher, school bus or car accident, acts of terrorism, and school shootings) can be disruptive and involve grief and loss, while also undermining the safety and stability of a campus (Gysber & Henderson, 2013). Professional school counselors utilize a range of leadership roles to support campus needs. They possess both the training and job roles to create schoolwide interventions addressing student behavior using a theoretical and development framework (Fecser, 2015; TEA, 2018). Professional school counselors, parents, school administrators, support staff, and other mental health workers should work collaboratively and listen to and support trauma-impacted students. Researchers (Gysbers & Henderson, 2013) suggest using the following pointers to assist traumatized students in diminishing feelings of isolation, increasing feelings of connectedness, and supporting students academically, personally, socially, and emotionally.

First, schools should organize and implement a campus-based crisis plan that can provide opportunities to galvanize social and emotional support within the school community. Schools should predetermine an action plan that assumes a proactive and preventive mode, train staff to respond with corrective intervention techniques, and offer a wide range of support that increases school stability in order to remain effective. Second, school administrators should obtain parental consent by sending a letter (or providing opportunities to do this via student handbooks) to parents at the beginning of each school year. This informs parents about student access to immediate counseling support services during and following school-related crises. Third, school and professional counselors should be trained on culturally sensitive, trauma-informed care and should train other school personnel on the effects and symptoms of trauma and grief with an understanding of how to respond using a cultural framework. Fourth, trusted adults whom students may contact to discuss their feelings, concerns, and frustrations regarding a traumatizing event should escort these students to the school counselor (Garbarino et al., 2002). Garbarino and colleagues further suggest that provisions be made to allow teachers and professional school counselors to participate in genuine classroom discussions about the importance of maintaining confidentiality and embracing diversity. Fifth, trauma-informed approaches and training must be put in place to support students and their overall personal safety and to provide resources aimed at student needs. In doing so, schools develop leaders who can assist students socially, emotionally, and academically. Sixth, professional school counselors should provide a variety of supportive, age-appropriate, and culturally sensitive activities or modes of expression (e.g., journal writing, drawing, cards or poster creations, music, brainstorm ideas to offer support, bibliotherapy, memory book). Finally, the school community should promote individual and small support groups facilitated by professional school counselors.

BUILDING CULTURE IN THE ENTIRE SCHOOL THROUGH SCHOOL-BASED INTERVENTIONS

In schools, negative behavior results in negative consequences typically in the form of punishment. Punishment-based discipline used on traumatized students triggers responses that exacerbate the matter (Garbarino et al., 2002). Students better regulate their brains when they feel safe with a sense of control and perceive predictable outcomes. Under perceived threatening or adverse conditions, the amygdala in a traumatized student sidesteps the prefrontal lobe inhibiting real learning (Fecser, 2015). A positive relationship between an adult and a traumatized student appears to be a powerful determinant in managing oppositional behavior. Consequently, this reorganizes the traumatized brain and promotes more productive student choices.

Fecser (2015) offers the following school-based strategies for traumatized students: (a) Encourage adults to demonstrate empathy and understand the function of traumatizing behavior. (b) Encourage adults to maintain a calm demeanor, which fosters more student compliance. A reactive and domineering adult creates oppositional and defiant behavior in a trauma-exposed student. (c) Provide structure, predictability, and routine. This minimizes unnecessary manipulation and defiance. (d) Give students opportunities to engage in frequent movement and rhythm breaks (i.e., done through music, dancing, drumming, or poetry). Traumatized students thrive on this in that this regulates the amygdala leading to better processing, increased focus, and learning in the prefrontal lobe (Perry & Szalavitz, 2006). (e) Provide acceptable choices whenever possible to instill a sense of control. This fosters a sense of power and minimizes motivation to exercise power in oppositional ways. (f) Inform traumatized children about the operation of their brains. This provides an understanding of why they feel so insecure or can so easily lose their tempers. Such an explanation provides comfort in knowing about options to calm the amygdala.

CHAPTER SUMMARY

Trauma work with children and adolescents remains challenging on all levels and becomes increasingly complex when violence permeates various domains of life. Although all traumatic situations can disrupt a child's life, understanding categories of trauma and their unique, yet at times interwoven, impact on children and adolescents allows counselors to select effective interventions. Counselors must also consider the reciprocal relationships between trauma and neurologic, psychological, social, cultural, and systemic factors that alleviate or exacerbate the experience of trauma. Early identification, assessment, and intervention remain critical components of trauma recovery. The inclusion of trauma-informed interventions such as emotional awareness and regulation, as well as mindfulness skills, can help children and adolescents diminish symptoms that overwhelm internal coping mechanisms. Other interventions found to effectively address trauma among children and adolescents include creative interventions and support groups. The author provided special considerations for professional school counselors in this book, with special attention to the link between social-emotional health and academic success, the role of professional counselors, and the importance of school-based interventions to address trauma among children and adolescents.

POINTS TO REMEMBER

- Children and adolescents may perceive an event as traumatic without actual or threatened death, serious injury, or sexual violence to oneself or others.
- Children and adolescents can experience acute, chronic, complex, and historical trauma.
- Trauma symptoms vary based on child's age and development, yet the pervasiveness of trauma can be seen physically, emotionally, socially, and psychologically.
- The brain's development and function may be altered by trauma and can be seen through the dysregulation of the stress response system.
- Trauma, especially of the sort arising from interpersonal violence and exploitation, can disrupt early attachment, which determines the youth's ability to develop and maintain relationships in their early and later years of life.
- Environmental and behavioral factors should be considered within schools and classrooms due to trauma's impact on learning.
- Psychological, social, physical, cultural, and systemic factors that occur before or after trauma may directly or indirectly affect a youth's vulnerability to traumatic stress and risk for mental health disorder.
- The most prevalent and concerning trauma experienced by today's youth includes abuse, bullying, community violence, exposure to violent crimes, and human trafficking.
- The inclusion of trauma-informed interventions such as emotional awareness and regulation, as well as mindfulness skills, can help children and adolescents diminish symptoms that overwhelm internal coping mechanisms.

OTHER HELPFUL INFORMATION FOR CONSIDERATION

OTHER TRAUMA BOOKS

- Duffey, T., & Haberstroh, S. (2020). *Introduction to crisis and trauma counseling.* American Counselor Association.
- Fisher, S. F. (2014). *Neurofeedback in the treatment of developmental trauma: Calming the fear-driven brain.* W. W. Norton & Company.
- Judith, H. (1992). *Trauma and recovery: The aftermath of violence—From domestic abuse to political terror.* Basic Books.

OTHER HELPFUL RESOURCES

- American Counseling Association (ACA) provides additional resources, articles, and books for counselor works with trauma: https://www.counseling.org/knowledge-center/mental-health-resources/resources-for-counselors-and-clients
- The SAMHSA provides Treatment Improvement Protocols (TIPs) for trauma-informed care: https://www.integration.samhsa.gov/clinical-practice/SAMSA_TIP_Trauma.pdf

QUESTIONS FOR FURTHER DISCUSSION

- In this chapter, we described neuroscience and trauma. What benefits for the counselor might there be for integrating neuroscience into clinical practice? What about benefits for the client?
- At the beginning of the chapter, we discussed Chelsea's case. What social, psychological, and cultural factors appear to be important to consider? How could you integrate interventions discussed in this chapter in your work with Chelsea?

KEY REFERENCES

Only key references appear in the print edition. The full reference list appears in the digital product on Springer Publishing Connect: connect.springerpub.com/content/book/978-0-8261-4764-6/part/part04/chapter/ch12

American School Counselor Association. (2019). *ASCA school counselor professional standards & competencies.* American School Counselor Association. https://www.schoolcounselor.org/getmedia/a8d59c2c-51de-4ec3-a565-a3235f3b93c3/SC-Competencies.pdf

Bremner, J. D. (2006). Traumatic stress: Effects on the brain. *Dialogues in Clinical Neuroscience, 8*(4), 445–461. https://doi.org/10.31887/DCNS.2006.8.4/jbremner

Cook, A., Spinazzola, J., Ford, J., Lanktree, C., Blaustein, M., Cloitre, M., DeRosa, R., Hubbard, R., Kagan, R., Liautaud, J., Mallah, K., Olafson, E., & van der Kolk, B. (2005). Complex trauma in children and adolescents. *Psychiatric Annals, 35*, 390–398. https://doi.org/10.3928/00485713-20050501-05

Fecser, M. E. (2015). Classroom strategies for traumatized, oppositional students. *Reclaiming Children and Youth, 24*(1), 21–24. http://www.icase.org/resources/Documents/Classroom%20Strategies%20for%20Traumatized,%20OppositionalStudents(1).pdf

Finkelhor, D., Tuner, H. A., Shattuck, A., & Hamby, S. L. (2015). Prevalence of childhood exposure to violence, crime, and abuse. *The Journal of the American Medical Association Pediatrics, 169*(8), 746–754. https://doi.org/10.1001/jamapediatrics.2015.0676

Polaris Project. (2010). Human trafficking power and control wheel. https://humantraffickinghotline.org/sites/default/files/HT%20Power%26Control%20Wheel%20NEW.pdf

Substance Abuse and Mental Health Services Administration. (2014b). *Trauma-informed care in behavioral health services. Treatment Improvement Protocol (TIP) Series 57*. HHS Publication No. (SMA) 13-4801. Substance Abuse and Mental Health Services Administration.

van der Kolk, B. A. (2003). The neurobiology of childhood trauma and abuse. *Child and Adolescent Psychiatric Clinics of North America, 12*(2), 293–317. https://doi.org/10.1016/s1056-4993(03)00003-8

van der Kolk, B. A. (2005). Developmental trauma disorder: Toward a rational diagnosis for children with complex trauma histories. *Psychiatric Annals, 35*(5), 401–408. https://doi.org/10.3928/00485713-20050501-06

van der Kolk, B. A. (2014). *The body keeps the score: Brain, mind, and body in the healing of trauma*. Viking.

CHAPTER 13

Techniques in Crisis Management Involving School-Age Children

Brenda Jones

LEARNING OBJECTIVES

After completing this chapter, the reader should be able to:

- Identify the elements for establishing crisis management, crisis responses, and crisis protocols.
- Demonstrate an understanding of the impact that critical incidents present to schools, children and adolescents, faculty and staff, parents, and the wider community.
- Establish an awareness of what needs to occur before, during, and after a crisis.

CACREP STANDARDS FOR THIS CHAPTER

- CACREP 2016: 2.F.1.b.c.d.e.j.k.l.; 2.a.d.g.h.; 3.e.f.g.h.i.; 5.b.e.f.h.i.j.k.; 7.d.j.; School Counseling: 5.G.2.a.b.d.e.f.g.j.k.; Clinical Mental Health Counseling: 5.C.2.f.g.j.
- CACREP 2009: II.G.1.b.c.d.h.i.j.; 2.a.b.f.; 3.c.f.; 5.a.b.e.f.g.; 7.f.; School Counseling: III.A.3.5.6.7.; C.6.; E.1.; A.2.; M.1.2.3.4.5.7.; O.1.2.4.; Clinical Mental Health Counseling: III.A.3.9.; C.1.6.8.9.; E.1.3.

INTRODUCTION

Children and adolescents spend a significant portion of their lives on school campuses. School professionals no longer perceive crisis experiences in schools and communities as rare occurrences. In today's world, schools and communities readily grasp the necessity for establishing crisis response protocols because the likelihood of critical incidents occurring on school campuses and in school communities appears to be inevitable. Crises come in many forms and magnitudes (small- and large-scale). Many events may spark a crisis. Catastrophic environmental occurrences (e.g., tornados, hurricanes, earthquakes, floods, and other natural disasters; acts of violence [including mass shootings on school campuses or in the community]; the accidental, natural, or unexpected death of a student, principal, teacher, or community leader; deployment in response to war or the threat of war; acts of domestic and international terrorism; suicide; and trauma, physical, and mental health concerns due to pandemics such as the coronavirus disease 2019 [COVID-19] pandemic) all presented as commonplace examples of critical incidents that may evolve into crisis experiences for children and adolescents. Crisis events may also come from shocking and disruptive occurrences in the lives of children (e.g., many children and adolescents across the United States archived in their memory the horrible experience of watching, in a gruesome and public display, an unarmed African American father, George Floyd, being suffocated by four police officers). Amid COVID-19, many experienced or witnessed profound disparities, sickness, hospital and death rates, food insecurities, academic disruptions, and intense fears of returning to face-to-face campus instruction. Countless watched loved ones die alone and bereaved in the absence of funerals or the opportunity to say goodbye. Mental health challenges (inaccessibility to adequate and immediate services) for many became as pronounced as academic and social challenges. Experiences such as these pose to the young observers serious and growing threats (real or vicarious) that may present far-reaching effects as they attempt to traverse their lived experiences.

Small-scale crises, as opposed to large-scale crises, usually involve fewer individuals with a much smaller magnitude. Although small-scale crisis events may not be profiled on national news, they warrant the attention from professionals who need to continuously recognize and respond to the reactions of trauma-exposed children and adolescents. School officials may manage small-scale crises without executing a schoolwide crisis plan. In contrast, it becomes necessary to implement this type of plan during large-scale crises. Regardless of the magnitude of the crisis, school professionals monitor the impacts that a crisis may have on emotions, psychological effects, behavior, and learning.

SCHOOL SHOOTINGS

As mentioned in Chapter 12, society no longer views schools as safe havens. Although today's youth live in an era of zero tolerance and gun-free school zones with security surveillance, print and visual media continues to unearth disruptions in academic and social environments in the form of high-profile gun violence and school shooting. Trends starting from the post-1970s continue on the increase, with 20 shootings in 1970 and 111 in 2019 (Statista, 2020). The frequent and intense publicity related to on-campus shootings of elementary, middle school, high school, and college/university-age students (coupled with the country's lack of consensus in adopting nationwide, commonsense gun control legislation and access to mental health services) appears to produce internalized desensitization in many individuals based on seemingly increasing numbing reactions. The shock value of such commonplace occurrences does not appear to be as strong and concerning as before.

NATURAL DISASTERS

The scientific world predicts that as climate warms, weather-related extremes may increase in frequency, intensity, timing, and magnitudes and may cause more natural disasters. Kousky (2016) indicates that children represent approximately half of those impacted by weather-related disasters (wildfires, floods, hurricanes, tornados) and may be more vulnerable and warrant more attention due to differing needs than adults. Natural disasters can present disproportionate, long-lasting harm to children and adolescents and may affect them through many interrelated pathways: loss of caregiver income; damage to physical health including injury and death; malnutrition caused by the disruption of food supplies; exposure to unhygienic conditions; lack of access to needed medical care and safe drinking water; psychological harm resulting from damage to homes and possessions; grief from loss of loved ones; neglect, abuse, and exploitation; breakdown in social networks; loss of sense of safety and security; and disruption to education through displacement (Kousky, 2016).

In their vulnerability, children and adolescents may depend on caregivers who, many times, may be unprepared or overwhelmed. Very young children lack the communication and cognitive processing skills needed in the absence of caregivers. Some require special care, nutrition, and supplies. The disaster may happen at a time in their development where health problems present long-term effects. Due to varying socioeconomic conditions, children may respond differently to the same circumstance, making crisis assessment difficult for campus professionals to systematically identify clear, causal linkages.

As mentioned in Chapter 12, whether being exposed to school violence, natural disasters, unexpected deaths, military deployment, or domestic and international terrorism, children may experience trauma through direct exposure, by witnessing occurrences, learning about occurrences, or through repeated exposure to disturbing details (American Psychiatric Association [APA], 2013). Counseling literature points to two important components of trauma exposure following a critical incident: physical proximity (varying degrees of closeness) and emotional proximity (individuals' closeness to victims or the perpetrator). *Emotional proximity* refers to relational connections with a friend, family member, or acquaintance of the victim or perpetrator who happens to be in the area during the event. Examples of *physical proximity* includes being in the building at the time of the violent act, sheltering in on-campus lockdown, or receiving care in areas of emergency response (Hughes et al., 2011). Deković et al. (2008) report that greater emotional proximity may result in grief and depression and greater physical proximity may result in bodily harm or death. Deković et al. also report that greater physical proximity may also cause internalizing reactions such as anxiety, depression, and avoidant coping. Research conducted by Brown and Goodman (2005) and Deković et al. found that more exposure to physical *and* emotional proximity to a traumatic event presents greater negative outcomes from the trauma.

WAR AND THREATS OF WAR

Brown and Goodman (2005) recap the various war engagements in the United States. During the first decade of the 21st century, America became consumed with two wars simultaneously—Iraq and the Afghanistan wars. Other wars included Enduring Freedom (2001–2011), Operations Iraqi Freedom (2003–2011), and New Dawn (2010–2011). These wars involved the largest call-up ever of American military troops and included an unprecedented number of women and members of the National Guard Reserve. Many lived in civilian communities and held civilian jobs.

Wars (and the threat of war) presented significant impacts on children and adolescents. Many family members experienced numerous deployments to meet the needs of these engagements. Barker and Berry (2009) revealed concerns relating to family reintegration. As mentioned in Chapter 10, changes in children's social environment may cause threats to healthy trajectories toward development. In young children, attachment problems became increasingly severe with each subsequent deployment. As mentioned in Chapter 1, as children's cognitive capabilities develop, they more clearly understand the danger and context of parental or other family members' combat deployment. Therefore, children's and adolescents' reactions to deployment and war vary depending on their level of development.

As mentioned in several other chapters in this book, counselors will need to implement effective support for youth impacted by war and deployment in order to reduce risks and strengthen protective and promotive factors. Many of these youth possess the internal capabilities to cope and adjust. Chapter 2 highlights the use of Bronfenbrenner's ecologic framework in the understanding of the cumulative and reciprocal influences of development. This approach may prove to be relevant and useful in assisting counselors in further understanding children and adolescents affected by deployment and war.

DOMESTIC AND INTERNATIONAL TERRORISM

Today's youth grow up in the shadows of domestic and international terrorism. Parents, school officials, and peers provide children information about most of these events; however, many of them learn about these events by watching live television or through various technological media. Whatever the learning format, the impact of terrorism differs from those of natural disasters.

Torabi and Seo (2004) state that both natural disasters and terrorist attacks, like most crises, usually come without warning and may present aftershock effects. The difference lies with the fact that meteorologists and other scientists may be able to recognize low points and signals for a clear ending for natural disasters. It becomes difficult, however, for officials to pinpoint an ending point when it comes to terrorist attacks. Terrorist attacks exacerbate situations in that they represent capricious deliberate acts characterized usually by political or ideological overtones with the goal of instilling fear and ongoing anxiety leading to wide-ranging consequences (Silver & Matthew, 2008). As mentioned throughout this book, exposures to disruptive events such as terrorist attacks elicit similar symptom responses as other critical incidents do—anxiety, generalized distress, reexperiencing of the event, and behavioral difficulties—and present detriments to healthy, normal development. As mentioned in Chapter 1, young children may be unable to process abstract concepts such as terrorism. Therefore, counselors should be mindful that children and adolescent's stress responses may be triggered by viewing the modeling of adult stress responses and reactions.

CRISIS, CRISIS MANAGEMENT, AND CRITICAL INCIDENTS

Slaikeu (1984) defines crisis as "a temporary state of upset and disorganization, characterized chiefly by an individual's inability to cope with a particular situation using customary methods of problem solving, and by the potential for a radically positive or negative outcome" (p. 13). Bundy et al. (2017) define crisis as "an organizational crisis—an event perceived by managers and stakeholders as highly salient, unexpected, and potentially disruptive—can threaten an organization's goals and have profound implications for its relationships with stakeholders" (p. 1661). Bundy et al. (2017) recognized that crises may be categorized into four primary characteristics: (a) They cause uncertainty, disruption, and change; (b) they can be harmful or threatening for organizations and stakeholders (Fediuk et al., 2012); (c) they can be described as behavioral phenomena where those affected construct their own meaning and responses (Coombs, 2010); and (d) they become parts of larger processes, rather than separate and distinct events (Jaques, 2009). These conditions may exert adverse effects on student learning and behavior, causing schools and communities to be in a state of unreadiness when children enter such states.

Crisis management broadly captures organizational leaders' actions and communication that attempt to reduce the likelihood of a crisis, work to minimize harm from a crisis, use their best professional judgment, and endeavor to reestablish order in the aftermath of a crisis (Bundy & Pfarrer, 2015). Schonfeld et al. (2002) describe three assumptions regarding managing crisis: (a) Even with ideal prevention plans in place, crisis will occur on school campuses; (b) crisis involves people (students, teachers, counselors, school administrators, support personnel, and the community) and individual or group responses to the rippling effect of the crisis event; and (c) the literature underscores the importance of advanced organizational preparedness where safety prevails as the utmost concern. (Schonfeld et al., 2002).

Clarke et al. (2014) and Valadez (2014) reveal that no national model for school-based crisis preparedness exists. Add to this, only 86.3% of U.S. school districts report developing a crisis plan, with only 25% indicating that their plans include provisions for children, adolescents, and adults with disabilities or special needs. All of this underscores the importance of the roles that professionals play in their work with children. In order to provide potentially urgent psychological, social, and emotional services that promote optimal physical and mental health, preparedness to meet the needs of all remains critical.

Northside Independent School District's [NISD] (2013) Guidance and Counseling Department Safe Schools Initiatives Program, San Antonio, Texas, developed an effective critical response plan and defined critical incidents as "any incident/situation, that potentially impacts or compromises the safety of the school, work setting, individuals, department, or community" (p. 7). The incident may occur at, in close proximity to, or far away from a school campus. NISD and Steele (2001) highlight two kinds of critical incidents: (a) *Acute* represents those that occur abruptly, unexpectedly, usually without warning (e.g., suicide; accidental, natural, or unexpected death of a student, principal, teacher, or community leader); and (b) *chronic*, which symbolizes a day-to-day problematic situation that in due course evolves into an unmanageable state (e.g., large-scale bullying and student fights). Either way, counselors characterize both as atypical situations that induce trauma and anxiety in students, teachers, counselors, school administrators, other support personnel, parents, and the community (Cowan & Rossen, 2013; Duffey & Haberstroh, 2020; Gysbers & Henderson, 2013; Jones et al., 2020). The focus of this chapter is on large-scale, acute crises, events, or incidents.

TRAUMA VERSUS GRIEF

Children and adolescents exposed to any critical incidents (small or large) may experience trauma and grief. Steele (2001) points to significant comparisons and contrasts between trauma and grief. Trauma reactions usually involve grief reactions. However, grief refers to a generalized reaction to sadness, whereas trauma connotes a generalized reaction to terror. Individuals' grief reactions may be displayed in public, while trauma reactions may not be so apparent in public. Grief-stricken individuals usually want to talk about what transpired. Trauma-exposed individuals typically do not. In grief, pain acknowledges the loss; in trauma, pain triggers immense terror, powerlessness, and loss of safety. Unlike grief, anger often becomes assaultive and destructive with trauma. Grief typically does not distort one's self-image, whereas trauma causes cognitive attacks and distortion to one's self-image. Lastly, grief usually does not involve trauma responses (e.g., flashbacks, shocking reactions, hyperarousal, and numbing effects), whereas trauma does. The counseling profession now offers many innovative trauma-informed strategies and techniques for counselors to use while intervening in the lives of trauma-exposed children. Chapter 12 covers in more detail these innovations for trauma- and grief-exposed children and adolescents.

Preparing for a crisis on a school campus includes implementing best practices prior to, during, and following an actual crisis (Gysbers & Henderson, 2013; Jones et al., 2020; NISD, 2013; Valadez, 2014). To optimize attempts to restore calmness in the aftermath of a crisis, schools and school districts must develop a crisis plan. Without this type of preparation, schools will encounter inconsistent and fragmented implementation measures and procedures resulting in many layers of ineffectiveness (Alba & Gable, 2011). Consequently, when addressing the matter of preparedness for any type of crisis, schools must adopt essential strategies to sustain a consistent state of readiness at all times, regardless of the size or location of the school district (Kano & Bourque, 2007). Professionals view members of the crisis team as key to effective implementation of the crisis plan. School district leaders, specifically the collaboration of campus principals, professional school counselors, school psychologists, and other professionals, play a critical implementation role and, if well prepared, will determine a school community's effectiveness in preparing for an inevitable crisis on campus.

ESSENTIAL CONSIDERATIONS FOR EFFECTIVE CRISIS PLANNING

Crisis response protocol teams usually include in the crisis plan certain fundamentals designed to effectively transmit strategic information into action. They include curriculum models, considerations for school culture and climate, threat assessment, and multiculturalism and diversity factors.

CURRICULUM

Although several curricula related to responding to critical incidents exist, the author advises counselor and school administrators to follow models deemed credible by the profession and those published in resources (e.g., textbooks and peer-reviewed journals) in the professional literature. NISD (2013) offers the following factors for an effective crisis protocol. (a) Prevention includes purposeful attempts to create and implement a healthy climate and a caring culture for a safe school environment. Prevention also involves the establishment of a sound system for effective communication. Schools must be open to the voices of diversity and promote inclusivity in the development of a culturally responsive, trauma-informed focus in the event of a crisis. Additionally, schools must promote a sense of safety by providing students access to mental health services conducted by professional school counselors. Professional school counselors represent possibilities for school community. They conduct needs assessments, which allows them to target areas for prevention and address them through individual or small-group counseling sessions, classroom guidance, and psychoeducation. Other areas to consider include positive discipline, effective behavioral interventions and support, and bullying prevention. (b) Preparedness involves assessing, in a timely manner, the crisis situation; developing an understanding of the emotional reactions so that an adequate conceptualization of the crisis can be made; informing campus principals who notify the district superintendent (or vice versa depending on who first receives notification); and convening and actively participating on the crisis team. Preparedness also involves coordinating the crisis protocols (checklists; rooms and logistical setups; preparation for faculty and staff; announcements; psychoeducational sessions; counseling for students, faculty, and staff; and handling inquiries from the media) and determining appropriate staff and parental notifications. Together, prevention and preparedness connect the actions and procedures that can be engaged prior to an event and foster effective responses to the crisis. (c) Response involves making preparations to stabilize the campus and reestablish normal routine. Approaching a response to crisis in this manner allows for an understanding of how and when all stakeholders can provide a holistic perspective of a comprehensive plan to decrease the chances of a crisis, handle an emergency with expertise should one occur, and stabilize the school for continued routine.

Brock (2011) offers another resource example: *PREPaRE,* a schoolwide crisis prevention and intervention training curriculum developed by the National Association of School Psychologists (NASP), which may be used in the development of a crisis team response plan. The PREPaRE model acronym outlines specific hierarchical and sequential steps: ***P***reventing and preparing for psychological trauma; ***Re***affirming physical health and perceptions of security and safety; ***E***valuating psychological risks; ***P***roviding interventions ***a***nd ***R***esponding to mental health needs; and ***E***xamining the effectiveness of crisis prevention and intervention (U.S. Department of Education, 2003). The PREPaRE model additionally stipulates specific response activities to assist students and staff instantaneously following a crisis. These activities include a three-pronged approach: (a) confirming physical health and perceptions of safety; (b) evaluating factors that induce psychological trauma such as exposure, threat perceptions, individual vulnerabilities, crisis responses, and coping behaviors; and (c) offering interventions that respond to the need of trauma-exposed individuals such as reestablishing social support systems, psychoeducation, instilling empowerment, and providing immediate first aid and mental health counseling (Brock, 2011). This curriculum may be adapted at the local level for varying school sizes and needs. The curriculum consists of training designed to assist schools in focusing on mental health needs during a crisis intervention and recovery and in creating systems to meet the safety and crisis prevention and preparedness needs of students, staff, and families. Additionally, the curriculum facilitates collaboration among school and community professionals and, in the aftermath of a critical incident, helps school leaders support school staff, parents, and the community in their caregiver roles.

SCHOOL CULTURE AND CLIMATE

When schools provide an emotionally healthy student body and staff access to supportive resources in times of need, they offer fewer chances for detrimental manifestations that lead to crisis (Cowan & Paine, 2013). Composed of many professionals trained with unique skills and experiences, school campuses retain the capability to purposefully create and implement a healthy climate and a caring culture for a safe school environment. This included school administrators, professional school counselors, school psychologists, classroom teachers (including those who teach students with disabilities and students with language barriers); school nurses, support personnel; the community (including parents and religious leaders to ensure culturally appropriate responses); and educational service centers, all working in collaboration with school district leaders and clinical mental health counselors. Most students and campus personnel do not understand, recognize, or know how to identify individuals' responses and reactions to a critical incident. Professional school counselors validate these experiences. They work collaboratively with the individuals listed earlier and provide instruction through curriculum, which addresses coping skills, self-esteem and resilience building, social skills development, conflict resolution, and violence prevention skills (Skiba et al., 2000). All of the individuals listed previously may deal with discontentment and conflict on campuses by addressing the needs of disgruntled students. They head initiatives that lead students to choose alternative strategies as outlets for their emotions as opposed to responding with self-defeating choices that produce undesirable outcomes (O'Neill et al., 2008). Upon completion of a crisis plan, the school should establish a sound system for effective communication.

THREAT ASSESSMENT

The practice of assessing threats in a rapidly changing environment on campus now becomes a fundamental course of action when preparing for a potential crisis. A threat assessment, executed by trained school staff, determines credible threats of self-harm or violence with the intent to harm others (National Association of School Psychologists [NASP], 2016). The NASP recommends that schools build threat assessment teams in a multidisciplinary manner and include mental health specialists in this effort. Comprehensive threat assessments should include an evaluation and categorization of a threat, as well as an appropriate response and intervention to the threat. The threat assessment should also be a part of a wide-ranging process in establishing and maintaining a safe school environment (NASP).

School culture also directly impacts how troubled students respond. It remains vital that this group of students be considered and served when creating a climate to prevent a school crisis (Madfis, 2013). As part of a threat assessment, schools should also make early efforts to identify potentially troubled or violent students, student bystanders, and those who experience prior victimization; identify deficits in student needs; involve families to collaborate in this effort; and provide students access to counseling services. Individuals or teams that implement threat assessments need intensive training to apply the essential skills for effectiveness (Harwood, 2007). These efforts promote a sense of belonging and promote effective communication and positive behaviors. Chapters 8 and 10 addressed other preventive measures for students at risk.

MULTICULTURAL CONSIDERATIONS

Society no longer views critical incidents as isolated events that happen only at urban schools. Large-scale, acute critical incidents occur in communities regardless of socioeconomic levels and ethnic or racial makeups, and include those in rural and suburban areas (Cowan & Rossen, 2013).

As mentioned in Chapter 12, counselors must consider the reciprocal relationships between trauma and culture. Statistics on rapidly changing demographics and cultural diversity in America underscores this point. According to the U.S. Census Bureau (2010), 40 million people classified themselves as foreign born. The overwhelming majority of the U.S. population (299.7 million, 97%) reported only one race. Of these, the largest group reported White alone representing 223.6 million (72%); Black or African American population totaled 38.9 million (13%); Asian Americans totaled 14.7 million (approximately 5%); American Indian and Alaska Native totaled 2.9 million (0.9%); and Native Hawaiian and Other Pacific Islander totaled 0.5 million (0.2%). The remaining population totaling 19.1 million (6%) classified themselves as "some other race." Of the total number of individuals who report only one race, 76.1 million (25.1%) classified themselves in categories other than non-Hispanic White. Add to this, 9 million (3%) reported more than one race, totaling 85.1 million (28.1%). Twenty-one percent of the U.S. population spoke a language other than English at home. The census identified over 40 religious affiliations. Of the socioeconomic brackets, 15.4% fell below the poverty level and 14% aged 18 and over reported not completing high school.

Marsella (2010) reminds us that culture facilitates the transmission of shared learned behavior from one generation to another. Culture promotes (through artifacts, roles, institutions, attitudes, epistemology, consciousness, and values and beliefs) individual and societal growth, adjustment, and adaptation in a cultural context. The U.S. Department of Veterans Affairs: National Center for PTSD (2014) reported that individuals may be more likely to experience posttraumatic stress disorder (PTSD) if they fall into the following categories: female, young, less educated, African American or Hispanic, little social support, and stressful life changes.

Culture may affect how individuals experience trauma including the severity of their symptoms. In the face of an acute critical event, experiences of trauma reactions differ from culture to culture. Linguistic, behavioral, and interpersonal practices derive from a constellation of a cultural socialization process and the storage of a response to stimuli that accumulated as a result of one's life experiences. Therefore, in the drafting, designing, and implementation of a crisis plan, the crisis team must strive to understand individuals in the context of life experiences and cultural backgrounds, recognize the impact of violence and victimization on development and coping skills, welcome the voices of diversity, and promote inclusivity of a culturally responsive, trauma-informed focus. Levels of diversity in the United States demonstrate the myriad of ways individuals and groups may construct their own meaning and reactions to a crisis situation. This also includes their thoughts and feelings about counseling and privacy. This requires relational collaboration (including trust and empowerment), input, and involvement in the designing and evaluation of the plan with all stakeholders in the community (Pow & Vladimir, 2015). In order to accomplish this, the school must take the stance of *cultural humility* (as mentioned in Chapter 3). Hook et al. (2013) define the construct of cultural humility as "having an interpersonal stance that is other-oriented rather than self-focused, characterized by respect and lack of superiority toward an individual's cultural background and experience" (p. 353). Taking the stance of cultural humility develops strong bonds in situations in which relationship partners may present a strong tendency to value their own perspectives regarding cultural differences. In order to develop strong partnerships (as mentioned in Chapters 3 and 4), the crisis team must be open to the beliefs, values, and worldview of stakeholders from diverse populations (Davis et al., 2013).

PREVENTING CRISES ON SCHOOL CAMPUSES

Critical incidents on school campuses hold a long-standing association with negative mental health outcomes. Many children and adolescents reveal scars and struggles that manifest in numerous ways (e.g., fear of attending school, recurring nightmares, the inability to focus, depressive symptoms, and substance abuse—all basically descriptions of posttraumatic stress; Connor, 2006; Su & Chen, 2015). Children now view differently the simple pleasure of playing with balloons and fireworks and respond quickly with startling reactions at the sound of loud, unexpected bursting blasts from these objects.

Preventive measures foster an environment in which students, faculty, staff, parents, and the community feel valued and empowered. These efforts also support optimal learning, access to mental health services, positive discipline, effective behavioral interventions and support, bullying prevention, and other school safety issues (Cowan & Rossen, 2013).

RELATIONAL CONSIDERATIONS

A crisis plan should include preventive measures as well as intervention measures needed to minimize the occurrence of a crisis. Gephart et al. (2009) and Bundy and Pfarrer (2015) identified two primary perspectives that focus on different aspects of crises and crisis management. The first perspective, *internal perspective* (leadership), concentrates on the within-organization dynamics of managing threats, potential complication, and technology. Additionally, they posit that crisis management involves the coordination of multifaceted methodologic and relational systems and organizational structural designs put in place to prevent the occurrence, minimize the impact, and discover knowledge from the crisis. Conversely, the second perspective, *external perspective* (stakeholder relationships), focuses on the interactions of school and community collaborators and engages in determining perceptions and collaborating with all involved stakeholders in a preventive, solution-oriented, and growth-fostering manner. It remains central to build and foster positive relationships with critical stakeholders and, if possible, develop strong alliances before a crisis occurs. Equally important, schools and school districts should be proactive, rather than reactive, in creating a culture of safety to achieve calmness among students, faculty, staff, parents, and community in times of crisis (Cornell & Sheras, 1998). This should be done by forming partnerships and engagements in consultation with school administrators, counselors, teachers, parents, and district guidance leaders. The need to be immediate should be the primary focus. All of these facilitate the school avoiding conditions that might escalate a crisis situation should one occur.

In order for the school to include built-in provisions that address preventive measures, certain components must be in place. Professionals must develop an understanding of the emotional responses experienced by those in crisis in order to conceptualize the dynamics of crisis situations (Cowan & Rossen, 2013). Zealberg et al. (1998) detail key components of crisis teams and staff training: The team (a) must be collaborative; (b) must be able to sustain school- and districtwide efforts; and (c) must include all stakeholders such as school staff and community. Leader experience with diverse student populations and cultures should be instituted. The school looks to leaders, according to Cohen et al. (2009), to create a positive school climate, which represents the quality and character of school life on campus and includes the campus learning environment as well as the relationships between those on the campus and the school environment. Blauvelt (1999) stresses that school leaders should possess traits such as being good listeners and communicators, be experienced negotiators and counselors, possess levelheadedness, be seen as someone whom students and staff trust to be fair and impartial, and hold experience in crowd control. Cohen et al. further state that the school climate encompasses a consolidation of values of individuals, shared school experiences, relationships, and learning practices. Consequently, school leaders would need to develop and implement a campuswide, comprehensive plan led by a crisis team that promotes a safe school environment. Erwin (2016), as one example, utilizes William Glasser's Choice Theory of Behavior, which endorses the premise that the school climate solution should strive to reduce disciplinary issues on a campus, increase graduation and attendance rates, and improve learning and achievement. Through this, many professional school counselors implemented the *Character Counts!* program and designated the six pillars (Trustworthiness, Respect, Responsibility, Fairness, Caring, and Citizenship) to serve as core ethical values, which appear to transcend culture, religion, and socioeconomic differences. These traits inspire a positive school climate and a culture of kindness, ultimately creating a safe environment for students to learn (Character Counts, 2021).

ESTABLISHING A CRISIS PLAN AND TEAM (PRIOR TO A CRITICAL EVENT)

Some school leaders may make the common mistake of waiting out a critical incident to see if the situation stops on its own. Cornell and Sheras (1998) label *a reflective mode*, which will delay a response to the point where a potential problem becomes a crisis (Cornell & Sheras, 1998). As mentioned earlier, recommendations call for *proactive mode*, rather than a reflective or *reactive mode* (Cornell & Sheras, 1998). When a crisis occurs, children and adolescents look to surrounding adults to understand their worlds; so preparedness starts with a plan developed by knowledgeable and trained staff members. Essential to the overall mission of learning, the school creates and maintains a culture of safety and makes arrangements for implementing a plan of action to be carried out at the onset of the crisis (Crepeau-Hobson & Summers, 2011). This allows for prompt and efficient responses, which may minimize or alleviate a crisis (Cornell & Sheras, 1998). Without this, children and adolescents and school personnel remain vulnerable when the school districts, school administrators, counselors, and the community fail to take a strategic stance toward safety for all (Crepeau-Hobson & Summers, 2011). Schonfeld et al. (2002) write that "while there is no ideal crisis preparation plan" (p. 6), "every school should develop the capacity to deal with crisis situations" (p. 7) to the greatest extent possible.

Cowan and Rossen (2013) stress that preparing for a crisis continues to be an ongoing and dynamic process. In preparation for a potential crisis, many school districts implement a crisis team model, which serves as the prevailing paradigm to address the needs of a school community during and following a crisis event (Nickerson et al., 2006). Additionally, this team of professionals must establish strong relationships between parents and the school and between the school and the community to create the opportunity to respond to school-based crises through partnerships instead of working in isolation (Cowan & Rossen, 2013; National Child Traumatic Stress Network, 2021). A school's ability to address the confluence of needs while mitigating trauma responses and reactions during a critical incident will always be a reflection of the functionality of the safety and mental health mechanisms and resources put in place prior to the crisis (Cowan & Rossen, 2013).

Fierman and Thrower (2011) list characteristics essential for practical solutions and best practices. Solutions must be secure, accessible, controlled, versatile, comprehensive, practical for normal operations, and spontaneous in emergency cases. The crisis plan must integrate interdisciplinary communication and information sharing, access to all essential information, teaching and training, professional networking, partnerships, and collaborations, and provide means for evaluating data collection, analysis, trending, and reporting. Therefore, the crisis team includes assigning staff with appropriate training to address the safety and mental health needs of students and adults to the team as well as assigning roles for each member. Additionally, the school district should provide these individuals with advanced training and resources. Nickerson et al. (2006) state that most schools establish typical crisis team models in a multidisciplinary fashion and organize teams by functions, not by discipline. This allows team members to serve in areas of their strength and offers a myriad of abilities, experiences, and skills. Parents should be included as partners who can assist in times of need (Cowan & Rossen, 2013).

The campus principal, working in collaboration with the head or lead counselor and the district's director of guidance, usually serves as the team leader on school-based teams. True leadership requires a vision, intentionality, and connections to others in order to accomplish a common goal during a critical incident goal (Maxwell, 2013; Northouse, 2010). The principal must possess ardent leadership skills and must understand the constituents in order to successfully determine a vision for the school and clearly communicate the mission while supporting staff, students, and parents. Cowan and Rossen (2013) indicate that planning efforts should "focus on minimizing effects and promoting recovery rather than only putting out fires. In other words, schools should be prepared, not scared" (p. 11).

Information presented in this section and going forward reflects the author's experience of facing and managing critical incidents, while working in collaboration with other professionals, as a professional school counselor leader in a former school district. This includes the author's roles as a professional school counselor in planning for culturally diverse ways of responding to grief and trauma before, during, and after a crisis event and collaborations with the campus principal, other staff members, parents, and the community in the development of a crisis team and crisis plan.

Professional school counselors play an important role in the development of district-/campus-/community-level crisis response planning and process. Elements of this planning include assessing, recognizing, and respecting cultural environments with specific instructions as to how the crisis team responds. Professional school counselors may invite clinical mental health counselors and school psychologists (depending on the magnitude of the crisis) to assume the task of ensuring that impacted students and staff receive individual and group counseling and other related services (Gysbers & Henderson, 2013; Nickerson et al., 2006; Valadez, 2014; Zealberg et al., 1998). They assume a major role in crisis management. They offer possibilities and instill optimism through the development and implementation of theory-based, developmentally appropriate, trauma-informed interventions. These include classroom guidance, group counseling, and psychoeducation sessions to respond to loss of life and other types of trauma experiences for children and adolescents, teachers, administrators, school nurses, and other adults who experience a close connection to the crisis. Their preparation includes planning for cultural diversity (ways of responding to grief and trauma) and for the most vulnerable populations by taking into consideration the diverse range of intellectual, social, emotional, physical, and language development of all students. They work in collaboration with campus administrators in designating rooms that may be used by visiting and campus-based counselors, and for check-ins, breakfast, snacks, and lunch breaks. Additionally, professional school counselors request that district leaders and campus administration or district-level guidance leaders provide a budget for counselors to order books, materials, and supplies to implement trauma-informed student response strategies, psychoeducation, and small-group or individual counseling during the critical incident. The budget should also include money for food and drinks and a crisis kit that will store all needed items in preparation for a crisis response. Schools may also establish a GoFundMe page as a financial resource to support these efforts.

Professional school counselors participate in other ways to prepare for a potential crisis. This includes assisting the administration in creating a checklist of items that will need to be implemented and in place should a critical incident occur. This also includes developing the referral process for students to see a counselor and a list of phone numbers of school administrators and professional school counselors (on and off campus) for quick use should an incident occur after school hours. They assist the principal in preparing a letter to be sent to parents regarding plans for providing safety, structure, and procedures that will be put in place for the well-being of children. Information about on- and off-campus counseling should also be included. Professional school counselors assist in developing debriefing plans that monitor and take care of caregivers (e.g., school administration, professional school and clinical mental health counselors, school psychologists, teachers, and support personnel). These individuals hold frontline positions, and a debriefing plan assists them as they deal with their own grief and trauma during a crisis event. This includes designating times and places where this will occur. Professional school counselors assist in other areas such as reminding principals to make provisions for utilizing substitute teachers for grief-stricken individuals (e.g., teachers, coaches, and school nurses who experience a close connection to the crisis) and assisting them in preparing guidelines for addressing the media.

Additionally, the school should include special education and English as a second language staff to work collaboratively with the crisis team. Because of their familiarity with these student populations, these individuals will provide crucial input to address the unique needs of these students. These individuals and the ones listed earlier hold the power to control the impact critical incidences present to students, staff, and community. Their decisions and reactions during a crisis may create long-term effects on a school community (Low, 2008). Aside from establishing systems and trainings, effective school leadership involves the ability to generate and maintain an optimistic culture and hope during and after a crisis situation to promote effective efforts from all involved stakeholders. As mentioned earlier, school leaders must demonstrate the capacity to facilitate open and trustworthy communications to and between all impacted members of the school community prior to, during, and in the aftermath of a crisis (Smith & Riley, 2012). The principal and professional school counselors may define roles with detailed responsibilities to support staff members and utilize these staff members to address other appropriate areas as needed. Moreover, when creating the response plan, school professionals must craft strategies and actions that align with the needs of the local community since each school community presents with its own unique needs. Therefore, these procedures may require modification in individual communities (National Child Traumatic Stress Network, 2021; Zealberg et al., 1998).

Research conducted on prior critical events points to preparedness as a characteristic of schools that function well. As mentioned earlier, preparedness includes systematic prevention measures, advanced planning, responding, and recovery from a potential catastrophic event through best practices by putting a crisis plan and team in place, expanding the role of mental health counseling, and training all involved so that they may become adept at responding. Given the prevalence of critical incidents in our world, schools, and communities, school and clinical mental health counselors nowadays become tasked with taking an active role in responding to potential crises similar to actions taken for academic and postsecondary preparedness; therefore, schools should expand the role of mental health counseling on campus.

All schools should follow a comprehensive developmental guidance and counseling program to meet a myriad of needs for all students. Most school counseling models address professional school counselors' roles in collaborating with the school's crisis plan. NISD (mentioned earlier in this chapter) represents one of the many school districts that follow the fifth edition of the Texas Model for Comprehensive School Counseling Programs for Texas public schools (Texas Education Agency, 2018). The Texas Counseling Association (TCA) recently revised the model in collaboration with the Texas Education Agency. The Texas model, based on the statutory description of Texas school counseling programs and school counselor responsibilities (Texas Education Code [TEC] §§33.005-33.007), delineates guidance and counseling services that span pre-K to 12th grade (Texas Education Agency, 2018). Other states (e.g., Florida) also offer a state-based comprehensive framework for professional school counselors. Some school districts opt to use the American School Counselor Association (ASCA) National Model (2016). This model, also recently revised, defines the role of professional school counselors in implementing comprehensive school counseling programs and aligns practices with ASCA mind-sets and behaviors for student success.

SYSTEMIC AND DIVERSITY CONSIDERATIONS

School leaders and appropriate staff must identify systems, procedures, and tangible physical barriers that may inhibit students during a crisis event. When planning and preparing for critical incidents, professional school counselors take into account and consider the needs of all individuals, not just those within the majority group. Critical events present scaffolding effects to vulnerable individuals; and judicious, proactive (as opposed to reactive) planning for the most vulnerable populations becomes crucial (Hoffman, 2009). Specifically, this includes the needs of students and adults with disabilities and language barriers. As mentioned earlier, schools must include in their crisis team plan a diverse range of intellectual, social, emotional, physical development, and cognitive and physical challenges relating to all individuals with disabilities on campus (Clarke et al., 2014; Council for Exceptional Children & Council for Children With Behavioral Disorders, 2021). Relying on translators during a crisis can be unpredictable. Professionals will need to discern if translators will be able to pay close enough attention to accurately interpret and ensure full comprehension of critical information (Hoffman, 2009). This compels school leaders to continuously reflect on and examine the language needs on their campuses while considering viable alternative ways of communicating vital information during a critical event.

Some individuals with special needs may face impediments that may get in the way of their ability to follow directives and safety guidelines during a crisis. They may not be able to (a) tolerate or possess the ability to be a part of large crowds during an evacuation; (b) process directives that must be quickly followed; (c) remain quiet during a lockdown situation; or (d) cope with scary noises such as sirens or shouting or (e) they may be inhibited by their physical limitations, thus leaving them incapable of complying on any level. Research presented by Clarke et al. (2014) indicates that students with special needs appear to face higher risks for acquiring health conditions and emotional trauma after a crisis than their typical peer counterparts.

All staff who serve students with disabilities, including substitute teaching staff members, must be aware of these measures and demonstrate capabilities to assist in times of emergency. Moreover, schools must provide an adequate number of special education and limited English speaking teachers along with other adults to ensure student safety during a crisis (Clarke et al., 2014). Tables 13.1 to 13.3 provide checklists of tasks for counselors to follow before, during, and after a critical incident.

TABLE 13.1 CRITICAL INCIDENT CHECKLIST—COUNSELOR TASKS TO PERFORM BEFORE A CRISIS

✓	CRITICAL INCIDENT CHECKLIST COUNSELOR TASKS TO PERFORM BEFORE A CRISIS
	Build and foster positive relationships with critical stakeholders and develop strong alliances before a crisis occurs.
	Assist schools and school districts in being proactive, rather than reactive, in creating a culture of safety to achieve calmness among students, faculty, staff, parents, and community in times of crisis. This should be done by forming partnerships and engagements in consultation with school administrators, counselors, teachers, parents, and district guidance leaders. The need to be immediate should be the primary focus.
	Participate in the development of district-/campus-/community-level crisis response planning and process to include assessing, recognizing, and respecting cultural environments with specific instructions as to how the crisis team will respond.
	Participate in the creation of a district-level and school-based crisis team at the school and the community levels—collaboration of school administrators, professional school counselors, school psychologists, classroom teachers (including those who teach students with disabilities and students with language barriers); school nurses, support personnel; the community (including parents and religious leaders to ensure culturally appropriate responses); and educational service centers all working in collaboration with school district leaders and clinical mental health counselors.
	Assist the school administration in providing training for teachers and staff. Develop research-based trauma-informed protocols, practices, strategies, and policies that align with best practices for student/clients with multiple needs including identifying tangible physical barriers that might inhibit a safe implementation of the crisis plan and grief and trauma strategies that teachers may use with students. Prepare to the fullest extent possible.
	Establish a sound communication system.
	Assist the administration in creating a checklist of items that will need to be implemented and in place should a critical incident occur. This includes developing the referral process for students to see a counselor and a list of phone numbers of school administrators and professional school counselors (on and off campus) for quick use should an incident occur after school hours.

(continued)

TABLE 13.1 CRITICAL INCIDENT CHECKLIST—COUNSELOR TASKS TO PERFORM BEFORE A CRISIS (*CONTINUED*)

✓	CRITICAL INCIDENT CHECKLIST COUNSELOR TASKS TO PERFORM BEFORE A CRISIS
	Develop and implement theory-based, developmentally appropriate, trauma-informed interventions. These include classroom guidance, group counseling, and psychoeducation sessions to respond to loss of life and other types of trauma experiences for children and adolescents, teachers, administrators, school nurses, and other adults who experience a close connection to the crisis. Their preparation includes planning for cultural diversity (ways of responding to grief and trauma) and for the most vulnerable populations by taking into consideration the diverse range of intellectual, social, emotional, physical, and language development of all students.
	Assist campus administrators in designating rooms that may be used by visiting- and campus-based counselors, and for check-ins, breakfast, snacks, and lunch breaks.
	Assist the principal in preparing a letter to be sent to parents regarding the critical incident. Include plans for providing safety, structure, and procedures that will be put in place for the well-being of children. Also include information about on- and off-campus counseling.
	Professional school counselors assist in developing debriefing plans that monitor and take care of caregivers (e.g., school administration, professional school and clinical mental health counselors, school psychologists, teachers, and support personnel). These individuals hold position on the front line; and a debriefing plan assists them as they deal with their own grief and trauma during a crisis event. This includes designating times and places where this will occur.
	Remind principals to make provisions for utilizing substitute teachers for grief-stricken individuals (e.g., teachers, coaches, and school nurses) and assisting them in preparing guidelines for addressing the media.
	Request that campus administrators or school district guidance leaders provide a budget so that counselors can order books, materials, and supplies (e.g., paint, clay dough, colored pencils, boxes of tissue, index cards, rolls of butcher paper) to implement trauma-informed student response strategies, psychoeducation, and small-group or individual counseling during the critical incident. The budget should also include money for food and drinks and a crisis kit for caregivers. The crisis kit includes the campus bell schedule, sign-in sheet for visiting counseling, name tags, list of rooms to be used for counseling, hall passes, copies of a map of the school campus; contact information for visiting counselors; schedules (including a schedule of the deceased student, if the crisis relates to the death of a student); resources and supplies for counseling; strategies for classroom teachers; checklist of tasks to perform; sample script for teachers to assist in responding to student grief. Schools may establish a GoFundMe page as a financial resource to assist in this effort.
	Assist the campus administration on preparing guidelines for the media relations and designate a spokesman for the campus.

Source: Data from Jones, B., Zambrano, E., & Haberstroh, S. (2020). Crisis intervention and prevention in K-12 schools. In T. Duffey and S. Haberstroh (Eds.), *Introduction to crisis and trauma counseling* (pp. 273–291). American Counseling Association; McKenzie, K. (2008). *School crisis and staff preparedness.* Proquest LLC; Northside Independent School District. (2013). *Critical incident management manual.* Northside Independent School District.

RESPONDING DURING A CRITICAL EVENT ON SCHOOL CAMPUSES

At the onset of an acute crisis, campus principals, professional school and clinical mental health counselors, school psychologists, teachers, support personnel, in partnership with district leaders, should immediately implement the procedures and actions outlined in the crisis plan developed by the school crisis team. A comprehensive preparedness to respond will allow them to effortlessly bring together a variety of members with a shared objective and a centralized mode of operation (U.S. Department of Homeland Security, 2016). As an example, responding to the death of a popular student, teacher, or campus principal, the team would administer to the family, peers of the student, the staff, and the rest of the student body as needed. The plan to provide space throughout the campus and the delivery of counseling services to those in need will be immediately implemented by trained counselors and school psychologists. In parallel, identified team members will carry out the responsibility for various related tasks such as monitoring the emotional levels and needs of students, staff, team members; providing resources such as food and drinks for caregivers; responding to the media and the proliferation of postings on social media; quelling rumors; and providing outreach to families (Aubert-Santelli et al., 2014; Brunner & Lewis, 2009; Cowan & Rossen, 2013; Gysbers & Henderson, 2013; Jones et al., 2020).

When schools respond to an acute critical event on campus, they should not do so in a random or haphazard manner. As mentioned earlier, a school's response to a crisis almost always reflects fundamental elements (e.g., the school climate, the level of preparation, a comprehensive and holistic approach, and the necessary resources needed to address the multifaceted needs for safety, crisis management, and mental health unique to each school community). The closer the connection of the school to the nexus of the critical incident (such as school shooting or the death of a student, teacher, or principal), the greater and more intense the impact will be on individuals' circle of diverse needs, which leaves the entire system vulnerable (Cowan & Rossen, 2013). Therefore, schools and mental health professional organizations recommend that campus leaders remain proactive in their actions concerning prevention, preparation for, and response to acute critical incidents. In essence, these elements should be in place prior to the crisis event (Cowan & Rossen, 2013).

Campus life becomes extremely hectic amid the implementation of a crisis response plan. School staff must first and foremost seek and confirm accurate information from the campus principal regarding the existing crisis. The district superintendent and public relation/communication director typically informs (as timely as possible) the campus principal of a community crisis occurrence. If the crisis happens on camps, the campus principal usually informs the district superintendent. The campus principal informs other campus administrators and the campus-based head or lead professional school counselors. The head or lead counselor informs the rest of the counseling staff. Sometimes this occurs during the school day. Other times, this notification may occur the night or weekend before. Regardless, the accuracy of the information surrounding the crisis must be confirmed before reacting and releasing. Potential harm may result if school officials do not make these confirmations.

Principals usually assign professional school counselors to work with grief-stricken individuals who struggle to respond to a death or critical incident on campus. After receiving confirmation of the crisis event, professional school counselors move immediately to assist the administrative staff in setting up a faculty meeting to remind faculty and staff of procedural information developed by the crisis team to respond to the crisis at hand. If possible and for time efficiency, school officials should do this the day before the actual campuswide intervention, leaving more time for implementing the actual crisis plan when the student body returns to campus. During this time, it remains imperative that counselors and campus principals work proactively in providing needed communication and consultation with other school administrators and teachers. They should make a continuous effort to reduce rumors regarding the event proliferated through social media, print and news media, and gossip.

At the start of the day of the crisis response intervention, a myriad of efforts will transpire. Professional school counselors (working in conjunction with the campus principal) should remind other campus administrators, counselors, and teachers of the roles and responsibilities assigned and the procedures planned for the day. In the case of a student death, the head or lead counselor should assign a professional school counselor to follow the deceased student's schedule and remain in the classroom to monitor students' and teachers' emotional responses at the start of each class period. During times of heightened emotions, classroom teachers prefer professional school counselors to be the spokesperson who addresses the student's death. Professional school counselors hold credentials, education, and training to be effective in meeting this need. Because no one can predict a student's emotional and psychological response to an ongoing crisis, students needing counseling services should never walk to the counseling center alone. After speaking to the teacher and class, the professional school counselor provides escorts to take grief-stricken students to the designated counseling areas when needed. If possible and for time efficiency, arrangements for escorts should be made the day before the actual campuswide intervention. Plans should also be in place to arrange for students experiencing immense grief to be picked up by parents or guardians. For safety reasons, the school should never allow students experiencing debilitating grief to ride home on a school bus.

Professional school counselors should also make provision for escorting grief-stricken teachers to the adult counseling areas. For time efficiency, the teachers' lounge should be reserved the day before the actual campuswide intervention and a clinical mental health counselor should counsel teachers. This avoids dual relationships involving professional school counselors counseling various campus staff members. The head or lead counselor should remind the principal the day before to provide several substitute teachers for grief-stricken individuals (e.g., teachers, coaches, and school nurses who experience closeness to the deceased individual).

As mentioned earlier, school officials count on advanced preparation in order to effectively get through the day. Professional school counselors recognize the importance of storing all needed items in a crisis kit located in the counseling office in the event of an acute crisis. They use the prepared crisis kits for easy implementation. They store sign-in sheets; name tags of on-campus and visiting counselors; list of rooms to be used for counseling; the campus bell schedule; hall passes; copies of the school campus map; staff telephone tree; list of members of the school crisis team with room numbers, telephone numbers, and extensions; a description of roles and expectations; list of staff trained in first aid and CPR; contact information for visiting counselors invited by the campus head or lead counselor; schedules (including a schedule of the deceased student if the crisis relates to the death of a student); resources and supplies for counseling (including boxes of tissue; strategies for classroom teachers in addressing student grief needs; checklist of tasks to perform; and sample script and helpful hints for teachers to use while responding to students' grief and/or trauma reactions); and computer file of forms and letters (including form letters for notification to parents); see Jones et al. (2020) and NISD (2013).

Professional school counselors should be mindful of other situations on campus that require immediate attention. In the case of a student's death, the head or lead counselor should assign professional counselors to visit clubs and organizations a deceased student participated in and respond to their grief and trauma needs. If possible, make plans to implement this the day before the actual campuswide intervention. Professionals recognize that individuals respond in varying ways to grief and loss. Professional school counselors may set up tables covered in butcher paper and include art supplies in an area (e.g., a courtyard or cafeteria) so that students can express their grief in diverse ways. Expect that not all students will be empathic; therefore, these tables should be monitored and checked for inappropriate expressions and contents. Also, plans should be made to respond to other individuals in the deceased student's immediate circle (i.e., contact the deceased student's former schools so that professional school counselors can get prepared to respond to family members or other students on their campus[es]). Contact other counseling offices where the deceased student and siblings attended as well. If possible, do this the day before the actual campuswide intervention (Jones et al., 2020; NISD, 2013).

After getting clearance from the principal, superintendent, and communications director, professional school counselors (usually designated by the campus principal) will need to prepare to respond to television reporters. They should advocate for the counseling profession and educate the media by informing them that the mystical characterization "grief counselors" primarily refers to professional school counselors working in collaboration with clinical mental health counselors and school psychologists. No grief counseling group stands idly waiting to enter schools to address counseling needs should acute crises occur. Rather, professional school counselors usually spearhead this effort. When interacting with the media, professional school counselors should use extreme caution in facilitating contact between the media and the campus. They should protect student and campus confidentiality and advocate for the campus against sensationalism (Jones et al., 2020; NISD, 2013).

Professional school counselors set up and implement theory-based, developmentally appropriate, trauma-informed classroom guidance, group counseling, and psychoeducation sessions to respond to loss of life and other types of trauma experiences for children and adolescents, teachers, administrators, school nurses, and other adults who experience a close connection to the crisis. Counselors meet the diverse needs of students by offering individual sessions or heterogeneous or homogeneous groups when appropriate. Plans should be made to allow students and staff members to respond to loss in a cultural, religious, or spiritual context (American Counseling Association Code of Ethics, 2014). Again, this approach may be comforting and reassuring to some individuals. Additionally, counselors should also include the most vulnerable populations by taking into consideration the diverse range of intellectual, social, emotional, physical, and language development of all students. Planning ahead makes this possible.

Professional school counselors implement a comprehensive school counseling model that addresses handling crisis on school campuses using various resources (e.g., Federal Emergency Management Association [FEMA], Texas Education Agency [2018], Florida School Counseling Framework [2010], other state standards for licenses and certification, and the ASCA Model [2016]). They should schedule time and rooms for individual and small-group counseling and assign counselors in each room. Also, they should use leadership and advocacy by being knowledgeable and ready to lead; being proactive in controlling the situation from the beginning; utilizing professional school and other mental health experts to provide a voice for students and others who experience grief, trauma, and loss. Counselors provide grief-informed and trauma-informed care and read grief and trauma reactions so that professionals respond correctly with specific services. They accomplish this by using books, materials, and supplies (e.g., including paint, clay dough, colored pencils, boxes of tissue, index cards, rolls of butcher paper, breathing techniques, grounding, and other creative, experiential interventions) to implement trauma-informed student response strategies, psychoeducation, and small-group or individual counseling during the critical incident. Many situations evolve and transpire over the course of the day. Professional school counselors, in coordination with the campus principal, should be proactive in providing needed communication and consultation with parents (via face-to-face contact, by phone, or via a letter sent home at the end of the school day). A quick checklist of tasks to perform during a crisis is provided in Table 13.2.

TABLE 13.2 CRITICAL INCIDENT CHECKLIST—COUNSELOR TASKS TO PERFORM DURING A CRISIS

✓	CRITICAL INCIDENT CHECKLIST COUNSELOR TASKS TO PERFORM DURING A CRISIS
	Seek and confirm accurate information from the campus principal (who receives confirmation from the district superintendent and public relation/communication director before reacting and releasing).
	Assist the principal in training faculty and staff (through a faculty meeting) on responding to a crisis on campus. If possible and for time efficiency, do this the day before the actual campuswide intervention.
	Continuously assist the administration in reducing rumors while living in the proliferation of social media during a critical incident.
	Be proactive in providing needed communication and consultation with school administrators and teachers.
	After getting clearance from the principal, superintendent, and communications director, prepare to respond to television reporters. Principals usually assign professional school counselors to respond to a death or critical incident on campus. Professional school counselors advocate for their profession. They educate the media by informing them that the term "grief counselors" connotes primarily professional school counselors working in collaboration with clinical mental health counselors and school psychologists. Counselors should use extreme caution in facilitating contact between the media and the campus and advocate for the campus against sensationalism.
	Remind campus administrators, counselors, and teachers of the roles and responsibilities assigned when responding to the crisis. Also remind them of the procedures planned for the day.
	In the case of a student death, assign professional school counselors to follow the deceased student's schedule and remain in the classroom to monitor students' and teachers' emotional responses. Provide escorts to take grief-stricken students to the designated counseling areas when needed. If possible, do this the day before the actual campuswide intervention.
	Assign counselors to visit clubs and organizations that the deceased student participated in and respond to their needs. If possible, do this the day before the actual campuswide intervention.
	Make arrangements for students experiencing immense grief to be picked up by parents. Never allow students experiencing debilitating grief to ride home on a school bus.

(continued)

TABLE 13.2 CRITICAL INCIDENT CHECKLIST—COUNSELOR TASKS TO PERFORM DURING A CRISIS (*CONTINUED*)

✓	CRITICAL INCIDENT CHECKLIST COUNSELOR TASKS TO PERFORM DURING A CRISIS
	Set up tables covered in butcher paper with art supplies on the side in an area such as a courtyard so that students can express their grief in diverse ways. These tables should be monitored and checked for inappropriate expressions and contents.
	Make provision for escorting grief-stricken adults (e.g., teachers, coaches, and school nurses) to the adult counseling areas. Reserve the teachers' lounge and use a clinical mental health counselor to counsel teachers and other staff members. This avoids dual relationships during counseling. Remind the principal to provide substitute teachers for these grief-stricken individuals. If possible and for time efficiency, do this the day before the actual campuswide intervention.
	In the case of a deceased student, make plans to respond to other individuals in the deceased student's immediate circle (i.e., contact the deceased student's former schools so that professional school counselors can get prepared to respond to family members or other students on their campus[es]). Contact other counseling offices where the deceased student and siblings attended as well. If possible, do this the day before the actual campuswide intervention.
	Use the prepared crisis kits for caregivers (including sign-in sheets; name tags of caregivers; list of rooms to be used for counseling; the campus bell schedule; hall passes; copies of the school campus map; staff telephone tree; list of members of the school crisis team with room numbers, extensions, or telephone numbers; a description of roles and expectations; list of staff trained in first aid and CPR; contact information for visiting counselors; schedules [including a schedule of the deceased student if the crisis relates to a student]; resources and supplies for counseling [including boxes of tissues; strategies for classroom teachers; checklist of tasks to perform; and sample script and helpful hints for teachers to use while responding to students' grief and/or trauma reactions]; and computer file of forms and letters [including form letters for notification to parents]).
	Facilitate ways that individuals may understand their grief responses. Set up and implement theory-based, developmentally appropriate, trauma-informed classroom guidance, group counseling, and psychoeducation sessions to assist students in responding to loss of life and other types of trauma experiences for children and adolescents, teachers, administrators, school nurses, and other adults who experience a close connection to the crisis. Meet the diverse needs of students by offering individual sessions or homogeneous and heterogeneous groups as appropriate. Include the most vulnerable populations by taking into consideration the diverse range of intellectual, social, emotional, physical, and language development of all students.
	Implement a comprehensive school counseling model that addresses handling crises on school campuses using various resources (e.g., FEMA; Texas Education Agency, 2018; Florida School Counseling Framework, 2010; other state standards for licenses and certification; and the ASCA model). Schedule time and rooms for individual and small-group counseling and assign counselors in each room. Use leadership and advocacy by being knowledgeable and ready to lead; being proactive in controlling the situation from the beginning; utilizing professional school and other mental health experts to provide a voice for students and others who experience grief, trauma, and loss. Provide grief-informed and trauma-informed care and read grief and trauma reactions so that professionals respond correctly with specific services. Use books, materials, supplies, and creative counseling interventions to implement trauma-informed student response strategies, psychoeducation, and small-group or individual counseling during the critical incident.

(*continued*)

TABLE 13.2 CRITICAL INCIDENT CHECKLIST—COUNSELOR TASKS TO PERFORM DURING A CRISIS (*CONTINUED*)

✓	CRITICAL INCIDENT CHECKLIST COUNSELOR TASKS TO PERFORM DURING A CRISIS
	Make plans to allow students and staff members to respond to this loss in a cultural, religious, or spirituality context. This may be comforting and reassuring to some individuals (American Counseling Association Code of Ethics, 2014).
	Be proactive in providing needed communication and consultation with parents (via face-to-face contacts, phone calls, or via a letter sent home at the end of the school day).

Source: Data from Jones, B., Zambrano, E., & Haberstroh, S. (2020). Crisis intervention and prevention in K-12 schools. In T. Duffey and S. Haberstroh (Eds.), *Introduction to crisis and trauma counseling* (pp. 273–291). American Counseling Association; McKenzie, K. (2008). *School crisis and staff preparedness.* Proquest LLC; Northside Independent School District. (2013). *Critical incident management manual.* Northside Independent School District.

THE AFTERMATH (FOLLOWING A CRISIS)

In the aftermath of a crisis, the pathway to recovery and healing begins. School officials should anticipate that the effects of trauma brought on by an acute critical incident may produce long-term and sometimes permanent effects (Cowan & Rossen, 2013). Research points to the occurrence of critical impairments to student learning and emotional development if adequate and appropriate support is not provided. As explained in Chapter 12, students and school officials may experience conditions such as PTSD, profound grief and bereavement, and other major mental health conditions. Again, schools and school districts must possess an awareness of the potential problems and concerns that trauma-exposed individuals may experience. Children and adolescents experience and express grief and trauma responses in diverse ways. Therefore, plans should be made to provide continuous counseling modalities through the length of time needed.

OTHER CONCERNS FOR STUDENTS AND PARENTS IN THE AFTERMATH OF A CRISIS

Meeting physical and psychological safety needs as well as prevention and recovery become crucial in the aftermath of a crisis. Mental health implications of crisis exposure emerge as critical challenges for school safety, and crisis response addresses potential psychological reactions associated with crisis experiences. As mentioned in Chapter 12, students may experience sudden mental health concerns (e.g., difficulties with concentration, aggression, and isolation and withdrawal). Others may experience anxiety, fear, guilt, or depression. Trauma-exposed students may experience these conditions even though they did not know the individuals who caused or directly encountered the trauma experience. They may also be affected even though they live in a city different from the one that the crisis occurred (Cowan & Rossen, 2013). Therefore, the crisis team should strive to achieve calmness among students and staff during and after a crisis event and respond effectively to allay anxiety and fear postcrisis (National Child Traumatic Stress Network, 2021).

Professional school and clinical mental health counselors should periodically perform risk assessments on students and staff after an acute critical incident. Additionally, counselors may provide helpful hints to parents, which include ways to observe their children's behavior that might signal continued distress to the critical incident. This includes monitoring children for difficulty concentrating, regression, unusual irritability, and changes in behavior (including changes in sleep and eating habits, increased withdrawal or aggression, loss of interest in once-desired activities, increased worrying and depressive mode, and decrease in school performances). Additionally, parents should monitor children's television and social medial use, especially those related to the critical incident. This exposure may increase stress and anxiety levels. Parents should be available to discuss the critical incident with the children in a developmentally appropriate manner. Professional school counselors do not conduct diagnostic assessments on students; therefore, as a reminder, the letter sent to parents from the school should include referrals and access to continued counseling on and off campus over the coming days. A quick checklist of tasks to perform after a crisis is provided in Table 13.3.

TABLE 13.3 CRITICAL INCIDENT CHECKLIST—COUNSELOR TASKS TO PERFORM AFTER A CRISIS

✓	CRITICAL INCIDENT CHECKLIST COUNSELOR TASKS TO PERFORM AFTER A CRISIS
	Continue ongoing monitoring of students and teachers for emotional support and counseling. Continue using visiting counselors if needed.
	Assist the school administration in providing structure and routine to get the campus back to normal. Be mindful that recovery may be short- or long-term depending on many factors.
	Provide referral resources for students and teachers who struggle to deal effectively with their bereavement.
	Assign a counselor to be with the grieving family members when they arrive on campus to secure the student's property from all lockers (those in classroom hallways and possibly those in the gymnasium).
	Assist the school in making plans to provide voluntary, homogeneous critical incident debriefing sessions (led by a debriefing counselor) that will attend to the emotional status of caregivers (e.g., a group for school administration, one for professional school and clinical mental health counselors, school psychologists, and one for teachers, and support personnel who assisted others in dealing with grief and trauma that occurred during the crisis event).
	Assist the school administration in evaluating and refining the crisis plan utilizing postsurveys that capture responses from all participants.
	Assist the school administration in evaluating and refining the effectiveness of training and the skills acquisition for caregivers—what worked and what did not.
	Assist the school administration in assessing, evaluating, and refining needs for ongoing training.
	Send thank-you notes to visiting school, clinical mental health counselors, parents, and others who assisted.

ASCA, American School Counselor Association; FEMA, Federal Emergency Management Association.

Source: Data from Jones, B., Zambrano, E., & Haberstroh, S. (2020). Crisis intervention and prevention in K-12 schools. In T. Duffey and S. Haberstroh (Eds.), *Introduction to crisis and trauma counseling* (pp. 273–291). American Counseling Association; McKenzie, K. (2008). *School crisis and staff preparedness.* Proquest LLC; Northside Independent School District. (2013). *Critical incident management manual.* Northside Independent School District.

School officials should be mindful that recovery from a critical incident may be short or long term depending on many factors (e.g., PTSD, anxiety, hyperarousal, hypervigilance, and depression). Professional school counselors continuously assist the school administration in providing structure and routine to get the campus back to normal. They continue implementing additional responsibilities after a crisis event and visiting counselors may be needed to assist in diminishing the magnitude of student and staff reactions to the critical incident. They continue to participate in ongoing monitoring of students and teachers for emotional support and counseling and provide referral resources for students and teachers who struggle to deal effectively with their bereavement. They assist the school in making plans to provide voluntary, homogeneous critical incident debriefing sessions (led by a debriefing counselor) that will attend to the emotional status of caregivers (e.g., a group for school administration, one for professional school and clinical mental health counselors, school psychologists, and one for teachers, and support personnel who assisted others in dealing with grief and trauma that occurred during the crisis event). Groups may also be formed heterogeneously.

CRITICAL INCIDENT DEBRIEFING PLAN

Acute critical incidents can be debilitating and hold the potential to disrupt one's capacity to function effectively. Some professionals describe debriefing as the process that puts the critical incidents and reactions to these events into perspective. Others define debriefing as a crisis intervention where facilitators provide a supportive process that allows group members to diffuse their emotional reaction to the crisis at hand, thereby mitigating the impact of the crisis experience (Johnson, 1993; Jones et al., 2020; Meichenbaum, 1994; NISD, 2013; Peterson & Straub, 1992). Debriefing differs from trauma-specific interventions. At the end of each day of the crisis, the school should offer critical incident debriefing groups for caregivers (those most exposed to the critical incident) as part of the recovery process. Professional counselors use debriefing to promote healing and mitigate long-term effects of the experience of vicarious trauma that may lead to chronic or acute stress.

A debriefing group (usually comprising 8–10 group members) differs from the group set up for assessing, evaluating, and refining the implementation of the crisis plan prepared by the crisis team. The group facilitators also do not consider this to be a counseling group, and confidentiality cannot be implied or guaranteed. Group facilitators strongly encourage group members, however, to avoid discussing information of a personal nature outside the group (NISD, 2013; Steele, 2001).

DEBRIEFING FOR TEACHERS, COUNSELORS, SCHOOL ADMINISTRATORS, AND SUPPORT PERSONNEL

Ground rules should be established for the group and should include the following: (a) allowing group members the right to pass or simply not speak; (b) allowing group members who choose to speak, to speak for themselves; (c) promoting respect for others including what others might say; and (d) encouraging group members to remain in attendance during the entire group time (NISD, 2013; Steele, 2001).

The school and school district set up this type of group for caregivers who worked during the time of the critical incident. Again, debriefing groups should not be led by the campus professional school counselors to avoid dual relationships. These groups include a debriefing counselor (usually a district director of guidance, district counseling staff, or a clinical mental health counselor not involved in the crisis response) to facilitate a small heterogenous or homogeneous group meeting to assist caregivers, in a structured way, in processing their thoughts and experience related to the critical incident and provide services, coping skills, and resources for crisis management. The debriefing counselor, while observing group members' body language and emotional responses, assists them in processing difficult moments that occurred during the day; identifying signs of stress and anxiety; and understanding that their grief reactions (cognitive, emotional, physical, and behavioral) may be typical for many. Referrals to the district's free Employee Assistance Program (EAP) may be made for those needing further counseling to deal with work-related stress and their own personal emotional health.

Additionally, head or lead counselors assign a professional school counselor to be with the grieving family members when they return to the campus to secure a deceased student's property from all lockers (those in classroom hallways and possibly those in the gymnasium). When time permits, professional school counselors should send thank-you notes to visiting school, clinical mental health counselors, parents, and others who assisted with managing the critical event.

EVALUATION OF THE CRISIS PLAN IMPLEMENTATION

The crisis team should reconvene in the aftermath of the crisis to assist the school administration in evaluating and refining the crisis plan utilizing postsurveys, which capture responses from all participants; to assist the school administration in evaluating and refining the effectiveness of training and the skills acquisition for caregivers—what worked and what did not; and to assist the school administration in assessing, evaluating, and refining needs for ongoing training.

OTHER DEVELOPMENTAL, SYSTEMIC, RELATIONAL, AND MULTICULTURAL CONSIDERATIONS

As mentioned in most chapters in this book, the family plays an important role in children's and adolescents' development and well-being. This chapter presents implications for schools (e.g., administrators, professional school counselors) and others who respond to critical incidents on school campuses. Schools should lend their expertise by providing psychoeducational sessions to assist parents, teachers, school administrators, and other support personnel in their efforts to raise productive and responsible youths. This includes teaching disaster- and trauma-exposed parents how to build emotional-focused coping and resilience skills that may be used to extend the learning at home with their children using developmentally appropriate methods. These may assist parents in becoming aware of physiologic and emotional states experienced during the time of crisis. Sessions may be presented on the efficacy of journaling, art, music, positive thinking, reframing, mindfulness, breathwork, guided visualization, grounding exercises, and yoga. These strategies provide present-moment connections and may assist them in tracking their thoughts and feelings developmentally, thereby allowing them to become more aware of emotional triggers (Agaibi & Wilson, 2005).

Although trauma resulting from critical incidents holds the capacity to challenge worldviews, the counseling literature suggests that many individuals convert adverse experiences from critical incidents into personal growth and reports that a considerable number of individuals may experience positive changes following a traumatic event (e.g., improved relationships with others, increased connections with spirituality and religion, resilience, gratitude, and a deeper appreciation for life; Calhoun & Tedeschi, 1999; Joseph et al., 2012).

The literature particularly highlights how the protective characteristics of *resilience* (the capability of growing, adapting, and thriving successfully after moments of risk or adversity) and *gratitude* (an affective, cognitive reaction that demonstrates gratefulness to a recognized benefit) serve as buffers and contribute to emotional and psychological growth (Connor, 2006; Meichenbaum, 1994; Moran & Nemec, 2013). Consequently, children and adolescents who exhibit resilience experience fewer anxiety, depressive, and readjustment-related symptoms and difficulties. Those without remain susceptible to greater vulnerability (Meichenbaum, 1994). Gratitude, which receives less attention in the literature, appears to be associated with increased spiritual growth and an intensified sense of value to one's life following a traumatic event (Vernon et al., 2009). This promotes deeper existential thoughts and questions that foster an individual's ability to step up with purpose and vision. All of the preceding protective characteristics coupled with the relational-cultural factors and interventions discussed in Chapter 3 may provide growth-fostering opportunities for children and adolescents.

CASE STUDY 13.1

Your community school (for which you serve as a professional school counselor) followed routine operational procedures, until school personnel receive notification that the entire community will shut down for shelter in home amid a health-threatening pandemic: COVID-19. This shelter-in-home situation lasted through the summer months. At the end of the summer, federal and state governments now see possibilities of schools to safely reopen. Students, teachers, administrators, and counselors at your school now struggle with fears of becoming severely ill if exposed to this virus. The school district developed a campuswide crisis plan before the shutdown.

Activity 13.1

Divide into small groups and process how counselors would demonstrate leadership and advocacy for their campus community considering developmental, systemic, relational, and multicultural aspects during this critical event. Include collaboration between professional school counselors, clinical mental health counselors, school psychologists, and other helping profession positions. Each group will report afterward.

CHAPTER SUMMARY

The likelihood of critical incidents occurring on school campuses and within school communities prompts schools and school districts to continuously work toward establishing crisis response protocols. Crises come in many forms and magnitudes (small- and large-scale) and wield significant effects on individuals. These conditions may exert adverse effects on student learning and behavior, causing schools and communities to be in a state of unreadiness when children enter such states.

Critical incidents evoke trauma and grief in individuals. In these states, children and adolescents look to adults to guide them in understanding and coping with crisis events. Significant contrasts exist between trauma and grief; and counselors need to remain mindful of these differences as they help students develop coping skills. The chapter provides crisis definitions and details, namely, crises involve four primary characteristics: (a) They cause uncertainty, disruption, and change; (b) they can be harmful or threatening for organizations and stakeholders; (c) they can be described as behavioral phenomena where those affected construct their own meaning and responses; and (d) they become parts of larger processes, rather than separate and distinct events.

Preparing for a crisis on a school campus includes implementing best practices prior to, during, and following an actual crisis. This includes built-in provisions that address preventive measures. Preparing for a crisis continues to be an ongoing and dynamic process. In preparation for a potential crisis, many school districts implement a crisis team model and develop a crisis plan, which serves as the prevailing paradigm to address the needs of a school community during and following a crisis event. Most students and campus personnel do not understand, recognize, or know how to identify individuals' responses and reactions to a critical incident. Professional school counselors validate these experiences and work collaboratively with other professionals (including clinical mental health counselors) in providing instruction through curriculum, which addresses coping skills, self-esteem and resilience building, social skills development, conflict resolution, and violence prevention skills.

The chapter highlights the important role that culture plays in the development of this plan. Culture may affect how individuals experience trauma, including the severity of their symptoms. In the face of an acute critical event, experiences of trauma reactions differ from culture to culture. Linguistic, behavioral, and interpersonal practices derive from a constellation of a cultural socialization process and the storage of a response to stimuli that accumulated as a result of one's life experiences. Therefore, in the drafting, designing, and implementation of a crisis plan, the crisis team must strive to understand individuals in the context of life experiences and cultural backgrounds, recognize the impact of violence and victimization on development and coping skills, welcome the voices of diversity, and promote inclusivity of a culturally responsive, trauma-informed focus. This requires relational collaboration (including trust and empowerment), input, and involvement in the designing and evaluation of the plan with all stakeholders in the community.

Critical incidents can be debilitating and hold the potential to disrupt caregivers' capacity to function effectively. Professional counselors use debriefing to promote healing and mitigate long-term effects of the experience of vicarious trauma that may lead to chronic or acute stress.

Schools should lend their expertise by providing psychoeducational sessions to assist parents in their efforts to raise productive and responsible youths. This includes teaching disaster- and trauma-exposed parents how to build emotional-focused coping and resilience skills that may be used to extend the learning at home with their children. These may aid parents in becoming aware of physiologic and emotional states experienced during the time of crisis.

POINTS TO REMEMBER

- Professional school counselors, working in collaboration with clinical mental health counselors, must develop and implement theory-based, developmentally appropriate, trauma-informed interventions when counseling children and adolescents.
- When working with children and adolescents, counselors need to be reminded that significant contrasts exist between trauma and grief.
- Crisis management broadly captures organizational leaders' actions and communication that attempt to reduce the likelihood of a crisis, work to minimize harm from a crisis, use their best professional judgment, and endeavor to reestablish order in the aftermath of a crisis.
- When counseling children and adolescents, counselors must remember that a reciprocal relationship exists between trauma and culture.
- A crisis plan should include preventive measures as well as intervention measures needed to minimize the occurrence of a crisis.
- Critical incident debriefing enables caregivers to mitigate the impact of the crisis experience and provides a supportive process that allows group members to diffuse their emotional reaction to the crisis at hand.
- Although trauma resulting from critical incidents holds the capacity to challenge worldviews, counseling literature suggests that some individuals may convert adverse experiences from critical incidents into personal growth; and reports that a considerable number of individuals may experience positive changes following a traumatic event.

OTHER HELPFUL INFORMATION FOR CONSIDERATION

USEFUL WEBSITES

- Adverse Childhood Experiences (ACEs) Connection: https://www.acesconnection.com/blog/models-training-for-developing-trauma-informed-systems-of-care-tisc-1
- American Academy of Child & Adolescent Psychiatry (AACAP): https://www.aacap.org
- American Counseling Association (ACA): https://www.counseling.org
- American Red Cross: https://www.redcross.org
- American School Counselor Association (ASCA): https://www.schoolcounselor.org
- Centers for Disease Control and Prevention: https://wonder.cdc.gov
- The Children's Bereavement Center of South Texas: https://cbcst.org
- Crisis Management Institute (CMI): https://cmionline.com

- Crisis Prevention Institute (CPI): https://www.crisisprevention.com
- Federal Emergency Management Agency (FEMA) for Kids: https://www.govtech.com/archive/FEMA-for-Kids--Lessons-in.html and https://wiki.kidzsearch.com/wiki/Federal_Emergency_Management_Agency
- International Critical Incident Stress Foundation (ICISF): https://icisf.org
- National Alliance for Grieving Children (NAGC): https://childrengrieve.org/resources
- National Center for Children Exposed to Violence (NCCEV): https://www.kidsmentalhealthinfo.com
- The National Child Traumatic Stress Network: https://www.nctsn.org
- National Education Association (NEA): https://www.neamb.com
- The National Institute for Trauma and Loss in Children: https://starr.org/programs/national-institute-for-trauma-and-loss-in-children-tlc
- National Organization for Victim Assistance (NOVA): https://www.trynova.org
- OSPI School Safety Center: https://www.k12.wa.us
- Suicide Prevention Resource Center—PREPaRE Training Curriculum: https://www.sprc.org
- The Texas Model for Comprehensive School Counseling Programs (5th ed.): https://tea.texas.gov/academics/learning-support-and-programs/school-guidance-and-counseling
- U.S. Department of Education: https://www.ed.gov
- U.S. Department of Homeland Security: https://www.dhs.gov

QUESTIONS FOR FURTHER DISCUSSION

- Considering the critical events involving the 2020 COVID-19 pandemic played out during racial and political unrest, what approach(es) would you use to address the impact of trauma on young clients?
- What roles will you play in mitigating trauma-related reactions and returning young clients to a sense of normalcy?
- What necessary resources will be required to make this happen?
- What stressors do critical incidents place on the teaching, learning, and support systems necessary to maintain "normalcy" and learning?
- What factors distinguish the differences between trauma and grief?
- What factors distinguish the differences between crisis, crisis management, and critical incidents?
- What features make critical incident debriefing necessary and beneficial?
- What multicultural or diversity factors would you consider in working with trauma-exposed children from your particular community?
- What other counseling-related factors would you take into consideration before, during, and after a critical incident?

KEY REFERENCES

Only key references appear in the print edition. The full reference list appears in the digital product on Springer Publishing Connect: connect.springerpub.com/content/book/978-0-8261-4764-6/part/part04/chapter/ch13

Bundy, J., & Pfarrer, M. D. (2015). A burden of responsibility: The role of social approval at the onset of a crisis. *Academy of Management Review, 40*, 345–369. https://doi.org/10.5465/amr.2013.0027

Clarke, L., Embury, D. C., Jones, R. E., & Yssel, N. (2014). Supporting students with disabilities during school crises: A teacher's guide. *Teaching Exceptional Children, 46*(6), 169–178. https://doi.org/10.1177/0040059914534616

Cowan, K. C., & Rossen, E. (2013). Responding to the unthinkable: School crisis response and recovery. *Phi Delta Kappan International, 95*(4), 8–12. http://journals.sagepub.com/doi/pdf/10.1177/003172171309500403

Jones, B., Zambrano, E., & Haberstroh, S. (2020). Crisis intervention and prevention in K-12 schools. In T. Duffey & S. Haberstroh (Eds.), *Introduction to crisis and trauma counseling* (pp. 273–291). American Counseling Association.

Kousky, C. (2016). Impacts of natural disasters on children. *The Future of Children, 26*(1), 73–92. https://doi.org/10.1353/foc.2016.0004

National Child Traumatic Stress Network. (2021). *The 3R's of school crisis and disasters: Readiness, response, and recovery.* National Child Traumatic Stress Network. https://www.tfec.org/wp-content/uploads/Murk_3Rs-ofSchoolCrises.pdf

Nickerson, A., Brock, S., & Reeves, M. (2006). School crisis teams within an incident command system. *The California School Psychologist, 11*, 63–72. http://files.eric.ed.gov/fulltext/EJ902519.pdf

Valadez, R. A. (2014). *The role of leadership in the time of crisis: Preventing, preparing for, and responding to crises on a school campus.* Proquest.

Zealberg, J. J., Hardesty, S. J., & Tyson, S. C. (1998). Mental health clinicians' role in responding to critical incidents in the community. *Psychiatric Services, 49*(3), 301–303. https://doi.org/10.1176/ps.49.3.301

PART V

Personal and Professional Concerns for Counselors

CHAPTER 14

Ethical and Legal Considerations in Child and Adolescent Counseling

Barbara Herlihy, Anita M. Pool, and Gretchen Eckhardt McLain

LEARNING OBJECTIVES

After completing this chapter, the reader should be able to:

- Identify ethical and legal issues with unique applications to counseling minors.
- Distinguish between parents' rights and the rights of minor clients.
- Describe best practices in securing informed consent, defining confidentiality, determining competence, managing crisis, and dealing with boundaries and value conflicts when counseling children and adolescents.
- Explain how to best address situations when a minor client appears to be at risk for suicide, nonsuicidal self-injury, or other dangerous behavior.

CACREP STANDARDS FOR THIS CHAPTER

- CACREP 2016: 2.F.1.b., c., d., g., i., j., k., l., m.; 2.a., c.; 3.e., f., g., h.; 5.b., c., d., e., f., k., l., m.; 7.c., d., e.; School Counseling: 5.G.2.a., b., c., e., g., k., l., m., n.; Clinical Mental Health: 5.C.2.a., f., j., k. l.
- CACREP 2009: II.G.1.b., c., d., e., f., g., h., j.; 2.a., e.; 3.c., f.; 5.b., e., f., g.; School Counseling: III.A.2., 7.; B.1.; D.4.; C.6.; E.1.; H.4.; M.7.; N.5.; Clinical Mental Health Counseling: III.A.2., 3., 9.; C.2.; C.6., 8., 9.; E.1; F.1.

INTRODUCTION

A number of unique ethical and legal considerations arise when counseling children and adults. Although the ethical issues involved in counseling minors are much the same as those that pertain to counseling adult clients, these issues can be complicated by the fact that children and adolescents cannot act and make decisions independently in the same ways as adults. Children and adolescents navigate their world while being embedded in and dependent on multiple systems, including their families and the schools they attend. Because minors may find it difficult to make positive changes in their lives without the support of these systems, effective counseling requires a systemic lens. As noted later in this chapter, ethical standards such as those provided by the American Counseling Association (ACA) in the *ACA Code of Ethics* (2014) and the American School Counselor Association (ASCA) in their ASCA Ethical Standards for School Counselors (2016a) speak to the rights of parents and guardians and the need to involve support systems when working with minor clients.

A systemic perspective must consider all the social systems in which minor clients navigate their lives, including the legal system. As a general rule, few conflicts exist between ethics and the law with respect to professional counseling (Remley & Herlihy, 2020). When conflicts do occur, however, they often involve counseling minors. According to Remley and Herlihy (2020), counselors who work with children and adolescents may be more likely than any other counselors to experience conflicts between what they perceive as their ethical obligations to their minor clients and what the law dictates. These conflicts seem to occur most frequently around issues of confidentiality and protecting clients from harm. Later in the chapter, as the authors explore each of these issues, they will address both their ethical and their legal aspects and provide guidance for counselors on how to best meet both sets of obligations.

To further complicate matters, counselors who work with minors in the school environment must be knowledgeable about school system policies. School district policies offer guidelines adopted by a school board to describe the organization of the school district (Oregon School Boards Association [OSBA], n.d.) to provide consistency, stability, and continuity. Regulations formalize directions developed by the school superintendent to put the school board policies into practice. Policies and regulations inform the school staff, students, and public on the school district's organization and daily operations (OSBA, n.d.). When professional school counselors decide on a course of action, they must refer to regulations and policies first. Counselors are responsible for bringing attention to any policies or regulations that contradict state or federal law, particularly those that pertain to student confidentiality, parents' rights, issues of gender equity, child abuse reporting, potential liability, and rights of exceptional students (Schmidt, 2008). Professional school counselors also need to understand the provisions of a federal law known as Family Educational Rights and Privacy Act (FERPA), which is explained in a later section, and counselors who work with minor clients in all settings need to understand the Health Insurance Portability and Accountability Act (HIPAA).

To summarize, counselors need to navigate multiple systems in their work with minor clients. When confronted with ethical and legal dilemmas, counselors always want to make decisions that represent the best interests of their child and adolescent clients. To meet this goal successfully, they must remember that minor clients do not exist in a vacuum; they remain embedded in and dependent on multiple, diverse systems including the family, the school, and the community.

ETHICAL DECISION-MAKING

Resolving an ethical dilemma can be difficult, and at times, even agonizing because a single "right" or best answer rarely exists. After wrestling with an ethical issue, counselors typically find that several possible resolutions seem to be equally acceptable. In the end, counselors need to exercise their professional judgment and utilize their ethical reasoning skills to resolve ethical dilemmas.

Counselors understand that ethical reasoning is grounded in certain moral principles that the counseling profession agrees are foundational to our work with all clients and in all settings. The counseling literature consistently identifies five moral principles: autonomy, non-maleficence, beneficence, justice, and fidelity. *Autonomy* means that counselors respect the rights of clients to choose their own directions and control their own lives. Although minor clients hold limited autonomy because most legal rights belong to their parents or guardians, counselors work to ensure that children and adolescents receive as much freedom of choice as possible in any given situation. *Non-maleficence* means to "do no harm." Of course, counselors never intentionally harm their clients, but harm can occur inadvertently. To avoid harm, counselors need to consider both the best and worst possible effects of their decisions, not only on their clients but on others who will be impacted. Systems theory reminds us that any change in one member of a system, such as a family, will cause changes in other members of that system. Thus, this principle carries particular importance when counseling children or adolescent clients embedded in multiple systems. *Beneficence* presents the "flip side of the coin" to non-maleficence. Because counselors are helping professionals, their obligation goes beyond that of the ordinary citizen to refrain from harming others. Counselors must do more (Remley & Herlihy, 2020). They must also seek to actively do good, by ensuring that their actions promote the mental health and well-being of their minor clients. *Justice* refers to fairness and reminds counselors to treat clients equitably and avoid discrimination in any form. As our society and our school populations continue to become more diverse, this principle takes on increased importance. Finally, *fidelity* refers to honoring commitments and keeping promises. This includes the counselor's pledge to uphold confidentiality. Because minor clients enjoy only limited confidentiality, counselors must take care to ensure that these clients understand the exceptions to this pledge.

Some ethics scholars suggest that ethical decision-making grounded in this "principle ethics" perspective may present a narrow and incomplete perspective. *Principle ethics* focuses counselors' attention on the question of "What should I do in this situation?" when faced with an ethical dilemma. *Relational ethics* presents a different and emerging viewpoint in the literature (Birrell & Bruns, 2016; Gabriel & Casemore, 2009), in which counselors ask themselves, "Whom should I be in this relationship?" In other words, this newer approach urges counselors to consider whether their decisions will maintain and strengthen the counseling relationship, rather to simply search for the applicable laws or ethical standards. A relational ethics perspective aims to empower clients by involving them in the decision-making process. Especially when working with minor clients, counselors sometimes assume that they need to be making ethical decisions *for* their clients rather than *with* the clients. Through examples the authors use throughout this chapter, they demonstrate how involving minor clients in ethical decisions can work to preserve and strengthen counseling relationships.

Ethical decision-making can involve complex and sometimes competing considerations. The principles-based and relational approaches to ethical reasoning provide a framework in which this process can take place. Beyond a general framework, however, counselors need concrete resources to assist them in their decision-making. Professional associations and scholars have made many such resources available. Ethical decision-making models and codes of ethics are indispensable resources.

Ethical decision-making models are important resources for counselors. The *ACA Code of Ethics* requires counselors to use a "credible model of decision making that can bear public scrutiny" (American Counseling Association [ACA], 2014, Purpose). The *Code* does not define what makes a model credible, so counselors should choose a model published in a respected resource such as a textbook or professional journal. Numerous published models exist, including some specifically for professional school counselors (Brown et al., 2017; Luke et al., 2017) and play therapists (Seymour & Rubin, 2006). Conscientious practice requires that counselors familiarize themselves with several models. A credible model will include certain steps such as identifying the nature of problem (e.g., Does the problem present an ethical, legal, or clinical issue?), consulting with experts or colleagues, reviewing codes of ethics and relevant literature, identifying possible outcomes and implications of those outcomes, involving the client in the decision-making process to the extent possible, and documenting carefully. If a client ever challenges a counselor's actions in a court of law or files a complaint with a licensing or certifying board, the counselor would be in a much better position to respond if they have used a credible decision-making model and documented their steps.

Codes of ethics present another vital resource. Most counselors pledge to uphold more than one code of ethics, depending on their license or certification and membership in professional organizations. Professional associations such as ACA, ASCA, the American Mental Health Counselors Association (AMHCA), and the Association for Play Therapy (APT) all provide codes of ethics or statements of best practices. Most state counselor licensure laws have ethical standards embedded in their rules and regulations, and licensed counselors must be familiar with those standards. Counselors who hold national certifications, such as National Certified Counselor and National Certified School Counselor, must adhere to the ethics codes of these certifying bodies. This means that practicing counselors need to have a solid understanding of multiple codes of ethics. Throughout the chapter, relevant standards in these various codes are highlighted as they apply to particular issues. It may be helpful to know that the standards in the codes rarely, if ever, conflict with one another.

LEGAL DECISION-MAKING

Making decisions when faced with legal questions involves an entirely different process from that used in ethical decision-making. Most counselors do not hold a law degree; therefore, they should not try to make decisions that involve legal considerations. When presented with a legal question, counselors should obtain legal advice unless the question involves an issue with which they deal routinely. Counselors employed by a school or agency probably have not been given direct access to the legal counsel retained by their employer, but they can ask their supervisor to refer their question to that attorney. Self-employed counselors should purchase professional liability insurance from a provider who will afford access to legal advice. Professional associations in which counselors become members often provide a "legal hotline" or otherwise provide access to an attorney. Two cautions are offered with respect to seeking legal advice. First, when presented with a legal question, counselors should get advice from an attorney and not from a fellow mental health professional. Second, when counselors receive legal advice, they should follow that advice even if they do not agree with that advice. If a licensing board should ever challenge a counselor's decision in a court of law, it would be difficult to justify seeking legal advice and then failing to follow it.

SUMMING UP AND LOOKING AHEAD

This introductory section provided general information about ethical and legal decision-making when working with children and adolescents. The following section expands on the systemic lens needed when working with minor clients, with a focus on understanding the rights of parents or guardians. The third section focuses on specific issues, including consent to receive counseling services, confidentiality, counselor competence, ensuring client safety, dealing with crisis and trauma, resolving value conflicts, managing multiple roles and relationships, social media, and consulting with significant adults in minor clients' lives.

PARENTS' RIGHTS

CUSTODIAL AND NONCUSTODIAL PARENTS

Children and adolescents come from many different types of homes. Some live with both of their biological parents while some live with stepparents. Many children live with adoptive families, grandparents, or other relatives. Others live with two moms or two dads, although only one member of the couple may be the legal parent. Counselors who work with minors must understand that only biological parents or court-appointed guardians hold the legal right to confidential information regarding a minor. When counselors work with nontraditional families, they should obtain a copy of the most current court order regarding custody of their client or student (Remley & Herlihy, 2020). Stepparents, grandparents, other relatives, and nonmarried partners do not hold the legal privileges held by biological parents or court-appointed guardians. Sometimes, biological parents do not reside with their children, but unless the court removes their rights, they hold the same rights and authority as the noncustodial parent. Situations like these can be complicated, as the following example illustrates.

> Christopher, an 11-year-old boy, lived with Jose, his biological father, and Nina, his stepmother. He stayed with Kristen, his biological mother, on the weekends. The elementary school that Christopher attended kept all the required court orders on file, as well as an affidavit giving Christopher's stepmother permission to act on behalf of the parents when necessary. Mr. Juarez, the professional school counselor, invited Christopher to join a counseling group for children with divorced parents. On the first day of the group, Mr. Juarez gave each participant an informed consent form for their parent to sign. When Christopher got home, he excitedly told Nina about the group and about how much he had enjoyed it. He showed her the informed consent and Nina signed it. The next weekend, Christopher went to Kristen's house. As he told his mother about his week, he mentioned that he had become a member in the counseling group. Kristen became upset that no one had informed her about the counseling. On Monday morning, she called Mr. Juarez.

Mr. Juarez: *It's nice to talk to you! How can I help you today?*
Kristen: *Mr. Juarez, I'm very frustrated. Why do you think my son needs counseling? And why do you think you can take him out of class without my permission?*
Mr. Juarez: *I'm so sorry to hear that you're upset. Let me tell you about the counseling group. Christopher's teacher asked me to talk to him after Christopher wrote in his journal about how he sometimes forgets his homework at your house when he needs it at his father's house. He expressed anxiety about the living situation. I have a few other students who have expressed many of the same feelings, so I thought that it might be a great way for them to connect with one another. I sent home a consent form, and it was signed by Christopher's stepmother. I apologize if that was not okay.*
Kristen: *I knew that he was not very happy about the living arrangement, but there's no other way for it to be right now. Nina doesn't have any right to sign that form. She is always sticking her nose in where it doesn't belong. You should have made sure either I or his dad knew about the group.*
Mr. Juarez: *You are so right! I can't tell you how sorry I am. I made assumptions about how things are done in your family. Christopher's dad signed a form that allowed us to speak to Nina and accept her signature, but I should have reached out to you as well to get your consent. If you would prefer that Christopher not participate in the group, I completely understand.*
Kristen: *Thank you for your apology. Now that I know more about the group and why he's in it, I think it is okay that he participates. He really liked the first meeting. When is he being pulled out of class?*
Mr. Juarez: *This group meets during the time that his class goes to music. He misses about half of his music time once per week.*
Kristen: *I guess that's okay. In the future, please let me know if something is going on with Christopher. Jose and Nina almost always forget to tell me about stuff like that.*
Mr. Juarez: *I sure will. Again, I apologize. I'm making a note right now to contact you as well as Christopher's dad.*

This scenario serves as a reminder to counselors that family systems can take many different forms and that counselors should be careful to avoid making assumptions about the empowerment of certain family members to make decisions on behalf of the children. Mr. Juarez handled this situation well; acknowledging and apologizing for his mistake helped him to secure Kristen's cooperation.

FAMILY EDUCATIONAL RIGHTS AND PRIVACY ACT AND HEALTH INSURANCE PORTABILITY AND ACCOUNTABILITY ACT

Whether counselors work in a school or clinical setting, they need to understand the federal laws pertaining to parents' rights to access educational and medical records. Professional school counselors, in particular, need to be familiar with FERPA of 1974, a federal law that protects the privacy of students' educational records (FERPA, 1997, 20 U.S.C. § 1232g; 34 CFR Part 99) and gives parents the right to review their child's records and seek to have records corrected in certain circumstances. The school holds the responsibility to inform parents annually of their FERPA rights.

According to FERPA, schools must obtain written parental permission to release students' educational records or personally identifiable information, except to certain parties such as school officials with legitimate educational interest or other schools to which a student is transferring. The exception also extends to conditions such as complying with a judicial order or lawfully issued subpoena or in cases of health or safety emergencies (FERPA, 1997, 34 CFR § 99.31). A student's educational records include health records maintained by the school nurse. Certain student information can be disclosed without parental permission, such as a student's name, address, telephone number, and honors or awards; however, the school must inform parents about the release of "directory" information and give them an opportunity to request that the information not be shared.

FERPA regulations pertain to any educational system that receives federal funding from the U.S. Department of Education (2014), which includes virtually all public schools and most public and private postsecondary institutions. Private and religious elementary and secondary schools generally do not receive federal funding and are, therefore, exempt from FERPA.

Counselors also need to understand the provisions of HIPAA of 1996. HIPAA ensures the privacy of an individual's medical records or protected health information (PHI). HIPAA also gives individuals the right to examine their health records and to request corrections. As with FERPA, a parent must give written consent for their child's PHI to be released to another individual or provider. Counselors working in clinical settings will likely operate under HIPAA guidelines, while those in school settings will fall under FERPA guidelines, although in certain circumstances both laws apply. Regardless of setting, counselors must be familiar with parental rights under both federal laws.

Mental health providers acting in good faith may disclose PHI to law enforcement or family members when providers believe that patients pose a serious danger to themselves or others and the disclosure may prevent or reduce the threat (FERPA, 1997, 45 CFR § 164.512[j][4]). For example, if a student makes a credible threat to cause bodily harm to another student, the counselor may alert school administrators, parents, or law enforcement if the counselor believes the chance of harm may be reduced or prevented (U.S. Department of Health and Human Services, 2014).

Although this information about FERPA and HIPAA may seem quite technical, counselors do need to understand the basic guidelines of both Acts. Because adhering to FERPA and HIPAA requirements is a legal obligation, civil and even criminal penalties can be imposed on counselors who fail to adhere to them (Remley & Herlihy, 2020).

ETHICAL AND LEGAL ISSUES

The remainder of the chapter focuses on specific ethical and legal issues that arise frequently for counselors who work with minor clients and that may be the most troublesome to resolve. Some of the questions explored include the following: Who can give consent for a child or adolescent to receive counseling services? What limits to confidentiality apply when clients are minors? What competencies do counselors need to work with children and adolescents, and how are these different from the competencies needed for working with adult clients? How can counselors demonstrate that they are competent? What ethical and legal issues arise when attempting to ensure a minor client's safety in a situation involving risk to the client or others, or when managing crisis and trauma situations? How have special ethical considerations been created by the extensive use of social media? How should counselors deal with conflicts in values? How can counselors ethically navigate the multiple and sometimes conflicting roles they are asked to play? The answers to these questions are complicated and involve simultaneous consideration of multiple factors.

CONSENT TO RECEIVE COUNSELING SERVICES

Counselors are ethically obligated to obtain informed consent from clients before beginning counseling services. According to the *ACA Code of Ethics*, "Clients have the freedom to choose whether to enter into or remain in a counseling relationship and need adequate information about the counseling process and relationship" (ACA, 2014, A.2.a.). Counselors can uphold this ethical duty with adult clients by providing adequate information about counseling, both orally and in writing. Obtaining consent with minors may not be as straightforward, however. Legal language defines consent as the ability to enter into a binding contract (Remley & Herlihy, 2020). The law allows only adults to give consent, thus making a minor client's parent or legal guardian the person who usually gives legal consent for counseling. Moreover, gaining informed consent is both a legal and an ethical obligation. From an ethical standpoint, counselors want to preserve the autonomy and respect the choice-making capacity of minor clients. Counselors can uphold both the letter and the spirit of informed consent by obtaining the assent of minor clients along with the legal consent of the responsible adult (Remley & Herlihy, 2020). The best practice is to hold informed consent discussions with the minor client and consenting adult both present, and to have both the adult and the child (if of school age) or adolescent sign the informed consent document. Although children's signatures carry no legal weight, this process does convey the message to minor clients that their voices matter.

Counselors who work with minor clients outside the school setting need to be familiar with state laws regarding the age of majority and minors' rights to access mental healthcare. Although the age of majority is typically 18 years, some state laws give those under 18 the right to consent to their own mental health treatment. For example, according to Illinois law, a minor between the ages of 12 and 17 can receive up to eight 90-minute outpatient counseling or psychotherapy sessions without a parent's consent (405 ILCS 5/3-5A–105a.). Because state laws differ, counselors need to be familiar with the laws regarding the age of consent for treatment in the state where they practice.

According to Remley and Herlihy (2020), professional school counselors generally are not required to obtain parental consent to provide counseling services to students. When children enroll in school, parents are expected to understand that their children will be participating in obligatory services as well as optional services such as school counseling. However, parents do possess a right to object to their child's participation in counseling, and they would likely prevail if they would make such an objection. Sometimes, professional school counselors can overcome parental objections by meeting with the parents and reassuring them that they will be informed if their child reveals information that they need to know; for instance, that the child is engaging in behavior that poses a risk to the child or others.

CONFIDENTIALITY

Counselors hold a fundamental belief that confidentiality is essential for creating trust and establishing an effective therapeutic relationship. All clients, whether adults or minors, need to understand that their counselors will not share information about them without their permission, but that exceptions to this pledge exist. Of the numerous exceptions, two seem particularly important when counseling children and adolescents and are discussed in further detail. First, from a legal perspective, the parent or guardian of the minor client holds the rights for confidentiality. Legally, a minor does not hold that right. From an ethical standpoint, however, counselors want to promise confidentiality to their child and adolescent clients. Counselors should keep in mind that confidentiality belongs to clients, not their counselors, so that the client's perspective always must be considered. Sometimes, young children tell an adult about a situation that troubles them in hopes that the counselor will intervene with their parents or teachers. In these instances, counselors are advised to ask the child directly whether they want these important adults in their lives to know the details and, if the child appears willing, to involve those adults in the counseling process. Adolescents, on the other hand, may be reluctant to disclose anything at all without assurances of confidentiality, which makes it vital that counselors thoroughly explain the limits to the disclosures they can keep confidential from others.

The second exception that can create difficult dilemmas for counselors arises when counselors must exercise their duty to warn and protect someone who may be in danger. The danger-to-self exception to confidentiality seems clear when minor clients express suicidal ideation; in these cases, counselors need to conduct a careful risk assessment and, from a legal standpoint, must take the least intrusive measure that will keep the client safe. In other instances, the danger-to-self exception seems less clear. When minor clients engage in nonsuicidal self-injury (NSSI), their counselors must exercise professional judgment in determining whether to breach confidentiality. Occasionally, the danger posed to a minor client may arise from the behavior of others, such as in cases of severe bullying or when an adolescent client, in the heat of anger, expresses the intent to seriously hurt someone. In these kinds of situations, counselors may breach confidentiality over a minor client's objections. Again, counselors should do this only after carefully explaining to the client that they need to ensure that no one gets hurt, and only after offering to let the minor tell someone, perhaps with the counselor present to support them. The best practice includes notifying a minor client's parent or guardian to inform them of the risk assessment and tell them the results. In the school setting, in cases where the risk appears minimal, the counselor can recommend that the student be watched and be referred for counseling. School districts require professional school counselors to provide referrals for free counseling services when needed.

Clearly, counselors may struggle with their responsibility to balance their ethical obligation to keep a minor client's confidentiality with the parent's or guardian's inherent right to know about their child (American School Counselor Association [ASCA], 2016a). The following example demonstrates how a counselor might work to achieve that balance.

> Lisa, a 16-year-old student, visited her school counselor, Ms. Grant. Ms. Grant greeted Lisa with a smile while observing that Lisa appeared distressed. Lisa, after trying for several minutes to avoid talking about her distress, confided that she took a pregnancy test that morning and the result was positive. The father of the baby broke up with her 2 weeks ago and she expressed her fear of telling her mother about the pregnancy. Ms. Grant knew Lisa and her mother from previous years and felt confident that Lisa's mother might be upset at first but would be supportive of Lisa. She broached the possibility of telling her mother:
>
> Ms. Grant: *Lisa, we have talked before about how there are certain things that parents have the right to know about their children. Do you remember what those things are?*
>
> Lisa: *Yes, they have the right to know when we are in big trouble, or making bad grades, or are hurting ourselves.*

Ms. Grant: *That's right! Which of those categories do you think your pregnancy falls into?*

Lisa: *None of them! Mom can't know! She would hate me!*

Ms. Grant: *Lisa, you're scared and worried about how your mother will respond. How do you think your mom would feel if she found out that you wouldn't tell her?*

Lisa: *Well, she'd be upset that I didn't trust her.*

This conversation paved the way for Ms. Grant to explore further with Lisa the possibility of telling her mother. Ms. Grant then suggested to Lisa, "How about if I ask your mom to come in and we can tell her together? How would that be?" When Lisa agreed, Ms. Grant affirmed the decision and replied, "You and your mom have a good relationship! I will call her today and see when she can meet with us." Ms. Grant treated Lisa's situation with care and sensitivity. She could not keep Lisa's disclosure confidential, but she helped her maintain a sense of control over how her mother would learn about the pregnancy, thus respecting her autonomy.

CASE STUDY 14.1: WHAT WOULD YOU DO?

You are a counselor in private practice who works with children and teenagers. A 17-year-old client reveals to you that he is smoking marijuana and drinking alcohol frequently. The use is affecting his grades and you are concerned that it will lead to addiction. His parents are aware that he has been smoking and drinking on occasion because this was discussed during the intake session you held with the parents and client present. You suspect the parents are not aware of the frequency, despite the adolescent's claims that they know about it.

Activity 14.1

Reflect on your values and beliefs about drinking and marijuana use. Are your beliefs influenced by any personal experiences, such as having a family member or close friend who has struggled with addiction? How might your values or beliefs influence your decision-making process in this scenario?

COUNSELOR COMPETENCE

Boundaries of Competence

Competence involves a combination of knowledge, skill, and diligence (Remley & Herlihy, 2020). Counselor competencies define the mind-sets and behaviors that must be met by counselors to fulfill the demands of the counseling profession (ASCA, 2019). Counselors are ethically obligated to practice within the boundaries of their competence (*ACA Code of Ethics*, 2014, C.2.a). Although this ethical standard seems straightforward, competence in counseling is difficult to define (Remley & Herlihy, 2020). Counseling, like many other professions such as medicine or law, can be described as a broad field that involves numerous specialties, and no counselor could be competent to counsel all clients in all settings. Because counselors need specialized competencies, many organizations identify competencies for different areas of counseling. The Council for Accreditation of Counseling and Related Educational Programs (CACREP) sets standards that must be followed for any counseling program they accredit. These standards include eight core standards and six specialty standards broken down into learning objectives for counseling students (CACREP, 2016; Sommers-Flanagan, 2015). ACA provides nine lists of competencies in the areas of counseling lesbian, gay, bisexual, queer, intersex, questioning, and ally (LGBQIQA) clients, competencies for counseling transgender clients, animal-assisted therapy competencies, and multicultural and social justice competencies for counselors. ASCA (2019) provides competencies for professional school counselors.

All of the documents just mentioned assist in identifying the requisite competencies needed by counselors, but they do not answer the question of who decides whether a counselor actually possesses these competencies. The question of who determines a counselor's competency depends on the counselor's level of training and experience. When prospective counselors are enrolled in their master's degree programs, their professors determine whether they meet a certain competency level to proceed to the next level of training. As students make progress through their training and enter their internships to gain supervised clinical practice, those who provide the supervision at the university and at the student's site are responsible for determining competence. Once mental health counselors acquire their master's degrees and seek licensure, their supervisors act as the "gatekeepers" to their entry into the profession until they complete the required number of supervised hours (which vary from state to state).

For counselors who acquire their master's degrees and start working in school settings, however, it is likely that no individual will be assigned to assess their competence. Unlike clinical mental health counselors, who must complete extensive post-master's-degree supervision, professional school counselors are not required to practice under supervision once they hold the master's degree. Many school districts, particularly larger ones, offer clinical and administrative supervision to professional school counselors. Counselors in small or rural districts may not receive supervision, however.

Researchers have found that professional school counselors who do not receive adequate clinical supervision are at high risk for burnout. Consequences of burnout include poor job performance and compassion fatigue, which often lead to impairment. Professional school counselors who are impaired may experience feelings of isolation and depersonalization, with the result that students are not adequately served.

Once counselors have obtained their license or have begun working as professional school counselors, the burden of determining competence shifts to the counselors themselves; they are obligated to maintain competence to work with the clients or students they serve (ACA, 2014; ASCA, 2016a). What is tricky about this obligation is that competence is not a static state; as the body of knowledge in our field grows, and as counselors find themselves serving new client populations in our diverse society, counselors must continue to learn and develop new competencies. They need to maintain a delicate balance, meeting the ethical obligation to practice within one's boundaries of competence and at the same time extending those boundaries without causing harm to clients. Strategies that are helpful to counselors in maintaining this balance include periodically reviewing the competencies that professional associations provide, seeking professional development on a regular basis, and finding mentors or supervisors who can monitor their work with clients whom they find challenging. A peer consultation group that meets regularly to discuss these challenges is helpful. Counselors in schools or other settings can form such a group if one does not already exist where they work.

Multicultural Competence

As mentioned in Chapter 4 and many other chapters in this book, multicultural competence may be one of the most difficult aspects of competence to define and maintain. The United States is a richly diverse society that is constantly changing, so that even the most experienced counselors are challenged to develop new skills and knowledge. The case of Miranda is relevant in this context.

CASE STUDY 14.2: WHAT WOULD YOU DO?

Miranda, a professional school counselor, had worked for over a decade in a suburb of a large city. The population of this suburb had been stable and relatively homogeneous (mostly White and Christian) until the area received a large influx of immigrants from a strife-torn, predominantly Muslim Middle Eastern country. As Miranda quickly realized, the children of these immigrants were dealing with multiple stressors including the trauma of having fled their home country, struggling to learn in a language they barely knew, and being visibly different from the majority of their peers. Miranda had much to learn. She began reading about the Islamic faith, sought out an Imam in the immigrant community who could help her better understand the struggles of the children of his congregants, developed psychoeducation programs to educate students about their new peers, and formed support groups for the new students.

Students who identify as LGBTQ often report experiencing harassment and bullying in schools (Kull et al., 2019). Professional school counselors routinely work with LGBTQ students regarding their sexual orientation and gender identity (ASCA, 2016b). They advocate and support students who are in the LGBTQ community to provide a safe space for them by encouraging staff training on best practices for inclusion (ASCA, 2016b). Professional school counselors also advocate for school policies that address discrimination and promote violence-prevention programs.

Competence and Credentialing

Counselors can demonstrate their competence through acquiring and maintaining professional credentials. The first step to becoming credentialed is to earn a master's degree. Counselors who graduate from a CACREP-accredited program in counseling can rely on their training program to have provided them with the necessary competencies. It should be noted, however, that variations exist among programs even when they are CACREP-accredited and that training may differ according to specialization areas. In programs where mental health counseling is the primary emphasis, school counselors-in-training may feel less valued and may receive fewer opportunities to gain knowledge and experience specific to their intended work setting (Pool et al., in press). For example, all coursework except for two courses, likely in school counseling and in child and adolescent development, may be geared toward preparing students for mental health counseling positions. This situation persists in part because relatively few counselor educators come from a school counseling background and because some may not be well versed in state models such as the Texas Comprehensive Model for School Counseling Programs (Texas Education Agency, 2018) and the ASCA National Model: A Framework for School Counseling Programs (2019).

As has been noted, counselors who work with children and adolescents in nonschool settings must become state licensed, which involves meeting standards established by each state's licensure board. Licensure laws establish the educational, examination, and supervised experience requirements. In most states, CACREP-accredited programs meet all educational requirements. The licensure exam requirement varies from state to state. According to the National Board for Certified Counselors (NBCC), states require applicants to take and pass the National Counselor Exam or the National Clinical Mental Health Counseling Exam (NCMHCE), although some states require both. The final requirement for licensure is the supervised experience requirement; counselors-in-training acquire direct counseling hours and indirect hours at an approved site while under the supervision of a board-approved supervisor. Just as licensing requirements vary by state, the titles used to identify professional counselors also vary. According to the ACA, the titles may include Licensed Professional Counselor (LPC), Licensed Clinical Mental Health Counselor (LMHC), and Licensed Mental Health Professional (LMHP), among others. A provisional or associate license is issued until the required number of supervised hours is obtained. Once licensed, counselors must meet ongoing continuing education requirements to maintain their license.

Public professional school counselors must meet the requirements set by their state's department of education. Although the ASCA website references "State Certification Requirements," some states refer to the school counseling credential as a "license" rather than a "certificate," which may lead to confusion (ASCA, n.d.). Professional school counselors do not have the same experience and supervision requirements post their master's degree as do mental health counselors. In addition to the difference in language around "license" and "certification," variations exist in the educational, experience, and exam requirements. For example, some states require prior teaching experience for professional school counselors plus specified number of hours in designated counseling-related courses, whereas others require coursework in special education. Although the required exam also varies by state, most states require the Praxis for Professional School Counselors exam (ASCA, n.d.). Some professional school counselors hold dual credentials, possessing both certification and license. Further, individuals may choose to seek an additional credential through NBCC to become a National Certified Counselor (NCC) or National Certified School Counselor (NCSC). According to NBCC (n.d.), counselors who earn one or both credentials "have met stringent education, examination, supervision, experience, and ethical requirements" and "offer the highest standards of practice."

CHILD AND ADOLESCENT CLIENT SAFETY

Mandatory Reporting

Counselors have a legal and ethical obligation to keep their child and adolescent clients safe from foreseeable harm. As mandatory reporters (mentioned in Chapter 11), school and mental health counselors are required by law to report incidents of child maltreatment, which may include physical, sexual, or emotional abuse, or neglect. Laws and reporting procedures vary by state; therefore, counselors should become familiar with the laws and statutes specific to their state of practice. Schools and agencies often require employees to complete mandatory reporter training as a term of employment. The best practice is to complete a training program even if it is not required. The Child Welfare Information Gateway (U.S. Department of Health and Human Services, n.d.) provides easy access to state laws regarding child abuse and neglect, child welfare, and adoption. Although variations exist from state to state, generally a mandatory reporter must make a report to their state's Child Protection Services department when neglect or abuse is known or suspected. It is important to note that the abuse or neglect does not need to be confirmed to be reported. Further, counselors should not "investigate" to determine if a report should be filed; rather, they should consult with a supervisor or colleague. In some settings, such as in a school or hospital setting, an institutional or organizational report must also be filed. The requirement to maintain confidentiality does not apply in cases of mandatory reporting because safety takes precedence over the protection of confidential information (ACA, 2014, B.2.a.).

CASE STUDY 14.3: WHAT WOULD YOU DO?

Your 10-year-old male client is worried and very angry because his mom is in an abusive relationship with a new boyfriend. He lives 3 hours away with his dad and does not visit his mom at the boyfriend's house. He expresses to you that he wants to burn the boyfriend's house down. You have worked very hard for months to gain the trust of your young client, and he has finally begun to open up to you. You are concerned about losing his trust if you report what he has said to you. You realize that he cannot get himself to the boyfriend's house 3 hours away; however, you are concerned that he may actually carry out the threat if he were to ever visit.

Activity 14.2

Work with a partner or in a small group to apply the steps of a credible ethical decision-making model to this scenario. Describe what you would do in the situation. Do all group members reach consensus as to the best way to proceed? Why or why not?

Suicide and Nonsuicidal Self-Injury

According to Corey et al. (2015), dealing with a suicidal client can be one of the most stressful situations counselors will encounter. As with adults, when minor clients appear to be at risk of hurting themselves or others, counselors must take swift and immediate action. The best practice involves conducting a thorough risk assessment if a client expresses suicidal ideation, reveals NSSI, or if the counselor suspects that the client may harm others. Additionally, best practice includes the notification of a minor client's parent or guardian to inform them of the risk assessment and tell them the results. Counselors also need to adhere to the policies and procedures of the setting in which they practice, which may include informing a supervisor of the assessment.

Remley and Herlihy (2020) recommend that counselors use an ethical decision-making model and document all steps in the process when assessing a client's risk of suicide. Based on the level of risk determined from the assessment, counselors must take "concrete measures" to ensure the child's safety (Kress et al., 2019). Such measures should include monitoring the child and implementing a safety plan. Additional measures may include a referral to a pediatrician, psychiatrist, or other medical professional for further evaluation. If a child or adolescent is determined to be at a high risk, an inpatient hospitalization may be necessary to ensure safety. Counselors should be aware of the laws in their state related to the hospitalization of minors (King et al., 2013). The actions taken to ensure a client's safety may be disruptive to their lives and should be the least intrusive to prevent harm. It is imperative for counselors to know the warning signs of suicide and accurately assess the level of risk (Remley & Herlihy, 2020).

Counselors should regularly assess NSSI, or the intentional injury of one's body without the intent of suicide, in terms of the frequency, duration, severity, and onset (Hoffman & Kress, 2010). Suicide risk should also be assessed; however, self-injury should be considered suicidal in nature only if the client expresses a desire to die (Kress et al., 2019). A challenge for counselors is to determine when to inform parents of self-injurious behavior. Although some counselors may feel inclined to inform parents every time a child or adolescent self-injures, they should keep in mind the possibility that the therapeutic alliance may be damaged due to loss of trust. At the same time, a counselor can be held liable if the child is harmed and parents are not informed. Consultation is critical when making the determination to inform parents. In cases when parents are informed of self-injurious behavior, the counselor strives to maintain the therapeutic relationship. Recommendations for informing parents include the counselor and child telling together, the child telling the parents, or the counselor informing the child that they will be telling (Remley & Herlihy, 2020).

TRAUMA, DISASTER, AND CRISIS RESPONSE

Counselors inevitably will encounter clients who need help during or after a traumatic event. The traumatic event could occur at a personal or a familial level, such as a death, abuse, or sexual assault, or an event might happen on a larger scale and involve a school, community, region, or the entire country. As mentioned in Chapter 13, examples of large-scale events include school or community mass shootings, weather-related events such as hurricanes, terrorist attacks, and pandemics. Regardless of the magnitude of the event, counselors respond with immediate intervention, and they will encounter situations that present ethical issues. A counselor's response to an individual or family event may not present complex ethical dilemmas because services are likely delivered in a controlled environment, like the counselor's office. Other disaster-related events may necessitate that services be delivered in a setting where privacy cannot be guaranteed or are delivered through a different format such as the computer or phone. These events and nontypical settings can create ethical situations for counselors to navigate.

Some crisis events that occur in a school setting can place professional school counselors in unaccustomed roles. When a crisis occurs in a school, the administrative team typically focuses on securing the physical safety of the students and staff. Professional school counselors, on the other hand, often carry out the task of securing the emotional welfare of the students, staff, and parents. During normal day-to-day operations, professional school counselors would not be ethically responsible for the emotional care of staff and parents;

however, a crisis may dictate otherwise until additional mental health providers arrive. After the crisis, the school counselor may be called upon to coordinate larger response and postvention efforts for the school community (Kerr, 2009). The immediate response and recovery efforts may require professional school counselors to function beyond their typical responsibilities as outlined in the Texas Model for Comprehensive School Counseling Programs and the ASCA National Model.

The response to man-made and natural disasters can create challenges to ethical practice. After a disaster or crisis event, counseling services may take place face to face in nontraditional settings such as cafeterias, gyms, shelters, makeshift offices, tents, or outdoor areas (Call et al., 2012). Other national emergencies involving quarantine or shelter-in-place orders may necessitate counseling via telemental health. Issues related to confidentiality may arise in nontraditional settings. Although counselors have an ethical obligation to ensure client confidentiality and privacy (ACA, 2014, B.1c), doing so may be difficult in settings such as a shelter or an outdoor tent. Telemental health practice inherently creates issues related to privacy because the counselor cannot see who is out of view of the camera, may not be aware if someone else enters the room, and has no control over the remote setting. Siblings and others in the shelter or house may "join" the session unexpectedly. Child and adolescent clients should be informed of the limitations associated with nontraditional settings and telemental health, and counselors should include them in the discussion of how to handle such situations. For example, if someone approaches or enters the room, an agreed-upon "code word" may be used to alert the counselor that privacy has been compromised.

Typically, the delivery of crisis counseling services and telemental health services requires specialized training and certification through state licensure boards and the NBCC. Requirements may be waived or adjusted by state licensing boards during a disaster or emergency situation, however, so that individuals can receive necessary services. Although requirements are waived, counselors should still make every effort to receive the appropriate and necessary training prior to delivering services.

A final consideration is that counselors have an ethical obligation to inform clients of their approach to counseling (ACA, 2014, A.2.). When counselors are responding to a crisis or disaster, they may use a different approach than they use in ordinary circumstances. Due to the nature of crisis counseling, counselors often find themselves being more directive and action oriented (Schmidt, 2008) because clients often experience diminished decision-making ability in the wake of the crisis. When counselors deliver counseling services for young children via telehealth, they may deviate from their usual approach. For example, a child-centered play therapist may be more directive, given the telehealth platform. Regardless of the setting or situation, the client's welfare and safety are imperative. Rules, ethical guidelines, and laws pertaining to mental health professions are not suspended during disaster response (Call et al., 2012). An ethical decision-making model and consultation should guide counselors' decisions during disaster and crisis events.

DEALING WITH VALUE CONFLICTS

A series of court cases (*Bruff v. North Mississippi Health Services, Inc.*, 2001; *Keeton v. Anderson-Wiley et al.*, 2011; *Walden v. Centers for Disease Control and Prevention*, 2010; *Ward v. Wilbanks*, 2010, 2012) established that counselors cannot refuse to counsel clients because the client's beliefs or behaviors conflict with the personal values of the counselor. This means that counselors must be aware of their beliefs and values and must be able to set aside or bracket those values (Kocet & Herlihy, 2014) when they enter the counseling session. The court cases mentioned previously all dealt with conflicts between conservative religious values (the belief that same-sex sexual and romantic relationships are sinful) held by the counselors or counselors-in-training and the beliefs and behaviors of clients who sought their services. Counselors who work with children and adolescents should familiarize themselves with the position statements provided by ASCA on working with LGBTQ youth, gender equity, cultural diversity, and equity for all students. Those position statements may be found on ASCA's website.

Although value conflicts related to counselors' personal beliefs regarding sexual or affectional orientation continue to be the focus of controversy, value conflicts can arise around numerous other issues when counselors work with children and adolescents. A counselor might perceive parents' methods of disciplining their children to be abusive, even when the parents' behavior might not be considered abusive by cultural, community, or legal standards. A counselor may disapprove of some forms of adolescent clients' experimentation with sexual behavior or drugs. In today's digital world, children and adolescents make use of social media in ways that may seem to adults to be ill advised and carry potential for harm (such as "sexting"). Clearly, counselors intervene when their concerns are based on potential risk of harm to a client; however, they avoid actions that are based solely on their own personal moral or religious opinions or beliefs.

When the ACA revised its *ACA Code of Ethics* in 2014, Standard A.11.a. was added to provide guidance with respect to value conflicts. This standard supplemented Standard A.4.b, which advised counselors to be aware of and avoid imposing their values on clients, by clarifying that counselors do not refer clients based solely on the counselor's personally held beliefs or values.

APT published Best Practice guidelines in 2020, which go into considerable detail regarding therapist personal values. The guidelines state, in part, that play therapists recognize the vulnerability of clients and do not impose personal attitudes and beliefs on their clients. This does not mean, however, that therapists attempt to conduct therapy free of values. Play therapists intervene when the client's behavior presents a danger to the client or others. Play therapists should also be aware of how their own values, attitudes, and beliefs affect their clients. Play therapists seek out supervision, consultation, personal therapy, or personal reflection/reading to make sure their own values, attitudes, and beliefs do not negatively impact treatment. Lastly, play therapists make every effort to understand clients' and legal guardians' values, attitudes, and beliefs (therapy is not about us) and convey to clients, and their legal guardians, if applicable, the system or basis on which they, as therapists, make value judgments and decisions in therapy (Association for Play Therapy [APT], 2020).

Counselors who work with children and adolescents in school settings should adhere to the statement in the ASCA Ethical Standards for School Counselors (ASCA, 2016a), that counselors "respect students' and families' values, beliefs, sexual orientation, gender identification/expression and cultural background; and exercise great care to avoid imposing personal beliefs or values rooted in one's religion, culture, or ethnicity" (Standard A.1.f.). These robust standards in codes of ethics for members of ACA, APT, and ASCA underscore the importance of being aware of and not imposing one's own values.

DUAL ROLES AND RELATIONSHIPS

Dual relationships occur when counselors hold more than one relationship or play more than one role with a client (Herlihy & Corey, 2015). Because the expectations and responsibilities associated with different roles may conflict with each other, ethics experts advise counselors to be cautious about entering into dual relationships due to a potential for harm. At the same time, dual relationships, in and of themselves, are not unethical. In fact, they often are unavoidable and may even be beneficial at times. The criterion that matters when examining dual roles and relationships is the potential for harm. To give some examples that range along the spectrum of possible harm, at one extreme would be a counselor entering into a romantic or sexual relationship with a minor client. Because of the clear potential for exploitation, this behavior is judged as both unethical and illegal. At the other end of the spectrum might be an instance when a counselor attends a client's special event such as a graduation or awards ceremony. For example, a graduating high school senior and the student's parents might feel grateful to a counselor who helped this student stay in school, and they might invite the counselor to a graduation party hosted by the parents. The potential for harm in this situation seems minimal, and it would be acceptable for the counselor to accept the invitation.

An abundance of literature exists regarding dual relationships; however, very little literature explores the occurrence of boundary issues with minors or with counselors working in the school environment. Yet dual relationships occur frequently and may even be inevitable when counselors work with minors in "small worlds" or rural settings. Multiple roles seem inherent in the jobs of professional school counselors. Professional school counselors often have relationships not only with minor clients, but also with others in the lives of those clients, including parents, teachers, other school personnel, and community members. Realistically, professional school counselors cannot always avoid dual relationships. Particularly in rural communities, or in small schools with only one counselor, the counselor's friends may also be their student clients' teachers, or parents, or other family members. Confidentiality considerations limit what the counselor can share and not only about what the student revealed in counseling. The counselor should also exercise caution about discussing such seemingly innocuous topics as a bad day at work, if identities could be discerned. These kinds of constraints can be isolating for counselors, so that it becomes important for them to have social connections apart from their work. Role conflicts can occur in unanticipated ways. Consider the case of Maria.

CASE STUDY 14.4: WHAT WOULD YOU DO?

Maria, who is in recovery from an addiction, takes a job as a professional high school counselor in an isolated rural area. She wants to attend a 12-step group, but one of her adolescent clients attends the only group in the area. Maria seems to be faced with an impossible choice, either to attend the same group as one of her clients or to jeopardize her own recovery by not attending the group.

Professional school counselors often play multiple roles that may not be compatible with their primary role as counselor. Sometimes, counselors are tasked with administrative or ancillary duties such as sponsoring a student group, hall monitoring, or bus duty. In any of these noncounselor roles, the possibility exists that the counselor may have to act as a disciplinarian. When the counselor, who is accepting and nonjudgmental during counseling sessions, behaves in a judgmental or punitive manner outside the counseling office, these situations can be uncomfortable for counselors and confusing for students. Counselors can be proactive in working to minimize these problems by educating teachers, administrators, and parents about the nature of their role.

The Ethical Standards for School Counselors (2016) provide extensive guidance to professional school counselors who want to manage boundaries and dual relationships appropriately. Counselors are advised to "avoid dual relationships that might impair their objectivity and increase the risk of harm to students (e.g., counseling one's family members or the children of close friends or associates)" (Standard A.5.a.).

The standards caution professional school counselors to establish and maintain appropriate professional relationships with students at all times. When professional school counselors consider extending current school counseling relationships beyond conventional parameters, such as attending a student's distant athletic competition, they weigh the risks and benefits (Standard A.5.b.). Further, the standards address counselors' potential dual relationships with school personnel, parents/guardians, and students' other family members. Counselors must avoid these relationships when they might infringe on the integrity of the school counselor/student relationship. The standards present some examples, such as providing direct discipline, teaching courses that involve grading students, and accepting administrative duties in the absence of an administrator. Finally, the standards identify safeguards that professional school counselors can employ, including informed consent, consultation, supervision, and documentation.

CASE STUDY 14.5: WHAT WOULD YOU DO?

As a professional high school counselor, the school assigned you a caseload composed of the tenth graders each year. Your best friend, Monique, works as a teacher at your school. Her son, Mark, also attends the same school. You know Mark personally through your friendship with Monique. Next year, Mark will be a 10th grader assigned to your case load. You want to prepare for any issues that might arise.

SOCIAL MEDIA

A host of new boundary issues have emerged from the use of social media by children and adolescents. Children and adolescents use social media to communicate in ways, and to an extent, that older generations could never have imagined. According to the U.S. Department of Health and Human Services (2016), over 94% of youth use some type of social media and 71% use more than one social media site. The burgeoning use of social media presents many new questions that counselors must be prepared to answer. What if a child or adolescent client wants to "friend" the counselor on Facebook? What if the counselor suspects that an adolescent client is engaging in "sexting"? What if a professional school counselor receives a report that a student is being cyberbullied but the student refuses to identify the perpetrators? All these questions require the counselor to consider boundary issues. Some are relatively easy to answer; for instance, it is not wise to accept a "friend" invitation from a client of any age. Also, counselors who participate on Facebook or similar sites need to pay careful attention to their privacy settings so that clients cannot access information about the counselors' personal, social, or familial life. Other questions are more difficult to resolve. For example, it might be possible for a counselor to ascertain the identity of perpetrators of cyberbullying by searching students' social media sites, but this would be ill advised and would be an invasion of their privacy.

The ASCA Ethical Standards for School Counselors (2016a) provide specific guidance in Standard A.5.d. for counselors working in school systems. Professional school counselors cannot use personal social media, personal email accounts, or personal texts to interact with students unless this is specifically encouraged and sanctioned by the school district. Technologies that professional school counselors use, including social networking sites and apps, should be endorsed by the school district and used appropriately. Because professional school counselors are embedded in complex systems, they are tasked with considering multiple constituencies in addition to their student clients.

Because social media and other forms of technology are changing so rapidly, counselors must work to remain media savvy so that they are aware of the ways their minor clients are using these technologies and the potential risks involved. Despite the increasing popularity and usage of social media among teens and adolescents, current literature regarding ethical issues related to social media is sparse. The *ACA Code of Ethics* (2014) and Government Affairs division of the ACA provide guidance for counselors regarding social media usage; however, additional guidance is needed as it relates specifically to child and adolescent clients and their social media usage. Even though a client and a counselor are not "friends" or "following" one another on social media, a counselor may inadvertently learn of suicidal ideation or threat to a client or may become privy to other information that may pose an ethical dilemma for the counselor. Until further recommendations are made by our professional organizations, counselors should continue to consult with fellow professionals and follow ethical decision-making models when faced with social media–related situations.

CASE STUDY 14.6: WHAT WOULD YOU DO?

You live in a small town where you practice as a counselor. One of your friends sends you a screen shot of an Instagram post shared by her neighbor, who happens to be your teen client. The post states that she plans to kill herself that night. You do not use Instagram, so you could not have "happened across" the post on your own. During recent sessions, you have asked your client about suicidal ideation because of her feelings of hopelessness, but she has denied being suicidal.

CONSULTATION WITH TEACHERS, PARENTS, AND OUTSIDE AGENCIES

When working with children and adolescents, counselors often find it necessary to consult with others involved in the youth's life. According to Remley and Herlihy (2020), "Counselors regularly consult with others for the benefit of their clients and to further their knowledge of a particular area of counseling" (p. 375). Teachers, parents, and other professionals may provide valuable information to give counselors a more holistic view of the child's world. This more comprehensive understanding may help guide intervention choices, treatment goals, and ensure accurate diagnosis. Consultation with others in the school setting may help address the academic concerns of students, as well as determine appropriate accommodations for students with disabilities.

As mentioned previously, counselors need to follow HIPAA and FERPA guidelines when sharing information with others. According to the *ACA Code of Ethics* (2014), counselors may share information during case consultations if discussed for professional purposes only and when "every effort is made to protect client identity and to avoid undue invasion of privacy" (Standard B.7.a.). In addition, if prior consent is not obtained and consultation with a colleague is necessary, counselors should not disclose information that could lead to the identification of the individual. The *ACA Code of Ethics* (2014) further advises that the counselor should "disclose information only to the extent necessary to achieve the purposes of the consultation" (Standard B.7.b.).

Consultation is important not only for the benefit of the client or to further one's professional knowledge; consultation is also critical when making ethical decisions. Both the *ACA Code of Ethics* (2014) and the ASCA Ethical Standards for School Counselors (2016a) provide guidance for ethical decision-making and include consultation with experts or colleagues as part of the process.

CHAPTER SUMMARY

Counselors who work solely with adult clients might believe that counseling children and adolescents is easy by comparison. Child and adolescent counselors would be quick to disabuse them of that notion, particularly with respect to ensuring legally and ethically sound practice. Whereas legal and ethical mandates generally support counselors in their work, law and ethics can conflict when clients are minors, sometimes leaving counselors torn between what they believe is an ethical thing to do and what the law demands. Counseling minors is a complex undertaking because children and adolescents are not able to make decisions as independently as adults and are embedded in multiple systems that always need to be considered. A section of this chapter addressed parent rights and provided suggestions for enlisting the cooperation and support of parents and guardians, and the multiple constituencies of professional school counselors were highlighted throughout.

When child and adolescent counselors are faced with legal issues, they should seek legal advice. In this chapter, guidelines were offered to assist counselors in obtaining legal advice. Ethical decision-making, by contrast, is the responsibility of the counselors themselves. Resources for ethical decision-making include decision-making models, codes of ethics, and consultation with experts and peers. Throughout the chapter, ways to make best use of each of these resources are suggested.

The ethical issues that child and adolescent counselors encounter are much the same as the issues that arise when counseling adults, but these issues are complicated by the fact that their clients are minors with few legal rights and comparatively less capacity for independent decision-making. This chapter presented a discussion of the ethical obligation to provide clients with informed consent as it applies to working with minor clients, whose legal rights are limited in this area but who have the same ethical right to understand what counseling entails.

Although counselors want to uphold the confidentiality of their minor clients, a number of exceptions exist. Child and adolescent counselors are called upon to exercise their professional judgment when minor clients engage in risky behaviors such as NSSI, sexual experimentation, or unsafe use of social media. The burgeoning use of social media by children and adolescents warranted special attention to this issue in the chapter.

Counselors are ethically obligated to practice within their boundaries of competence; however, it can be difficult to determine exactly where those boundaries lie. Issues related to developing and maintaining competence were discussed, along with the obligation of counselors to be multiculturally competent in today's diverse society.

As the entire world has experienced the upheavals created by the coronavirus disease 2019 (COVID-19) pandemic, attention to ethical and legal issues related to trauma and crisis counseling has become vital; these issues are addressed in this chapter. Additional issues that were addressed in depth include value conflicts and dual relationships, two issues that have received limited attention in the literature on counseling children and adolescents. The chapter concluded with a discussion of consultation with adults who are important in the lives of minor clients. The material in this chapter has provided readers with a sense of the complexity and challenges of maintaining legal and ethical practice when counseling children and adolescents.

POINTS TO REMEMBER

- A systemic lens is required when counseling children and adolescents, because minor clients are embedded in multiple systems.
- Counselors should always obtain legal advice when faced with legal questions. When ethical questions arise, counselors should utilize resources such as decision-making models, code of ethics, the literature, and consultation with experts and peers.
- Although minor clients have few legal rights, they have the same ethical rights as adult clients (such as the right to understand and consent to counseling services, to have their confidentiality upheld to the extent possible, to receive competent services, and to have counselors who put their welfare first).

OTHER HELPFUL INFORMATION FOR CONSIDERATION

- American Counseling Association (ethical decision-making): https://www.counseling.org/knowledge-center/ethics/ethical-decision-making
- American Counseling Association (trauma and disaster mental health): https://www.counseling.org/knowledge-center/mental-health-resources/trauma-disaster
- American School Counselor Association (legal and ethical guidance): https://www.schoolcounselor.org/school-counselors-members/legal-ethical
- Child Welfare Information Gateway (state statutes): https://www.childwelfare.gov/topics/systemwide/laws-policies/state
- National Institute of Mental Health (suicide): https://www.nimh.nih.gov/health/publications/suicide-faq/index.shtml

QUESTIONS FOR FURTHER DISCUSSION

- What kinds of training do you think child and adolescent counselors need to have, in order to assure that they are able to practice at the highest ethical and legal standards? How would you describe the ideal preparation for this work?
- What do you foresee as the most challenging for you, of all the legal and ethical issues that are involved in counseling minor clients?
- How can you determine the extent of your responsibility in helping to keep children and adolescents safe when they engage in risky behaviors such as drug and alcohol use, sexting, cyberbullying, and NSSI?

- If you are counseling a child and you believe that the behavior of the child's parent or guardian is a primary reason for the child's problems but the parent or guardian refuses to cooperate in the counseling process, what should you do?
- How would you respond if the parent or guardian of one of your child clients accuses you of unethical behavior? Realizing that such events are very stressful, how would you practice self-care during this time?

KEY REFERENCES

Only key references appear in the print edition. The full reference list appears in the digital product on Springer Publishing Connect: connect.springerpub.com/content/book/978-0-8261-4764-6/part/part05/chapter/ch14

American Counseling Association. (2014). *ACA code of ethics*. Author.

American School Counselor Association. (2016a). *ASCA ethical standards for school counselors*. Author. https://www.schoolcounselor.org/getmedia/f041cbd0-7004-47a5-ba01-3a5d657c6743/Ethical-Standards.pdf

Association for Play Therapy. (2020). *Play therapy best practices: Clinical, professional, & ethical issues*. Author. https://cdn.ymaws.com/www.a4pt.org/resource/resmgr/publications/apt_best_practices_-_june_20.pdf

Birrell, P. J., & Bruns, C. M. (2016). Ethics and relationship: From risk management to relational engagement. *Journal of Counseling & Development, 94*, 391–397. https://doi.org/10.1002/jcad.12097

Brown, T., Armstrong, S. A., Bore, S., & Simpson, C. (2017). Using an ethical decision-making model to address ethical dilemmas in school counseling. *Journal of School Counseling, 15*(13). http://www.jsc.montana.edu/articles/v15n13.pdf

Corey, G., Corey, M., Corey, C., & Callahan, P. (2015). *Issues and ethics in the helping professions* (9th ed.). Brooks/Cole.

Luke, M., Gilbride, D., & Goodrich, K. M. (2017). School counselors' approach to ethical decision making. *Journal of Counselor Leadership and Advocacy, 4*(1), 1–15. https://doi.org/10.1080/2326716x.2016.1223569

Remley, T., & Herlihy, B. (2020). *Ethical, legal, and professional issues in counseling* (6th ed.). Pearson.

U.S. Department of Education. (2014). Family Education Rights and Privacy Act (FERPA). http://www2.ed.gov/policy/gen/guid/fpco/ferpa/index.html

U.S. Department of Health and Human Services. (2014). Health information privacy. http://www.hhs.gov/ocr/privacy

CHAPTER 15

Other Special Topics in Counseling Children and Adolescents: Program Identity, Essential Skills, and Counselor Wellness

Rhonda M. Bryant, Le'Ann Solmonson, Beth Durodoye, and Tracy M. Knighton

LEARNING OBJECTIVES

After completing this chapter, the reader should be able to:

- Identify trends and issues in school counseling programs.
- Discuss empathy and related counseling concepts and their applicability to teaching and learning.
- Explain the importance of counselor wellness.

CACREP STANDARDS FOR THIS CHAPTER

- CACREP 2016: 2.F.1.e., l.; 2.F.2.h.; School Counseling: 5.G.1.b., 5.G.2.a., 5.G.3.o.; Clinical Mental Health Counseling: 5.C.2.a., 5.C.3.b.
- CACREP 2009: Professional Identity: II.G.1.d., i., II.G.2.e., II.G.5.a.; School Counseling: A.5.; B.2.; D.1., 5.; E.3.; F.3.; J.3.; K.2.; O.4.; Clinical Mental Health Counseling: D.9.; F.2.

INTRODUCTION

The scope of responsibility for counselors, counselor educators, and counseling supervisors who counsel children and adolescents continues to evolve. Counseling professionals consider the prioritization of child and adolescent success in academic and social settings as a common thread in their work. Similarities also exist in the opportunities and challenges available to develop programs that meet students' needs and reflect counseling professionals' maintenance of their self-care and personal well-being. This chapter explores special topics for counseling professionals who work in diverse settings with children and adolescents. Specifically, this chapter identifies the barriers that impede the implementation of excellent school counseling programs and clinical mental health counseling programs with this population; the use of empathy in counseling and counseling supervision; and wellness and counselor self-care. Principles of development and relational, systemic, and multicultural approaches characterize this chapter's strategy.

SCHOOL COUNSELING PROGRAMS

Decades of research evidence that school counseling programs contribute to positive and measurable influences on students' learning in and out of the classroom (Carey & Dimmitt, 2012; Jones et al., 2019; Lemberger et al., 2018). The American School Counselor Association (ASCA), one of the professional organizations for professional school counselors, publishes numerous studies on school counseling efficacy. In particular, the ASCA National Model outlines components that characterize a comprehensive school counseling program for some school districts. First published in 2002 and now in its fourth edition, the National Model presents a framework that not only delineates essential aspects of a school counseling program but also posits the school counseling program as collaborative and beneficial to many stakeholders. The model identifies students, their families, educators, school leaders, the school community, and the communities that house them as stakeholders (ASCA, n.d.).

Not all states implement the ASCA National Model, however. In the United States, any given state can develop and codify its educational laws and policies that relate to professional school counseling. Examples of this include states such as Texas and Florida, which designed and implemented a statewide comprehensive model of school counseling codified by state law. Of note, in 2004, the state of Texas codified into law the *Texas Model for Comprehensive School Counseling Programs* in collaboration with the Texas Counseling Association; the agencies updated the model in 2018. Similar to Texas, the state of Florida also utilizes a state-codified model for school counselors. Clearly, state law and practice have influenced national conversations and planning about school counseling. In fact, parts of the ASCA National Model include excerpts from the Texas Model (e.g., the four delivery components—curriculum, responsive services, individual planning, and system support). The integration of state policy into the National Model illustrates the collaborative nature of the profession.

The value of school counseling programs becomes even more pronounced as discussions on the quality of K–12 schooling dominate national conversations about how to spend school funding dollars. For example, the Education Trust (2019, para. 1) notes that "as a part of a school support team, professional school counselors provide critical social-emotional and academic supports" and that the delivery of a comprehensive school counseling program can set students on a pathway to success after high school.

Further, a study by Lapan et al. (2012) found that lower student-to-school counselor ratios seemed linked to better student graduation rates and decreased disciplinary rates in high-poverty schools. Even with evidence supporting the value of school counseling, barriers still exist that prevent the implementation of quality school counseling programs nationwide. The next section of this chapter discusses three critical barriers for readers' consideration.

BARRIER ONE: PROFESSIONAL LEGITIMACY

Hatch (2008) and the Texas Education Agency (2018) presciently note that the field of school counseling historically and continuously struggles for professional legitimacy at local, state, and national levels. Hatch further maintains that a triad of theoretical constructs frames school counseling's *legitimacy* or perceived value and credibility in organizations and society (Table 15.1). *Organizational legitimacy* of school counseling refers to the profession's accountability and consistency of outcomes. *Institutional legitimacy* of the field includes professional school counselors' success in influencing policy and expectations that reflect the profession's standards and expectations for professional behavior and duties. *Political legitimacy* refers to the profession's reputation as integral to the educational process and tactical use of "political clout" and "social capital" (Hatch, 2008, p. 6) to manage bureaucracy and morass, which often interfere with the implementation of a robust school counseling program.

TABLE 15.1 PROFESSIONAL CHALLENGES OF SCHOOL COUNSELING: ORGANIZATIONAL, INSTITUTIONAL, AND POLITICAL

Theoretical Construct	Professional Challenge Facing the School Counseling Profession	How Has the Challenge Manifested Itself?	How Can the Challenge Be Addressed?	Desired Outcome
Organizational	Meeting effectiveness (predictive, desired, and intended goals and outcomes)	No measurements of impact of activities and do not know whether they work or not	Through program evaluations	Measure results Know what works and what does not work
	Internal efficiency (greatest output for least energy and resource)	Status quo Inefficiency Random acts of guidance	Program Improvement	Do more of what works, less of what does not Program refinement Time efficiency

(continued)

TABLE 15.1 PROFESSIONAL CHALLENGES OF SCHOOL COUNSELING: ORGANIZATIONAL, INSTITUTIONAL, AND POLITICAL (*CONTINUED*)

Theoretical Construct	Professional Challenge Facing the School Counseling Profession	How Has the Challenge Manifested Itself?	How Can the Challenge Be Addressed?	Desired Outcome
Institutional	Operational legitimacy	No structural elements institutionalized (e.g., rules, norms and routines, policies, procedures) Unaware of standards or models	Reporting program results Social and cultural pressure Educate on standards and model programs	Indispensability Influence policy actors to create institutionalization of structural elements, laws, policies, handbooks, routines, and procedures reflecting appropriate role of school counselor
	Social legitimacy	Not involved in site leadership No legitimate voice in programs or policies	Becoming involved in decision-making Systems change Student advocacy	Becoming a policy actor Influencing policy actors by contributing to the cultural pressure that leads to the creation of structures Partner with school leadership for systems change
Political	Value versus resource Social capital Political clout	Reduction in force Undervaluing profession Increase in nonschool counseling responsibility	Reporting program results Marketing	Seen as integral Valued Performing school counseling activities

Source: Reprinted with permission from Hatch, T. (2008). Professional challenges in school counseling. https://files.eric.ed.gov/fulltext/EJ894793.pdf

This section of the chapter applies organizational theory in exploring the professional legitimacy of school counseling. However, a broader application of Hatch's theory relates to the counseling profession on the whole. The profession continues to face similar challenges as professional school counseling, particularly when considering the disparate state licensing and credentialing processes for other types of counselors. For example, national counseling organizations, including the American Counseling Association (ACA) and the American Association of State Counseling Boards, continue to press for seamless licensure portability between states for clinical mental health counselors. For context, the ACA (2021) observes a "crisis" in licensure portability exists, given that the United States has "currently over 45 counselor licensure titles, no two scopes of practice are the same, minimum graduate credit hours vary from none stated to 60, and supervision requirements vary from 500 to 4,500 hours" (para. 4).

Establishing standards of preparation and professional behavior unifies and strengthens the counseling profession by creating a solid framework for professional identity (20/20 Vision for the Future of Counseling, 2020). The 20/20 Vision for the Future of Counseling (2020) further indicates that professional standards protect the public by ensuring that professionals who enter and continue in the counseling profession meet a minimum standard of training and practice. Similarly, Bobby (2013) writes that the Council for Accreditation of Counseling and Related Educational Programs (CACREP) established codified standards of preparation that "unify" the counseling profession by providing a "common professional identity" (p. 35), placing professional counselors first and emphasizing counseling specialties second. The CACREP standards, then, systematize counselor preparation standards for various counseling specialties, including school counseling.

To date, 262 master's level school counseling programs hold CACREP accreditation; 328 master's level clinical mental health programs hold CACREP accreditation (CACREP, 2019). CACREP outlines the following steps for the accreditation process. College or university master's level counseling programs seeking CACREP accreditation must apply for this recognition by first submitting a thorough electronic self-study detailing how the program's curriculum meets the CACREP criteria, which the organization updates periodically and last revised in 2016 (CACREP, 2016). Program submissions include program syllabi mapped to applicable CACREP standards and full- and part-time faculty curriculum vitae, which outline faculty professional backgrounds and activities that reflect professional identity as counseling professionals. Program and institutional leaders sign the self-study prior to submission to CACREP to indicate institutional support. If the submission meets initial screening criteria, a site visit from a group of counseling professionals trained in the CACREP standards takes place. The site visit team provides a written report on the programs and after review by the CACREP Board a program can receive a 2-year or 8-year accreditation approval or denial of CACREP status.

CACREP assesses fees associated with initial certification, which includes a review, a site visit, and, upon earning the CACREP distinction, the cost of ongoing program accreditation renewals (CACREP, 2020). Moreover, CACREP publishes a recertification calendar that outlines accreditation renewal requirements that usually require an updated self-study and program evaluation. Evidence-based principles remain integral to the CACREP standards for professional school counseling. These standards draw from several professional organizations. These organizations include the ACA, the ASCA, the College Board National Office for School Counselor Advocacy, the Southern Regional Education Board: Go Alliance, and the Texas Model for Comprehensive School Counseling Programs.

BARRIER TWO: NOT ENOUGH PROFESSIONAL SCHOOL COUNSELORS

Numerous sources recognize the impact of limited access to professional school counselors on students, families, educators, and communities. For example, Topete (2019) observes that the lack of professional school counselors affects the safety of students and their mental health. To support this observation, Topete (2019) cites data from the American Civil Liberties Union and the U.S. Department of Education, which show that American schools provide 7,000,000 students access to school police officers but no access to professional school counselors. The ASCA (2020a) recommends a ratio of 1 professional school counselor for every 250 students. A joint report from the National Association for College Admission Counseling (NACAC) and the ASCA using data from 2014 to 2015 shows that students-per-counselor ratios increased by 1% with 482 students to 1 counselor (NACAC & ASCA, 2020, p. 6).

BARRIER THREE: LACK OF DIVERSITY

Another barrier to implementing quality school counseling programs in the United States stems from the lack of diversity among the corps of professional school counselors. White women comprise 70% of the nation's professional school counselors (DataUSA, 2020a; Jones, 2019; Miller, 2020; U.S. Census Bureau, 2020). Yet research consistently documents the significant influence of counselors of color on students' decision-making about going to college (e.g., Cholewa et al., 2019; Mulhern, 2020). Similarly, professional school counselors cannot critically address the schools' responses to students' mental health needs until these students can get connected to more intensive outside resources (Erickson & Abel, 2013). The ASCA school counseling competencies advise that professional school counselors should support all students' mental health (ASCA, 2020b; Croft et al., 2020).

Historically, "White men" have "presented the face of the counseling profession and largely dictated its focus and direction" (Meyers, 2017, para. 1). Steadily, though, multiculturalism and social justice shaped the profession's trajectory, becoming counseling's "fourth" and "fifth" forces, respectively (Ratts & Pedersen, 2014, p. x). The code of ethics for counselors in general, and also for professional school counselors, guides counselors to implement interventions illustrative of clients' cultural needs and strengths. However, gaps remain, especially in the school environment. Holcomb-McCoy (2007) defines the achievement gap as "when groups of students with relatively equal ability don't achieve in school at the same levels . . . even when parents' income and wealth are comparable" for students of color (p. 6). The expectations gap refers to the different expectations of educators for individual students (Quaglia et al., 2010). Research shows that students' keen awareness of educators' expectations significantly predicts students' engagement in school across multiple domains (Rosenthal & Jacobson, 1968; Tyler & Boelter, 2008).

Lack of diversity in school counseling likely negatively affects students' postsecondary choices, school attendance, and graduation rates. Barnum (2019) found that the chance of graduating for students of color jumped by almost 4 percentage points when assigned a counselor of color. A research collaboration between Reach Higher, Education Trust, and the ASCA (2019) found that students of color who live in low-income communities in 38 states cannot adequately access professional school counselors. Moreover, this collaboration reported that the students in these schools systemically appear "overlooked and underserved" (p. 1) and that 11 million high school students attend schools without enough professional school counselors.

REMOVING BARRIERS

Removing barriers that stand in the way of implementing excellent school counseling programs seems rooted in establishing and maintaining the legitimacy of the profession and creating a pipeline of professional school counselors equipped to manage the complexities of counseling diverse children and adolescents. A substantial nexus exists between providing school counseling that emphasizes support of students' academic, social, and career success, along with meeting students' emotional and developmental needs, and ultimately their mental health needs. Nationally, school leaders, districts, and communities face an enduring struggle about how to meet the mental health needs of students and identify how school counseling programs and community partners can assist.

MENTAL HEALTH AND SCHOOL COUNSELING

In considering the developmental tasks associated with childhood and adolescence, Erikson (1950) theorized that people go through eight distinct stages of life that reflect a psychosocial crisis that must be resolved before moving forward to the next stage. For school-age children, Erikson's theory identifies two important developmental tasks: learning to become involved with their environment to initiate interactions with others, and simultaneously gaining a positive sense of self. Children who lack confidence about their environment and feel guilty when they do not achieve independence or mastery of physical and cognitive skills cannot move to the next stages of developing their self-understanding, values, and identity. The inability to develop self-understanding and personal identity results in role confusion and problems creating warm and meaningful relationships with family and friends, for example.

Professional counselors understand that different life events shape a young person's progression through developmental stages. For students who experience mental health concerns, though, meeting the rigors of K–12 schooling, which include navigating academic, peer, and family concerns, can feel overwhelming. Clinical mental health counselors can work in schools or community-based settings. The American Mental Health Counselors Association (AMHCA, 2017, para. 7) states that "clinical mental health counseling is a distinct profession with national standards for education, training and clinical practice. Clinical mental health counselors are highly-skilled professionals who provide flexible, consumer-oriented therapy." Clinical mental health counselors utilize "traditional" psychotherapy approaches in practical ways (AMHCA, 2017, para. 7); moreover, a strengths-based wellness paradigm provides the bedrock of clinical mental health counseling.

UNMET MENTAL HEALTH NEEDS OF CHILDREN AND ADOLESCENTS

So et al. (2019) report that research shows one in six children aged 2 through 8 years of age experiences a diagnosed mental, behavioral, or developmental disorder not treated fully by available counseling services. Whitney and Peterson (2019) observe that disparities in child and adolescents' access to mental health specialists will persist, particularly for those under-served and never-served. For example, DeKruyf et al. (2018) argue the necessity of professional school counselors shifting to a "conjoint professional school counselor identity that includes the roles of both educational leader and mental health" (p. 271). The authors note further that adopting this identity "positions school counselors to better respond to all students, including those with mental health needs" (p. 272).

Accessing therapy remains difficult, if not impossible, for some families. Bringewatt and Gershoff (2010) note that children living in poverty and their families face tremendous barriers to getting mental health treatment. Fiscella et al. (2000) found that disparities in getting mental health treatment for African Americans and working-class persons exist even when controlling for health insurance coverage. Kugelmass (2016) explored the effect of the race and gender of persons seeking mental health counseling on the accessibility of therapists, and her results showed that middle-class persons seeking mental health treatment received appointment offers at three times the rate of working-class persons. The study also found a difference among race, with therapists offering statistically fewer appointments to middle-class Black persons seeking treatment. Not surprising, then, is the fact that mental health service utilization reveals lesser engagement and early termination on the part of American Indian, Asian American, Black, and Hispanic clients (Sue, 2010).

Thus, similar to Black persons seeking treatment, attitudinal, financial, and access issues also exist for Asian American, Latinx, and Native American clients according to the U.S. Surgeon General (Office of the Surgeon General, 2001). In the years following the Surgeon General's landmark report, additional research documents the importance of minoritized communities having access to quality preventive and responsive mental healthcare (e.g., American Psychiatric Association, 2020; Bussing & Gary, 2012; Nelson, 2002). For children and adolescents, even greater barriers to mental healthcare exist and seem rooted, at the very least, in socioeconomic disadvantage and implicit bias on the part of practitioners (American Psychological Association, 2017). Other factors that can shape children and adolescents' mental health can include neighborhood level stressors found in urban communities, limited access to clean air and water, and limited opportunities to engage with nature and the environment (Greenleaf & Bryant, 2012).

Sue et al. (2019), similar to the American Psychological Association (2017), note that racial/ethnic minority children and adolescents continue to experience numerous inequities in mental healthcare that stem from racism. For example, Gibson (2020) writes about "racialized disparities in K–12 schools' application of discipline" (p. 133). The American Psychiatric Association (2020) indicates that when compared to White youth, referral patterns for racial/ethnic minority youth with behavioral concerns tend toward the juvenile justice system, as opposed to a primary care specialist. The American Psychological Association (2017) and Gibson (2020) note that uneven and disparate applications of discipline and school policies can disproportionately place racial/ethnic students in out-of-school suspension or expulsion. School discipline policies seek to manage and control students' problematic behaviors. Often, schools attempt to support students with mental health needs using "patchwork" (Walker, 2018, para. 6) crisis response approaches. The limited benefits of short-term interventions continue to predominate, even though ample evidence supports the implementation of "system-based, evidence-based, whole-school" programming for students and teachers (para. 18).

As stated in other chapters in this book, professional school counselors' training and expertise uniquely position them to intervene with students with unmet mental health needs and to collaborate with community-based colleagues and organizations to connect students with appropriate services. Counselors based in school and community settings can facilitate students' access to mental health counseling by collaborating with school-based mental health professionals such as clinical mental health counselors or social workers, who can provide services in schools. Clinical mental health counselors who work in school-based mental health interface with professional school counselors, who provide student referrals to the mental health program.

Many professional organizations emphasize that professional school counselors do not provide ongoing individual therapy but rather provide dynamic, responsive services to students, their families, and school communities that teach healthy functioning based on expected developmental milestones. Kaffenberger and Rorke-Trigiani (2018) further assert that professional school counselors and community-based clinical mental health counselors working together in school to community partnerships can address mental health service gaps that support referrals of students. Furthermore, professional school counselors create programming that provides direct services to students including individual and group counseling. These services teach mental health skills such as emotional regulation, psychoeducation, and coping strategies in response to grief and loss.

ACCESS TO CLINICAL MENTAL HEALTH COUNSELING

The managed care marketplace for mental health treatment caps the number of counseling sessions and can dictate the type of treatment children or adolescents receive. Ali et al. (2019) explored differences in children's and adolescents' utilization rates of mental health based on Medicaid coverage or private insurance. The researchers chose to study this topic because clinicians know little about how children and adolescents use mental health treatment regardless of their insurance coverage. They found the following most common mental health treatment for children and adolescents, regardless of insurance: psychiatric medication, reflecting "43% of young children with Medicaid and 39% of those with private insurance, and 55% of adolescents with Medicaid and 49% of those with private insurance" (Ali et al., 2019, para. 1).

EMPATHY AND SCHOOL COUNSELING

One of the hallmarks of the counseling profession involves the demonstration of empathy. Indeed, the term empathy pervades the literature, and a recent meta-analysis conducted by Hall and Schwartz (2019) found discrepancies between the conceptual definition of empathy and how mental health clinicians operationalize empathy in the profession. Fabi et al. (2019) define empathy in simple terms: the ability to understand and respond to the emotional state of another being. Exploring whether empathetic concern and personal distress lie rooted in dispositional traits or situation variables, Fabi et al. (2019) found that participants' perceptions of another person's psychological pain evoked compassionate consideration and empathy. The researchers also discovered that participants' perceptions of another person's physical pain led to higher ratings of participants' reports of physical distress (Fabi et al., 2019).

Carl Rogers, the founder of person-centered counseling, believed that the counseling relationship drives change between the counselor and client. Rogers (1963) theorized that counselors who demonstrated genuineness and empathy, predicated on unconditional positive regard and nonjudgment, created conditions necessary for change to occur. As mentioned in Chapter 1, children's and adolescents' brains develop through adulthood. Consequently, any counselor, regardless of specialty, must understand how to counsel children and adolescents to guide them through difficult concepts in developmentally appropriate ways.

TEACHING COUNSELING PROFESSIONALS EMPATHY AS A FRAMEWORK FOR SOCIAL JUSTICE ADVOCACY

In today's world, many live in a time in which deeply held beliefs contribute to a divided society. While surrounded by social media attacks, protests, and disrespectful discourse, many face challenges in developing and utilizing important advocacy competencies in a volatile cultural climate. Counselors should carry out these duties in a manner that encourages respectful dialogue and a deeper understanding to increase the effectiveness of social justice activities. Practicing social justice may call for challenging discourse when individuals appear limited in their capacity to consider another perspective on an issue and see the world from an opposing viewpoint of right and wrong.

William Perry, an educational psychologist who researched the intellectual development of college students, postulated the theory of epistemic cognition based on personal reflections on how individuals obtain and accept facts, beliefs, and ideas. "When mature, rational thinkers reach conclusions that differ from those of others, they consider the justifiability of their conclusions. When they cannot justify their approach, they revise it, seeking a more balanced, adequate route to acquiring knowledge" (Berk, 2014, p. 358). Perry conducted a longitudinal study of undergraduate students who participated in interviews at the end of each year of college. He found that the students' reflections on knowing changed as they matriculated through the university. He suggested that intellectual development begins with a dualistic mind-set, characterized by dividing information, values, and ideas into right or wrong, good or bad, one side or the other with no middle ground option. The reasoning at this stage of development includes a fundamental approach to knowledge with little room for ambiguity (Ambrose et al., 2010). As the students matured, they began to exhibit the ability to engage in relativistic thinking, which allowed for a diversity of opinions, no absolute truth, and consideration of the contextual framework of information and ideas. As individuals mature in the ability to engage in relativistic thinking, they often seek out different perspectives to increase their knowledge and develop their views (Berk, 2014).

Palmer (2016) suggests dualistic thinking lays the foundation for oppression, racism, misogyny, homophobia, and discrimination. Deeply held dualistic beliefs leave no room for critical thinking or reflection, which remains vital to the ability to actively listen to the perspectives of those with whom one disagrees. An individual must possess the ability to engage in relativistic thinking to challenge their views; this facilitates an honest examination of personal thinking to reveal biases and to consider a different point of view. The ability to feel the perspective or experience of others continues to be critical to developing empathy.

The word "empathy" evolved from the German psychological term *Einfühlung*, which means "feeling into" (Bloom, 2013). Two psychologists developed the word in 1908, deriving the word from the Greek *em pathos*, which translates to "in feeling" (Lanzoni, 2015). The definition of the word grew and developed as a result of a century of research, with some suggesting two categories of empathy: affective empathy and cognitive empathy (McLaren, 2013). Clinicians describe *affective empathy* as a visceral feeling and *cognitive empathy* as an objective understanding. Affective and cognitive empathy can exist within a dualistic mind-set as long as the other stays on the same side of the argument. However, relativistic thinking remains necessary to empathize with someone with whom one disagrees.

Daniel Batson, a social psychologist, conducted empathy research for several decades. He suggests that empathy refers to eight concepts: knowing another's thoughts and feelings; adopting the posture of another; feeling as another does; projecting oneself into another's situation; imagining how another feels; imagining how one would feel or think in another's place; feeling distressed at another's suffering; and feeling for another's suffering (Batson, 2009). Batson et al. (2015) suggest that the empathy–altruism hypothesis can motivate and propel individuals to act out of concern for the welfare of others. This motivational state results in the ultimate goal of acting on behalf of others to reduce the level of need. These concepts remain critical to moving from empathy to advocacy.

ADVOCACY

Professionals see advocacy as a natural outgrowth of empathy that occurs when an individual can no longer tolerate a perceived injustice or imbalance of power. Advocacy becomes a call to action rooted in underlying respect for others. Empathy acknowledges the plight of others, humanizes the issues, and gives the issue a face. Clinicians view empathy as a critical element in developing a culture of advocacy. Advocates work as translators between the "insiders" and "outsiders" to create a greater understanding of the other. Advocates must display intolerance for injustice but possess the ability to stand up without alienating the other side. Advocates persuade and possess the ability to engage others in caring about the cause (Mullican, 2015).

In 2003, the ACA endorsed a set of advocacy competencies developed by Lewis et al. (2003) in response to the growing need for counselors' influences on policy and clients' well-being in the community. While the advocacy competencies relate specifically to counselors and counselor educators, Toporek et al. (2009) applied the competencies to systemic change efforts, which the field can generalize outside of the profession. The authors found it essential to develop the requisite knowledge and skills to engage ethically and effectively in advocacy work. When possible, the advocate benefits from direct exposure to those for whom one advocates to understand another's perspective. If direct exposure cannot happen, aligning oneself with others with possible direct exposure or more knowledge will assist in developing awareness and understanding related to the needs and perspectives of the group facing societal disadvantage. Toporek and Daniels (2018) recently updated the competencies to reflect changes and multiple considerations of diverse counselors (Figure 15.1).

FROM ADVOCACY TO SOCIAL JUSTICE

Specific elements, rooted in social justice, comprise advocacy efforts and interface with multicultural counseling competencies. Social justice advocacy takes into consideration the needs and perspectives of the disadvantaged group for which one advocates and employs systemic change to increase the power of the disadvantaged group (Klugman, 2010). In essence, social justice advocacy "tackles the root and avoidable causes of inequities for those who are systematically and institutionally disadvantaged by their race, ethnicity, economic status, nationality, gender, gender expression, age, sexual orientation, or religion" (Klugman, 2010, p. 2).

Klugman (2010) goes on to identify three values related to social justice advocacy: "The redistribution of resources so that everyone can live a decent life; Human beings all have equal human rights, and diversity is worthy of recognition; All people should be represented and have the ability to advocate on their behalf" (p. 3). Klugman's values hinge upon core assumptions about human life. The first value offers that society can and should redistribute its resources (e.g., human, financial, ecologic), so that persons can have meaningful and safe lives free from poverty and unmet needs. Second, Klugman offers that diversity characterizes the human experience and deserves recognition as essential to humanity. Finally, Klugman's third value

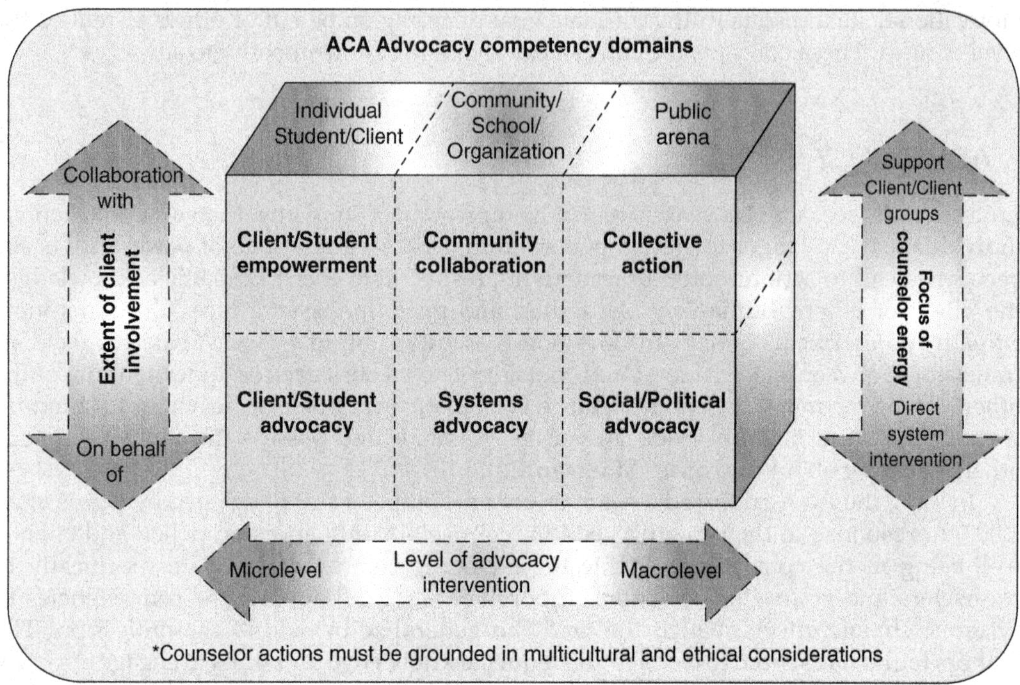

FIGURE 15.1 American Counseling Association Advocacy Competencies.

ACA, American Counseling Association.

Source: Reproduced with permission from *2018 update and expansion of the 2003 ACA Advocacy Competencies: Honoring the work of the past and contextualizing the present* by Toporek and Daniels (2018). Copyright 2018 American Counseling Association.

maintains that while advocacy on behalf of someone has value, providing space and time for persons to advocate for themselves renders them visible and not marginalized by others speaking for and about their needs. Interestingly, Klugman's three values of social justice advocacy mirror the assumptions of the ACA's Advocacy Competencies outlined previously in this chapter.

ADVOCACY AND SOCIAL MEDIA

Social media increases our ability to connect with others and engage in personal campaigns based on our set of beliefs and values. However, social media also contributes to a lack of empathy through what Manney (2015) refers to as confirmation bias. Individuals connect with others who validate their prejudices and empathize with those with whom they agree and who support their attacks and demonization of those with whom they disagree. Manney (2015) suggests that people demonstrate empathy better with an individual than with a larger group, especially one that embraces a value or trait with which they disagree. In his work on storytelling as a pathway to empathy, when individuals see the real-life observation of another's plight through the use of storytelling, they often develop empathy for the individual. However, through technology, people may find those stories repetitive and overwhelming to the point of reaching a saturation rate and shutting down. These continue as essential considerations in engaging in social justice advocacy.

Transformative experiences include activities designed to create some level of change within an individual. From a social justice standpoint, those activities should assist persons in expanding their worldview and increase their awareness of privilege and bias. These experiences should take persons outside of their comfort zone and increase the ability to take on the perspective of others. A well-designed experience can place persons in the shoes of others and facilitate a greater understanding of diverse views to develop empathy.

In applying Perry's theory of intellectual development (Berk, 2014), education presents the potential of moving an individual from dualistic thinking to relativistic thinking. Relativistic thinking does not necessarily result in a change in personal values. Persons can continue to hold fast to their values and accept the rights of others to hold a different set of values. Empathy facilitates acceptance without judgment. This type of knowledge can provide the necessary scaffolding for the growth and development needed before engaging in any advocacy activity.

Advocacy can occur both informally and formally, individually or collectively. Advocacy can focus on changes within the individual or at a systemic level. Regardless of the level of advocacy, professional school counselors must possess the skills necessary to present a case for change while continuing to be respectful of the multiple perspectives their stakeholders bring. Empathy not only motivates professional school counselors to advocate but also assists them in developing a more in-depth understanding of those with whom they disagree. This mind-set facilitates respectful discourse and can potentially address societal divisions.

PROFESSIONAL SCHOOL AND CLINICAL MENTAL HEALTH COUNSELOR WELLNESS AND SELF-CARE

Thus far, this chapter explored the roots of the counseling profession across multiple domains. The authors explored counselor preparation standards and the benefits the field offers children and adolescents in reaching their potential as students and members of their communities. The chapter also considers the stark disparities that exist related to access to mental healthcare. It highlights how advocacy and social justice continue to shape the profession currently while looking forward to the future. Counselor wellness and self-care remain integral to counselor effectiveness with clients (Barnett, 2014; Blount et al., 2016; Myers & Sweeney, 2005). Kerulis (2018) conceptualizes counselor wellness that includes counselors' connection to the community and emphasizes communication and personal responsibility with the family. Kerulis also stresses the importance of relationships with romantic partners that facilitate independence and equality and the benefit of work satisfaction that involves meaning, stamina, and connections with coworkers. As a final thought, Kerulis (2018) discusses counselors' need for flexibility in accessing support and changing personal attitudes when learning new information and seeking mentorship.

The research by Newsome et al. (2006) shows that not many counseling programs address how vital self-care reduces burnout, even though the literature shows the value of teaching counselors the principles of self-care. Similarly, the CACREP (2009) standards do not identify wellness as a core concept for counseling trainees regardless of specialty. Newsome et al. (2006) also observe that mental health professionals, in particular, face severe levels of stress due to working in emotionally exhaustive environments. Thus, counselors must learn to deal with occupational stress that can lead to compassion fatigue and burnout as a critical dimension of their professional development.

Without self-care, counselors may find themselves unable to fulfill their duties to their full potential (Bradley et al., 2013). The ACA deemed counselor well-being such an essential issue that the organization charged a task force on counselor wellness and impairment to identify self-care activities that enhance counselor and client well-being (ACA, 2006). Bradley et al. (2013) further suggest that the literature supports general self-care strategies for counselors that include eating a balanced diet, exercising, getting enough sleep, and seeking support from other professionals as appropriate. Similarly, Mayorga et al. (2014) report that although documented concerns exist regarding occupational stress and burnout in the field of counseling, practicing self-care may help prevent or lower the levels of stress and burnout in counseling professionals. Additionally, counselors who focus on personal self-care can likely help their clients focus on wellness behavior through modeling. As noted previously in this chapter, empathy undergirds the counseling process, and counselors must first experience empathy to model and teach empathetic skills to clients (Fulton, 2016). Fulton (2016) also found that self-compassion correlates positively with tolerance for ambiguity in counseling.

With regard to the preceding discussion, counselors must remember that wellness occurs within a milieu of diversity. Given this, counselors should also take care to continuously attend to their cultural selves for optimal personal and professional interactions. Hays (2016) implores clinicians to individually assess their backgrounds via an ADDRESSING perspective, which serves as an acronym encompassing the identities of "Age and generational influences; Developmental or other Disability; Religious or spiritual orientation, Ethnic and racial identity; Socioeconomic status; Sexual orientation; Indigenous heritage, National origin; and Gender" (p. 8). Counselors must also consider how their privilege and background impact their interactions with clients. Lastly and "equally important is a willingness to seek out new sources of information that will help you learn *from* and *with* (not simply *about*) people of diverse cultures" (Hays, 2016, p. 59).

The counseling profession views the concept of resilience as essential to preventing burnout and as a prerequisite to implementing self-care strategies (Skovholt & Trotter-Mathison, 2011). Skovholt and Trotter-Mathison (2011) consider the dichotomy between caring for others and caring for oneself and the anxiety that can arise as a result. Expanding on this dichotomy, Skovholt and Trotter-Mathison (2011) maintain that people who naturally care for others face physical and emotional exhaustion when saying "yes" to others and guilt when choosing to care for themselves over caring for others. As a guide, the *ACA Code of Ethics* indicates that "counselors engage in self-care activities to maintain and promote their own emotional, physical, mental, and spiritual well-being best to meet their professional responsibilities" (2014, Section 8). The code briefly mentions self-care in the introduction to Section C but does not mention the concept again in the document. Although the code includes a section on handling counselor impairment (C.2.g) after the manifestation of physical, mental, or emotional issues, the code lacks a section on the importance of primary intervention. Areas of the code include guiding counselors to comply with standards, monitoring their effectiveness; stressing the importance of ongoing professional development to maintain and learn new skills; the need for preparing a succession plan in case they cannot work due to illness or death; and outlining parameters by which they will see clients pro bono. The writers infer that the *ACA Code of Ethics* treatment of the subject speaks to the need for counselor self-care while simultaneously revealing the discrepancy between what we, as a profession, value and expectations for our professional practice.

The conflict between counselor roles, assigned duties, and job satisfaction can predict life satisfaction even when controlling for years of experience and practice location

(Bryant & Constantine, 2006) and burnout (Huat et al., 2018). Worry, exhaustion, feelings of unfinished business, long work hours, lack of support, and counseling duties unrelated to counseling form a perfect storm of burnout for counselors—especially those working in school settings (Huat et al., 2018; Kim & Lambie, 2018). Further, highly stressful professional school counselor jobs with poorly defined requirements and inconsistencies between job expectations and school counseling practice result in professional school counselors' stress and burnout, which potentially negatively influences job satisfaction (Mullen et al., 2018). These authors continue by noting that professional school counselors can face multiple and competing demands, leading to symptoms of stress, empathy, fatigue, emotional exhaustion, counselor impairment, and eventual departure or resignation from their jobs. Simultaneously, role expectations demand that professional school counselors deliver career education modules in the classroom and consult with parents and teachers while attending to non-counseling-related administrative tasks such as lunch duty. Professional school counselors may feel stressed, exhausted, and eventually burned out by attempting to balance these various professional requirements. Finally, Mullen et al. (2018) observe that the experiences of burnout can lead to a severe diminishment of professional school counselors' abilities to deliver adequate services to students and their families and exhibit negative self-concepts, impaired job attitudes, a devaluing of clients, and personal discouragement.

To support counselor wellness, Davis (2018) offers the following considerations. School counselor trainees must possess skills in working with parents and families in underserved communities. Professional school counselors should identify and tap community resources sufficient for serving clients and moving through possible bureaucratic red tape in advocating at the individual, school, and systemic levels. Also, Davis (2018) states that professional school counselors benefit from using a variety of skills to remain engaged in the profession. These skills range from applying ethical standards to difficult professional situations, utilizing self-care resources, and honing mediation/conflict resolution skills. Professional school counselors must also demonstrate competencies in advocacy models and theories that facilitate forming partnerships and collaboration across disciplines. Lastly, counselors must consistently use basic counselor skills such as communication, problem-solving, organization, and self-care principles to stay engaged professionally.

CASE STUDY 15.1: AMELIA'S WAY FORWARD

Amelia enjoys her high school counseling position, which she obtained after completing her master's studies in a CACREP-approved program 10 years ago. Her principal relies on her expertise as a professional school counselor to implement a counseling program, based on the field's best practices, that meets the needs of students in a high-needs, high-poverty, rural community. Natural disasters over the past 3 years include dangerous floods and a category three hurricane, all of which led to catastrophic loss of life and economic ruin for businesses and families. Historical racial inequities and hostilities remain rooted in the community, and the region recently made national news for holding its first racially integrated high school prom. Despite marginal progress in access to better wages and the presence of three colleges, upward mobility remains elusive, particularly for persons of

(*continued*)

CASE STUDY 15.1 (*continued*)

color. As a professional school counselor in this school, Amelia teaches students mental health wellness strategies. These strategies assist the students to cope with and overcome inequities to facilitate high school completion and readiness to enter postsecondary or career pathways poised to succeed.

During the recent coronavirus disease 2019 (COVID-19) pandemic, Amelia's community saw the second highest density of cases of this infectious disease nationwide, making the city a "hot spot" of infection (Lewis, 2020, para. 5). African Americans comprise the majority of the community at 72.5%, with 22.2% White, and 2.36% Latinx (DataUSA, 2020b). The area struggles with entrenched generational poverty, as reflected by a poverty rate of 33.2% and a median household income of $31,843 (DataUSA, 2020b). The current distribution of land ownership and low educational attainment rates for African Americans stem from the vestiges of African American enslavement on the economy, which still influence the community's contemporary functioning (similar to the United States at large, according to Bertocchi and Dimico [2014]). Because success in the town falls along deeply ingrained racial lines, residents already living in poverty found their lives even harsher following the recent natural disasters.

Farooqi (2019) laments that although the town's Black citizens hold elected positions, accessing resources remains ensconced along racial lines. Farooqi (2019) states that in the town, the wealthy "White elite" predominates and drives economic development and political power (para. 7). The imbalance of resources and attendant educational and health disparities follow de facto segregation patterns established decades before. Racial unrest characterizes the town's history, and notably Dr. Martin Luther King's leadership of the region's Civil Rights Movement in the 1950s catapulted the area into notoriety for its relentless effort to maintain segregation de jure. All of these factors serve as a backdrop for Amelia's counseling work in the community.

In addition to counseling at the high school, Amelia also teaches school counseling courses as an adjunct professor at the local university's CACREP-accredited school counseling program. Having completed the requirements for state licensure as a professional clinical mental health counselor, Amelia recently opened a private practice that provides in-home counseling to children and adolescents. While she does not offer direct services in the private practice, Amelia supervises other clinicians. Amelia's guiding principles rely on teaching self-advocacy and tenets of educational and social justice that prepare counselors to develop counseling interventions and programs that support students' and families' well-being.

Amelia's work in different settings sharpened her keen awareness of students and their families' unmet mental health needs and the challenges in overcoming these barriers at micro- and macrolevels. In the school setting, Amelia determines crisis response and interventions with students whose behavior disrupts learning and instruction. She recognizes, though, that students who do not disturb the classroom may still evidence unmet mental health needs, as noted by frequent absences and lack of engagement. Acknowledging Amelia's effective advocacy for the students at the classroom, building level, and community levels with parents and families, the central office published program assessment results that suggest Amelia's

(*continued*)

CASE STUDY 15.1 (*continued*)

program reduced the number of students dropping out and addressed disparities in suspension rates for underrepresented students. The program's evaluation data also indicated that it improved attendance for students with low attendance. Impressed with Amelia's efforts, her superintendent advises that a new position at the district will open soon. Amelia's new role will create new opportunities for professional school counselors and community-based organizations to collaborate. While Amelia's position no longer requires her to provide direct services to students, she will use her consultative skills and understanding of counseling practice with children, adolescents, and families to facilitate access to preventive mental health services and earlier counseling interventions.

Amelia finds the new opportunity exciting and welcomed it, particularly given her growing concern about personal and occupational stress and juggling the ethical considerations and demands of performing multiple professional roles in a small community. For example, Amelia's days last 12 hours easily, and recent events required the county's professional school counselors and educators to deliver all services via the internet. The area's demand for stable broadband connections eclipsed the capacity of the local internet service provider, and many students lack internet access at home. Amelia's adjunct teaching and supervision moved to an online environment as well. With the responsibilities of running the school counseling program, teaching and supervising master's students, and running a private practice, Amelia finds herself strategizing how to serve a community effectively given its great and complicated needs.

Previous research outlines the gender-related challenges that female school counselors face in managing various professional and life role expectations and the importance of balancing these roles in ways that support well-being. For example, Bryant and Constantine (2006) note that "role conflict and role ambiguity are two specific occupational stressors that school counselors experience with regard to the multiple roles they assume in schools" (p. 265). In this same study, Bryant and Constantine (2006) found that female professional school counselors experience more life satisfaction when they feel a "strong sense of personal control, experiencing role quality across various professional and personal roles, and having some professional autonomy" (p. 269).

Accordingly, Amelia remains aware that she must address the different needs of her employer, students, clients, and private practice staff to support their learning, development, and ethical practice. Concerned that she aligns her professional behaviors with ethical guidelines, Amelia consults the codes of ethics of the ACA, the ASCA, and the Association for Counselor Education and Supervision. She also obtains professional clinical supervision and professional peers' support to prioritize and handle her responsibilities to students, colleagues, and employees.

Of note, Amelia happens to be the only professional school counselor of color in her building. As she considers the new position, Amelia feels guilt and dissonance because she wants her team and community to feel supported and not abandoned. After discussing her concerns with her partner and activating her faith tradition, Amelia decides to accept the district position that moves her from direct service to one that develops systemwide policy for students and families with unmet

(*continued*)

CASE STUDY 15.1 (*continued*)

mental health needs. In deciding to leave direct service, Amelia recognized that she must trust the families and colleagues with whom she worked to implement the self-advocacy tools they learned from the counseling program. As a result of Amelia's and her team's efforts, Amelia expects these families to find success in their quest for well-being, and to secure educational and social justice. Amelia utilized her faith, family, and professional supports to reposition herself to avoid burnout and compassion fatigue. She came to understand that new strategies that helped her manage her time and personal commitments did indeed honor her deep commitment and served and preserved her sense of professional integrity and personal well-being.

Activity 15.1

Form small groups of five to think about and answer the following questions. At the completion of the small-group work, all groups will come together to share their answers. Before you begin, choose a recorder, who will be responsible for noting two main points for each question. Each recorder will then present these points to the larger class for a broader discussion.

1. Amelia moved from a school counseling position to one that involves school counseling and community partnerships. Discuss what ways you see the school counselor role evolving in the future to meet the needs of students living in diverse communities.
2. Think about Amelia's salient cultural identities and their intersections. How might they impact her personal and professional views? How might they impact how others see her and expect her to lead?
3. How might Amelia and the work she does be perceived by the school/town's various constituents?
4. What additional strategies might Amelia think about to avoid compassion fatigue and support her self-care?

CHAPTER SUMMARY

In this chapter, the authors draw from the literature, professional counseling and educational organizations, and their professional experiences to discuss the multifaceted areas associated with counseling children and adolescents. The chapter also details the evolving requirements to enter the school counseling profession and the standards that guide professional preparation and ongoing professional, ethical practice. Additionally, the chapter explores the challenges associated with balancing multiple roles and the benefits associated with using the literature to engage in the ethical practice of counseling that meets the needs of diverse stakeholders and supports personal well-being and professional excellence. Professional standards that undergird counselor preparation programs, such as those offered by CACREP, help school counselors-in-training learn how to make professional and self-care choices that support their personal and professional well-being. As these counselors-in-training move to professional practice, competencies and professional expectations further frame how to make self-care choices that protect the professionals from burnout and compassion fatigue. The authors offer this chapter as a resource to counselors-in-training and persons in professional practice to remain engaged in the profession. Durodoye and Bryant (2020) observe that professionals who engage in "solution-focused discourse and strategies" and who start and continue "challenging conversations" create opportunities and mind-sets that "serve as a basis for change" (p. ix–x). As this chapter comes to a close, the authors encourage readers to ponder the convergence of counselor training, professional standards, empathy, advocacy and social justice, and wellness on their work, well-being, and contributions to their communities and the profession.

POINTS TO REMEMBER

- Over the past few decades, societal shifts and needs changed the course of the counseling profession to place more emphasis on diversity and the various concerns that clients can bring to therapy.
- Despite the profession's change of focus, persons living in underserved communities lack access to counseling services, even when limited insurance coverage does not restrict access.
- Similar to the counseling profession overall, school counseling lacks the diversity of the communities in which professional school counselors serve. Research consistently documents the impact on student achievement and educational outcomes.
- Empathy, advocacy, and wellness provide the foundation of the counseling profession. Counselors who experience compassion fatigue and insufficient balancing of professional roles may find performing the counseling duties arduous, if not impossible.
- Strategies for counselors to care for themselves should begin in graduate school and continue as professionals continue in their careers.
- Understanding one's community, the social and political aspects that affect the community, and the strengths and limitations of clients' resources helps counselors tap multiple resources that support their work and prevent burnout.

OTHER HELPFUL INFORMATION FOR CONSIDERATION

- American Association of State Counseling Boards: https://www.aascb.org/aws/AASCB/pt/sp/about
- American Counseling Association Advocacy Competencies: https://www.counseling.org/docs/default-source/competencies/aca-2018-advocacy-competencies.pdf?sfvrsn=1dca552c_6
- American Counseling Association Code of Ethics: https://www.counseling.org/docs/default-source/default-document-library/2014-code-of-ethics-finaladdress.pdf?sfvrsn=96b532c_2

- American School Counselor Association Templates and Resources: https://www.schoolcounselor.org/About-School-Counseling/ASCA-National-Model-for-School-Counseling-Programs/Templates-Resources
- Multicultural Counseling and Social Justice Competencies: https://www.counseling.org/docs/default-source/competencies/multicultural-and-social-justice-counseling-competencies.pdf?sfvrsn=20#:~:text=The%20Multicultural%20and%20Social%20Justice%20Counseling%20Competencies%20%28MSJCC%29%2C,justice%20competencies%20into%20counseling%20theories%2C%20practices%2C%20and%20research.
- Self-Care
  a. Article on avoiding burnout: https://files.eric.ed.gov/fulltext/EJ1165683.pdf
  b. Self-Care Wheel: A tool to manage stress and achieve happiness: https://cmhanl.ca/app/uploads/2019/09/Self-Care-Wheel-Handout-2019.pdf
- Empathy and Counseling
  a. Article that discusses empathy and counseling caring: https://ct.counseling.org/2013/02/the-paradox-of-empathy-when-empathy-hurts/
  b. Article and videos of Carl Rogers discussing empathy and helpers: http://cultureofempathy.com/References/Experts/Carl-Rogers.htm#Empathic:_An_Unappreciated_Way_of_Being
- Disparities in Mental Healthcare
  a. Article on disparities in mental healthcare: https://www.nami.org/Blogs/NAMI-Blog/July-2017/Disparities-Within-Minority-Mental-Health-Care
  b. Substance Abuse and Mental Health Services Administration resources on behavioral health equity for diverse groups: https://www.samhsa.gov/behavioral-health-equity

QUESTIONS FOR FURTHER DISCUSSION

- How do professional school counselors balance multiple professional roles to provide ethical and quality counseling to their students?
- What resources exist that can assist professional school counselors to maintain empathy for their clients and avoid burnout?
- Numerous professional associations provide guidelines on counselor preparation and training. How do professionals utilize these guidelines to promote the profession of school counseling and prepare the next generation of professional counselors?
- The concept of wellness dominates the professional literature. What specific strategies can counselors use to promote their well-being and promote the wellness of colleagues?
- How can professional school counselors, clinical mental health counselors, social workers, and other professionals collaborate effectively on behalf of children and adolescents?

KEY REFERENCES

Only key references appear in the print edition. The full reference list appears in the digital product on Springer Publishing Connect: connect.springerpub.com/content/book/978-0-8261-4764-6/part/part05/chapter/ch15

American School Counselor Association. (n.d.). *Templates & resources*. Author. https://www.schoolcounselor.org/About-School-Counseling/ASCA-National-Model-for-School-Counseling-Programs/Templates-Resources

Berk, L. (2014). *Exploring lifespan development* (3rd ed.). Pearson.

Blount, A. J., Lambie, G. W., & Kissinger, D. B. (2016, November). Wellness matters. *Counseling Today*. https://ct.counseling.org/2016/11/wellness-matters

Council for the Accreditation of Counseling and Related Educational Programs. (2009). *2009 Standards*. Author.

Council for the Accreditation of Counseling and Related Educational Programs. (2016). *2016 Standards*. Author.

Erikson, E. (1950). *Childhood and society*. W. W. Norton & Company.

Lewis, J., Arnold, M., House, R., & Toporek, R. (2003). *American Counseling Association Advocacy Competencies*. American Counseling Association.

Rogers, C. (1963). The concept of the fully functioning person. *Psychotherapy, Research & Practice, 1*(1), 17–26. https://doi.org/10.1037/h0088567

Texas Education Agency. (2018). *The Texas Model for Comprehensive School Counseling Programs* (5th ed.). Texas Education Agency.

Toporek, R., & Daniels, J. (2018). *American Counseling Association Advocacy Competencies* (Updated). American Counseling Association.

Index